PEDIATRIC CLINICS
OF NORTH AMERICA

Scientific Foundations
of Clinical Practice, Part II

GUEST EDITORS
Ellis D. Avner, MD
Robert M. Kliegman, MD

October 2006 • Volume 53 • Number 5

SAUNDERS

An Imprint of Elsevier, Inc.
PHILADELPHIA   LONDON   TORONTO   MONTREAL   SYDNEY   TOKYO

W.B. SAUNDERS COMPANY
A Division of Elsevier Inc.

1600 John F. Kennedy Boulevard • Suite 1800 • Philadelphia, Pennsylvania 19103

http://www.theclinics.com

THE PEDIATRIC CLINICS OF NORTH AMERICA
October 2006
Editor: Carla Holloway

Volume 53, Number 5
ISSN 0031-3955
ISBN 1-4160-3897-3

The ideas and opinions expressed in *The Pediatric Clinics of North America* do not necessarily reflect those of the Publisher. The Publisher does not assume any responsibility for any injury and/or damage to persons or property arising out of or related to any use of the material contained in this periodical. The reader is advised to check the appropriate medical literature and the product information currently provided by the manufacturer of each drug to be administered to verify the dosage, the method and duration of administration, or contraindications. It is the responsibility of the treating physician or other health care professional, relying on independent experience and knowledge of the patient, to determine drug dosages and the best treatment for the patient. Mention of any product in this issue should not be construed as endorsement by the contributors, editors, or the Publisher of the product or manufacturers' claims.

The Pediatric Clinics of North America (ISSN 0031-3955) is published bi-monthly by Elsevier Inc. 360 Park Avenue South, New York, NY 10010-1710. Months of publication are February, April, June, August, October, and December. Business and Editorial Offices: 1600 John F. Kennedy Blvd., Suite 1800, Philadelphia, PA 19103-2899. Customer Service Office: 6277 Sea Harbor Drive, Orlando, FL 32887-4800. Periodicals postage paid at New York, NY and additional mailing offices. Subscription prices are $125.00 per year (US individuals), $260.00 per year (US institutions), $170.00 per year (Canadian individuals), $340.00 per year (Canadian institutions), $190.00 per year (international individuals), $340.00 per year (international institutions), $65.00 per year (US students), $100.00 per year (Canadian students), and $100.00 per year (foreign students). To receive students/resident rare, orders must be accompanied by name of affiliated institution, date of term, and the signature of program/residency coordinator on institution letterhead. Orders will be billed at individual rate until proof of status is received. Foreign air speed delivery is included in all Clinics subscription prices. All prices are subject to change without notice. POSTMASTER: Send address changes to *The Pediatric Clinics of North America*, Elsevier Periodicals Customer Service, 6277 Sea Harbor Drive, Orlando, FL 32887-4800. **Customer Service: 1-800-654-2452 (US). From outside of the US, call 1-407-345-4000**. E-mail: hhspcs@harcourt.com.

The Pediatric Clinics of North America is also published in Spanish by McGraw-Hill Inter-americana Editores S.A., Mexico City, Mexico; in Portuguese by Riechmann and Affonso Editores, Rua Comandante Coelho 1085, CEP 21250, Rio de Janeiro, Brazil; and in Greek by Althayia SA, Athens, Greece.

The Pediatric Clinics of North America is covered in *Index Medicus, Excerpta Medica, Current Contents, Current Contents/Clinical Medicine, Science Citation Index, ASCA, ISI/BIOMED,* and *BIOSIS.*

Printed in the United States of America.

GUEST EDITORS

ELLIS D. AVNER, MD, Associate Dean for Research, Medical College of Wisconsin; Director, Children's Research Institute, Children's Hospital and Health System of Wisconsin, Wauwatosa, Wisconsin

ROBERT M. KLIEGMAN, MD, Muma Family Professor and Chairman, Department of Pediatrics, Medical College of Wisconsin; Executive Vice President, Children's Research Institute, Children's Hospital and Health System of Wisconsin, Wauwatosa, Wisconsin

CONTRIBUTORS

ELLIS D. AVNER, MD, Associate Dean for Research, Medical College of Wisconsin; Director, Children's Research Institute, Children's Hospital and Health System of Wisconsin, Wauwatosa, Wisconsin

JOYDEEP BASU, PhD, Senior Scientist, Institute for Genome Sciences & Policy, Duke University, Durham, North Carolina

STUART BERGER, MD, Professor, Department of Pediatrics, Division of Pediatric Cardiology, Medical College of Wisconsin, Children's Hospital of Wisconsin, Milwaukee, Wisconsin

ULRICH BROECKEL, MD, Department of Medicine, Medical College of Wisconsin; Human and Molecular Genetics Center, Medical College of Wisconsin; Department of Pediatrics, Children's Hospital of Wisconsin, Milwaukee, Wisconsin

F. SESSIONS COLE, MD, Park J. White Professor of Pediatrics; and Director, Division of Newborn Medicine in the Edward Mallinckrodt Department of Pediatrics, Washington University School of Medicine and St. Louis Children's Hospital, St. Louis, Missouri

JIANG FAN, MD, Assistant Professor of Pediatrics, Division of Infectious Disease, Medical College of Wisconsin, Milwaukee, Wisconsin

DEBEBE GEBREMEDHIN, PhD, Department of Physiology; Cardiovascular Research Center, Medical College of Wisconsin, Milwaukee, Wisconsin

AARON HAMVAS, MD, Professor of Pediatrics; and Medical Director, Division of Newborn Medicine in the Edward Mallinckrodt Department of Pediatrics, Washington University School of Medicine and St. Louis Children's Hospital, St. Louis, Missouri

DAVID R. HARDER, PhD, Professor, Department of Physiology; and Director, Cardiovascular Research Center, Medical College of Wisconsin, Milwaukee, Wisconsin

KELLY J. HENRICKSON, MD, Professor of Pediatrics and Microbiology, Division of Infectious Disease; and Director of Respiratory Diagnostic Laboratory, Medical College of Wisconsin, Milwaukee, Wisconsin

JULIE R. INGELFINGER, MD, Senior Consultant in Pediatric Nephrology, MassGeneral Hospital for Children at Massachusetts General Hospital; Professor of Pediatrics, Harvard Medical School, Boston, Massachusetts

DENISE B. KLINKNER, MD, Resident in General Surgery, Children's Research Institute and Medical College of Wisconsin, Milwaukee, Wisconsin

GIRIJA G. KONDURI, MD, Professor, Department of Pediatrics, Division of Neonatology, Medical College of Wisconsin, Children's Hospital of Wisconsin, Milwaukee, Wisconsin

ANDREA J. KRAFT, MS, Laboratory Supervisor, Department of Pediatrics, Division of Infectious Disease, Medical College of Wisconsin, Milwaukee, Wisconsin

SUBRA KUGATHASAN, MD, Department of Pediatrics, Children's Hospital of Wisconsin, Milwaukee, Wisconsin

GERALD M. LOUGHLIN, MD, Nancy C. Paduano Professor and Chair of Pediatrics, Weill Medical College of Cornell University, New York, New York

KAREN MARESSO, MPH, Human and Molecular Genetics Center, Medical College of Wisconsin, Milwaukee, Wisconsin

YOHEI MATSUZAKI, MD, Department of Pediatrics, School of Medicine, Keio University, Tokyo, Japan

MICHAEL E. MITCHELL, MD, Assistant Professor of Surgery, Division of Cardiothoracic Surgery, Children's Hospital of Wisconsin, Medical College of Wisconsin, Milwaukee, Wisconsin

ANNE MOSCONA, MD, Professor of Pediatrics and of Microbiology and Immunology, Vice Chair of Pediatrics for Research, Weill Medical College of Cornell University, New York, New York

JAYASHREE NARAYANAN, MS, Department of Physiology; Cardiovascular Research Center, Medical College of Wisconsin, Milwaukee, Wisconsin

LAWRENCE M. NOGEE, MD, Associate Professor of Pediatrics, Division of Neonatology in the Department of Pediatrics, Johns Hopkins University School of Medicine, Baltimore, Maryland

PHILLIP F. PRATT, PhD, Department of Anesthesiology and Pharmacology and Toxicology, Medical College of Wisconsin, Milwaukee, Wisconsin

TARA L. SANDER, PhD, Assistant Professor of Surgery, Division of Pediatric Surgery, Cardiovascular Research Center, Children's Research Institute and Medical College of Wisconsin, Milwaukee, Wisconsin

WILLIAM E. SWEENEY, JR, Operations Manager, Children's Research Institute; Childrens' Hospital Health System of Wisconsin; Assistant Professor, Department of Pediatrics, Division of Pediatrics, Medical College of Wisconsin, Milwaukee, Wisconsin

MARIA TERASHVILI, PhD, Department of Physiology; Cardiovascular Research Center, Medical College of Wisconsin, Milwaukee, Wisconsin

AOY TOMITA-MITCHELL, PhD, Assistant Professor of Surgery, Biotechnology and Bioengineering Center, Human and Molecular Genetics Center, Milwaukee, Wisconsin

JEFFREY A. WHITSETT, MD, Professor, Department of Pediatrics, Division of Pulmonary Biology, Cincinnati Children's Hospital Medical Center and the University of Cincinnati College of Medicine, Cincinnati, Ohio

HUNTINGTON F. WILLARD, PhD, Director, Institute for Genome Sciences & Policy, Duke University, Durham, North Carolina

ANTHONY WYNSHAW-BORIS, MD, PhD, Professor of Pediatrics and Medicine, Vice Chair for Research, Department of Pediatrics Director, Center for Human Genetics and Genomics, University of California San Diego School of Medicine, La Jolla, California

CONTENTS

> Technological development in genetics and genomics provides un-
> precedented possibilities to identify the underlying molecular basis
> of many common diseases. With the availability of the human gen-
> ome sequence and growing information on the most frequent DNA
> variations combined with the molecular analysis on the RNA ex-
> pression and protein level, diseases might be characterized in the
> future at the molecular level. Describing gene function and the spe-
> cific role of DNA, RNA, and proteins in the disease process pro-
> vides novel diagnostic tools and treatment. Ultimately, the goal is
> to provide optimal therapy for each patient. Understanding how
> the unique genetic signature of an individual influences the risk
> and prognosis of disease will be the basis for individualized med-
> icine in the years to come.

> Bioterrorism is the calculated use of violence against civilians to at-
> tain political, religious, or ideologic goals using weapons of biolo-
> gical warfare. Bioterrorism is particularly concerning because these
> weapons can be manufactured with ease and do not require highly
> sophisticated technology. Moreover, biologic agents can be deliv-
> ered and spread easily and can affect a large population and
> geographic area. The terrorist attacks occurring around the world

necessitate society's continued investment in adequate defense against these unpredictable and irrational events.

Human Artificial Chromosomes: Potential Applications and Clinical Considerations

Joydeep Basu and Huntington F. Willard

Human artificial chromosomes demonstrate promise as a novel class of nonintegrative gene therapy vectors. The authors outline current developments in human artificial chromosome technology and examine their potential for clinical application.

Inborn Errors of Development: Disruption of Pathways Critical for Normal Development

Anthony Wynshaw-Boris

Traditionally, congenital birth defects have been classified descriptively based on the observed defects. As the genes important for some birth defects have been identified, it is clear that several of the genes mutated in malformation syndromes or genes whose expression is disrupted by environmental agents or teratogens are part of conserved signal transduction pathways. One can consider malformations to be inborn errors of development whereby pathways important for controlling development throughout evolution have been disrupted. This article focuses on three highly conserved pathways and their interactions and provides a framework that allows pediatricians to relate the phenotype of humans who have developmental disorders to the functions of genes in a signal transduction pathway.

Transcriptional Regulation of Perinatal Lung Maturation

Jeffrey A. Whitsett and Yohei Matsuzaki

Respiration at birth depends on maturation changes in lung tissue architecture, cell differentiation, and gene expression. At the transcriptional level, maturation is controlled by the actions of a group of transcription factors mediating gene expression in the lung. A network of transcription factors regulates gene expression in the respiratory epithelium, which then influences cell maturation throughout the lung. Glucocorticoids (via the glucocorticoid receptor), acting primarily in the pulmonary mesenchyme, influence maturation in the respiratory epithelium. Elucidation of the intersecting pathways controlling perinatal lung function may provide opportunities to induce pulmonary maturation in preterm infants at risk for respiratory distress syndrome before birth, and will help identify genes and processes important for various aspects of lung function.

Renal Cystic Disease: New Insights for the Clinician

Ellis D. Avner and William E. Sweeney, Jr

This article cannot comprehensively cover the enormous strides made in defining the molecular and cellular basis of renal cystic diseases over the last decade. Therefore, it provides a brief overview and categorization of inherited, developmental, and acquired renal cystic diseases, providing a relevant, up-to-date bibliography as well as a useful list of informative Internet Web sites. Its major focus is the translational biology of polycystic kidney disease. It demonstrates how emerging molecular and cellular knowledge of the pathophysiology of particular diseases such as autosomal dominant polycystic kidney disease (ADPKD) and autosomal recessive polycystic kidney disease (ADPKD) can translate into innovative therapeutic insights.

Defects in Surfactant Synthesis: Clinical Implications

F. Sessions Cole, Lawrence M. Nogee, and Aaron Hamvas

Since the original description of deficiency of the pulmonary surfactant in premature newborn infants by Avery and Mead in 1959, respiratory distress syndrome has most commonly been attributed to developmental immaturity of surfactant production. Studies of different ethnic groups, gender, targeted gene ablation in murine lineages, and recent clinical reports of monogenic causes of neonatal respiratory distress syndrome have demonstrated that genetic defects disrupt pulmonary surfactant metabolism and cause respiratory distress syndrome, especially in term or near-term infants and in older infants, children, and adults. In contrast to developmental causes of respiratory distress, which may improve as infants and children mature, genetic causes result in both acute and chronic (and potentially irreversible) respiratory failure.

The Cell Biology of Acute Childhood Respiratory Disease: Therapeutic Implications

Gerald M. Loughlin and Anne Moscona

Respiratory syncytial virus (RSV), the recently identified human metapneumovirus (HMPV), and the human parainfluenza viruses (HPIVs), cause most cases of childhood croup, bronchiolitis, and pneumonia. Influenza virus also causes a significant burden of disease in young children, although its significance in children was not fully recognized until recently. This article discusses pathogens that have been studied for several decades, including RSV and HPIVs, and also explores the newly identified viral pathogens HMPV and human coronavirus NL63. The escalating rate of emergence of new infectious agents, fortunately meeting with equally rapid advancements in molecular methods of surveillance and pathogen discovery, means that new organisms will soon be added to the list. A section on therapies for bronchiolitis addresses the final common pathways that can result from infection with diverse pathogens, highlighting the mechanisms that may be amenable to therapeutic approaches. The article concludes with a discussion of the overarching impact of new diagnostic strategies.

volved in blood pressure regulation is enormous, and dissecting those factors that are most important in hypertension has proven challenging. This article discusses molecular mechanisms of hypertension in several conditions in which mutations in a single gene give rise to hypertension and then considers the contribution of these and other genes to essential hypertension.

Reactive oxygen species (ROS) are a family of oxygen-derived free radicals that are produced in mammalian cells under normal and pathologic conditions. Many ROS, such as the superoxide anion (O_2^-) and hydrogen peroxide (H_2O_2), act as cellular signaling molecules within blood vessels, altering mechanisms mediating mechanical signal transduction and autoregulation of cerebral blood flow. This article focuses on the actions of ROS, such as $O_2^{\cdot-}$ and H_2O_2, and how they influence mechanisms responsible for the modulation of pressure-induced myogenic tone in the cerebral circulation and blood flow autoregulation in response to elevated arterial pressure. ROS may be a key target for therapeutic interventions in pediatric patients who have hypoxic injury or altered cerebral metabolism induced by trauma or infection.

FORTHCOMING ISSUES

RECENT ISSUES

PEDIATRIC CLINICS OF NORTH AMERICA OCTOBER 2006

GOAL STATEMENT
The goal of *Pediatric Clinics of North America* is to keep practicing physicians and residents up to date with current clinical practice in pediatrics by providing timely articles reviewing the state-of-the-art in patient care.

ACCREDITATION
The *Pediatric Clinics of North America* is planned and implemented in accordance with the Essential Areas and Policies of the Accreditation Council for Continuing Medical Education (ACCME) through the joint sponsorship of the University of Virginia School of Medicine and Elsevier. The University of Virginia School of Medicine is accredited by the ACCME to provide continuing medical education for physicians.

The University of Virginia School of Medicine designates this educational activity for a maximum of 15 *AMA PRA Category 1 Credits*™. Physicians should only claim credit commensurate with the extent of their participation in the activity.

The American Medical Association has determined that physicians not licensed in the US who participate in this CME activity are eligible for 15 *AMA PRA Category 1 Credits*™.

Credit can be earned by reading the text material, taking the CME examination online at http://www.theclinics.com/home/cme, and completing the evaluation. After taking the test, you will be required to review any and all incorrect answers. Following completion of the test and evaluation, your credit will be awarded and you may print your certificate.

FACULTY DISCLOSURE/CONFLICT OF INTEREST
The University of Virginia School of Medicine, as an ACCME accredited provider, endorses and strives to comply with the Accreditation Council for Continuing Medical Education (ACCME) Standards of Commercial Support, Commonwealth of Virginia statutes, University of Virginia policies and procedures, and associated federal and private regulations and guidelines on the need for disclosure and monitoring of proprietary and financial interests that may affect the scientific integrity and balance of content delivered in continuing medical education activities under our auspices.

The University of Virginia School of Medicine requires that all CME activities accredited through this institution be developed independently and be scientifically rigorous, balanced and objective in the presentation/discussion of its content, theories and practices.

All authors/editors participating in an accredited CME activity are expected to disclose to the readers relevant financial relationships with commercial entities occurring within the past 12 months (such as grants or research support, employee, consultant, stock holder, member of speakers bureau, etc.). The University of Virginia School of Medicine will employ appropriate mechanisms to resolve potential conflicts of interest to maintain the standards of fair and balanced education to the reader. Questions about specific strategies can be directed to the Office of Continuing Medical Education, University of Virginia School of Medicine, Charlottesville, Virginia.

The authors/editors listed below have identified no financial or professional relationships for themselves or their spouse/partner: Ellis D. Avner, MD (Guest Editor); Stuart Berger, MD; Ulrich Broeckel, MD; F. Sessions Cole, MD; Jiang Fan, MD; Debebe Gebremedhin, B.Pharm., PhD; Aaron Hamvas, MD; David R. Harder, PhD; Carla Holloway (Acquisitions Editor); Julie R. Inglefinger, MD; Robert Kliegman, MD (Guest Editor); Denise B. Klinkner, MD; Girija G Konduri, MD; Andrea Kraft, MS; Subra Kugathasan, MD; Gerald M. Loughlin, MD; Karen Maresso, MPH; Yohei Matsuzaki, MD; Jayashree Narayanan, MS; Lawrence M. Nogee, MD; Phillip F. Pratt, PhD; Tara L. Sander, PhD; William E. Sweeney, Jr.; Maia Terashvili, PhD; Jeffrey A. Whitsett, MD; Huntington F. Willard, PhD; and, Anthony Wynshaw-Boris, MD, PhD.

The authors/editors listed below identified the following professional or financial affiliations for themselves or their spouse/partner:
Joydeep Basu, PhD is a patent holder for and owns stock in Athersys, Inc.
Kelly J. Henrickson, MD owns stock and holds a patent with Prodesse, Inc., and is a consultant for MedImmune, Merck, and GlaxoSmithKline.
Michael Mitchell, MD owns stock and holds a patent with Fossa Medical, Inc. and owns stock with MDInteractive. com.
Anne Moscona, MD is employed by OptionCare; is on the speaker's bureau for Medimmune; and is on the advisory committee for GlaxoSmithKline and Roche.
Aoy Tomita-Mitchell, PhD owns stock and holds a patent with Fossa Medical, Inc. and owns stock with MDInteractive.com.

Disclosure of Discussion of Non-FDA Approved Uses for Pharmaceutical and/or Medical Devices:
The University of Virginia School of Medicine, as an ACCME provider, requires that all authors identify and disclose any "off label" uses for pharmaceutical and medical device products. The University of Virginia School of Medicine recommends that each physician fully review all the available data on new products or procedures prior to clinical use.

TO ENROLL
To enroll in the Pediatric Clinics of North America Continuing Medical Education program, call customer service at **1-800-654-2452** or visit us online at www.theclinics.com/home/cme. The CME program is available to subscribers for an additional fee of $195.00.

PEDIATRIC CLINICS
OF NORTH AMERICA

Pediatr Clin N Am
53 (2006) xv–xvi

Preface

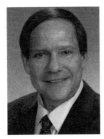 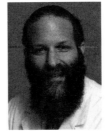

Ellis D. Avner, MD   Robert M. Kliegman, MD
Guest Editors

Genomic medicine has rapidly changed the practice of pediatrics. In this second of two issues of the *Pediatric Clinics of North America*, the authors continue to translate a new vocabulary of scientific terminology into a meaningful framework for the practicing pediatrician.

In the previous issue (Avner ED, Kliegman RM. Scientific Foundations of Clinical Practice, Part I. *Pediatric Clinics of North America* 2006;53:559–806), authors introduced new diagnostic modalities (preimplantation genetic diagnosis, microarrays), discussed the application of functional genomics to our understanding of common pediatric diseases (immunological disorders, bacterial infections, asthma, inflammatory bowel disease, ocular disorders, psychiatric disorders, obesity), and described the potential and pitfalls of new genomic therapies (gene therapy, pharmacogenomics, hematopoietic cell transplantation). In the current issue, a talented group of translational investigators continue to review specific methodologies that form the basis of this revolution in clinical practice, and then further describe the new scientific foundations of pediatrics. In these articles, laboratory bench findings are rapidly translated into mechanisms of disease, and subsequently provide the basis for innovative therapies to treat acute and chronic childhood diseases.

The editors know that a deeper understanding of the new scientific foundations of clinical practice will lead to improvements in child health and welfare. During these difficult times when children are threatened daily by man-made and natural complex humanitarian emergencies, may we have the wisdom to always use this knowledge to protect the children we serve.

0031-3955/06/$ - see front matter © 2006 Elsevier Inc. All rights reserved.
doi:10.1016/j.pcl.2006.08.011

In closing, the editors wish to thank Mrs. Marcia Barrett and Mrs. Susan Newlin for their excellent administrative support, and Ms. Carla Holloway for her patience and editorial assistance. Finally, we thank Jane, Sharon, and our families for their love and support.

Ellis D. Avner, MD
Medical College of Wisconsin
Children's Research Institute
Children's Hospital and Health System of Wisconsin
Children's Corporate Center
999 North 92nd Street
Wauwatosa, WI 53226, USA

E-mail address: eavner@mcw.edu

Robert M. Kliegman, MD
Department of Pediatrics
Medical College of Wisconsin
Children's Research Institute
Children's Hospital and Health System of Wisconsin
Children's Corporate Center
999 North 92nd Street
Wauwatosa, WI 53226, USA

E-mail address: rkliegma@mcw.edu

ELSEVIER
SAUNDERS

Pediatr Clin N Am
53 (2006) 807–816

PEDIATRIC CLINICS
OF NORTH AMERICA

Functional Genomics and Its Implications for Molecular Medicine

Ulrich Broeckel, MD[a,b,c,*], Karen Maresso, MPH[b], Subra Kugathasan, MD[c]

[a]Department of Medicine, Medical College of Wisconsin, 8701 Watertown Plank Road,
Milwaukee, WI 53226, USA
[b]Human and Molecular Genetics Center, Medical College of Wisconsin,
8701 Watertown Plank Road, Milwaukee, WI 53226, USA
[c]Department of Pediatrics, Children's Hospital of Wisconsin, 9000 W. Wisconsin Avenue,
Milwaukee, WI 53226, USA

Novel technological developments have always lead to fundamental changes in our understanding of disease mechanisms, ultimately changing the way we diagnose and treat patients. For example, the invention of the microscope lead to unprecedented discoveries that direct diagnosis and treatment, as demonstrated by the important role of a histologic characterization in cancer. It is not be surprising, therefore, that the identification of DNA, genes, and their downstream products, and the understanding of the molecular mechanisms leading to disease give us new tools for a novel molecular view of health and disease. As the Human Genome Project provides us with an unprecedented knowledge about all genes of the human genome, we now know the building blocks that determine biologic processes in humans [1]. The knowledge about DNA sequence, however, only provides a first glimpse, because RNA and ultimately proteins carry forward the information coded in genes. Consequently, extensive research efforts focus now on an integrated view linking all these components together to describe biologic systems. In large part this is enabled by the development of technologies for sequencing, expression analysis, and improved protein analyses. This global view of integrative systematic and comprehensive analysis to identify and describe processes and pathways involved in normal and abnormal states is summarized by the term functional genomics. With a specific

* Corresponding author. Human and Molecular Genetics Center, Medical College of Wisconsin, 8701 Watertown Plank Road, Milwaukee, WI 53226.
 E-mail address: broeckel@mcw.edu (U. Broeckel).

0031-3955/06/$ - see front matter © 2006 Elsevier Inc. All rights reserved.
doi:10.1016/j.pcl.2006.08.007

focus on disease, this analysis extends on the molecular level as a description of how DNA variation contributes to disease susceptibility. Ultimately, this molecular view of disease should provide us with novel molecular diagnostic tools and targets for improved treatment and drug development. In this article the authors review briefly the necessary technologies, focus specifically on the analysis of DNA as a first step to identify causal gene mutations that can be used for diagnostic tests in a clinical setting, and expand on key issues to bring the understanding of genetics of complex disease into clinical practice.

Tools and infrastructure

As an emerging discipline, functional genomics builds critically on the development and the availability of molecular technologies. At each step in the cascade from gene to protein, various methods have been developed and refined to address specific analytic needs. These include, on the molecular level, the development of cost-efficient sequencing and high-throughput analysis of DNA variants. For RNA analysis, with the development of chip-based expression profiling, the analysis of hundreds and thousand of RNAs enables us to analyze comprehensively the expression pattern of a large number of genes in cells or diseases of interest. Finally, the emerging area of proteomics has progressed significantly to permit simultaneous analysis of large numbers of proteins with increased accuracy and sensitivity. The next sections provide a brief review of some of the most widely used technology platforms for functional genomics.

DNA analysis

With regard to DNA analysis platforms, methods can be separated based on overall goal. Sequencing represents a well-established platform that allows the identification of novel DNA variants—also known as single nucleotide polymorphisms (SNPs)—and the determination of previously identified mutations by resequencing analysis. Over the years, the technology has been optimized with regard to reagents and further development of high-throughput sequencers. In part, the progress in sequencing technology was a critical component for the Human Genome Project to establish the full sequence of the human genome. Currently, direct sequencing as a means of DNA analysis is used mainly for the identification of novel mutations or the analysis of rare mutations that cannot be analyzed easily and cost-efficiently using other, more targeted platforms [2]. Significant research efforts are focused toward reducing the cost of sequencing, however, ultimately leading to analysis of an individual's entire genome sequence for a target cost of $1,000 [3].

For the analysis of a set of known and predefined mutations, a variety of genotyping platforms have been established and the technology has matured significantly over the last few years. The decision of which platforms would be most appropriate for a project depends on several factors. The different genotyping platforms vary in throughput, genotyping cost, and the ease of establishing an assay. For studies focusing on the analysis of a limited number of markers or the testing of defined and previously identified mutations, lower-throughput methods, such as the ABI TaqMan method, would be most appropriate. These lower-throughput methods are performed mainly in single reactions and assay one SNP or mutation at a time. With improved automation, these methods allow for the analysis of hundreds to thousands of samples for a limited number of markers. One advantage of the ABI Taq-Man platform is also the availability of established assays for a large number of previously identified SNPs. This availability allows for a rapid analysis of known DNA variants without the need for establishing and evaluating the assay performance. For a large number of diseases, however, risk mutations have not yet been identified and substantial efforts are geared toward improving our understanding of the genetic architecture of a disease and the identification of mutations that predispose to disease.

Identification of genes for common diseases leading toward DNA disease markers

In comparison to other specialties, genetics already plays a significant role in the field of pediatrics. Most diagnostic tests that are currently in use focus on rare diseases, often with a Mendelian mode of inheritance. Single-gene disorders, however, may account for only a small percentage of the overall diseases in patients seen by pediatricians. Consequently, the focus has expanded toward improving our understanding of how genes and genetic factors contribute to common pediatric diseases, such as asthma, diabetes, or obesity. In addition, pharmacogenetics and genomics also can be added to this list as we aim to understand how variation of genes involved in drug metabolism affect the therapeutic response to commonly used drugs. It is generally accepted that most common forms of pediatric diseases likely result from the interaction of several genetic and environmental factors. Such diseases therefore are multifactorial (genes and environment) and polygenic (multiple genes required in each patient) in nature.

Over the years, there has been an intensive discussion about the methods to map and identify genes for such polygenic, common diseases. Although the classical linkage approach has been successful for diseases with Mendelian forms of inheritance, this approach has been more challenging for polygenic diseases. The genes typically identified with this linkage strategy have been those with low-frequency mutations causing a substantial effect on the phenotype [4]. Conversely, the gene variants that underlie common disease are likely to have smaller effects. Under these circumstances, it is well known that the linkage approach alone might not be sufficient to identify possible loci [5]. Consequently, there is a need to develop further strategies to overcome these limitations. Using a high-density set of markers in an association study is likely to have greater power to localize genes with moderate effects on multifactorial disorders. With the development of highest-throughput analysis methods coupled with advanced bioinformatic data analysis, the association study approach has gained substantial interest [6].

With this in mind, there is still significant discussion about the best approach for association mapping. This discussion mainly is based on the uncertainty about what one might call the allelic architecture of polygenic diseases: how many genes contribute to the disease risk, how many mutations in a gene are present, what is their frequency, and what is the effect of each mutation? Because only a few disease genes actually have been identified for common diseases, our understanding of the underlying allelic architecture relies on these examples and simulation studies. The "common disease—common variant" hypothesis builds the basis for the newly initiated HapMap project aiming to develop genomewide haplotype information for whole genome association scans. Based on simulations incorporating evolutionary processes, such as selection, mutation, and genetic drift, there is also support for models that favor the notion that alleles with lower frequency can contribute significantly to polygenic diseases [7]. The frequency of disease alleles might also depend on whether an association study starts by looking at a priori functional candidate genes or whether the analysis starts from a linkage signal. In any case, following the seminal work by Risch and Merikangas [6], genomewide association analyses are likely to be a powerful approach for disease mapping. There has been encouraging progress overall, as illustrated by the recent successes of locating functional variants associated with such common diseases as non–insulin-dependent diabetes mellitus, inflammatory bowel disease, asthma, prostate cancer, and coronary artery disease [8–14].

Genomewide association studies for disease marker identification

The proposed technology of genomewide association (GWA) scanning builds critically on the technological platform for high-throughput genotyping. Over the last few years, this technology has matured significantly and several platforms have been made commercially available. Currently, two main platforms are commercially available from Affymetrix (http://www.Affymetrix.com) and Illumina (http://www.Illumina.com) allowing for the analysis of 500,000 or more SNPs at a time. The methodologies differ in the actual assay method. Although the Affymetrix chip uses oligonucleotides built on an array, the Illumina platforms uses beads labeled with oligonucleotides that are placed on an array. Currently, the markers that are selected on the platforms differ based on different selection criteria and in some part because of technical constraints of the method. Although it is difficult at this moment to assess advantages of one platform over the other, a recent comparison between these two techniques comes to the conclusion that both methods can be used for GWA [15,16]. With this technology available, several studies currently are underway to identify genes for common diseases. As these methods are novel, only a few reports have been published recently showing the feasibility and power of this approach. Most recently in a genomewide screen using the Affymetrix 100k SNP chip, Klein and colleagues [17] identified complement factor H (*CFH*) as a gene influencing the risk for age-related macular degeneration. A second recent example focused on obesity as a common disease with polygenic nature. Herbert and coworkers [18] used an association study approach with a 100,000 SNP chip and identified a common variant in the INSIG2 gene as a risk factor influencing BMI. Although the initial association was detected in a population sample from the Framingham Heart Study, the significant effect of a marker in this gene was replicated in a second white population sample, in African Americans, and in a pediatric cohort. These findings provide strong support that GWA can identify genes with significant effects. The finding that a gene that has been identified in an adult population can be replicated in a pediatric cohort is of significant importance also. Although caution is necessary and exceptions exist, the results from adult studies clearly warrant confirmation in pediatric patients for diseases that evolve from childhood to adulthood. Conversely, evidence from pediatric studies clearly should be tested in adult cohorts.

Taken together, these examples demonstrate that GWA is a promising approach to identify genes for common diseases. The identification of disease-causing genes is, however, only a first step in identifying markers for a disease process, improving our understanding of novel disease mechanisms, and describing the function and effect of these genes.

DNA mutations as markers of disease progression

Although large-scale linkage and association studies will uncover the genetic underpinnings of complex diseases, the question ultimately remains whether these methods identify genes with significant clinical or prognostic relevance. The authors recently demonstrated an association of the 3020insC polymorphism of the CARD15/NOD2 gene to pediatric-onset Crohn disease (CD) in a prospective cohort of white children. The CARD15/NOD2 gene was one of the first genes to be positionally cloned for a complex disease based on a prior genomewide scan. Particular SNPs within this gene have been associated previously with adult-onset Crohn disease, and the authors have extended these findings to children with the disease. As a subset of children who have CD progress to severe disease requiring surgical intervention, the authors' goal was to determine if the 3020insC SNP could identify a subset of children at high risk for surgery who would benefit from early aggressive therapy. This study also demonstrated that the disease identification paradigm actually can result in the discovery of clinically relevant genes that can be used to improve risk prediction.

In a prospective study, 163 white children who had CD were recruited with parents and followed for up to 70 months. The authors used a Cox proportional hazards model, stratified according to the presence or absence of the 3020insC allele, to determine the effect of this mutation on surgery-free survival.

The unadjusted hazard ratio carrying the 3020insC variant was 6.07 (95% CI 2.76–13.37, $P < .0001$), indicating that the hazard for surgery is six times greater in children with this SNP compared with those without (Fig. 1). This finding suggests that this variant could be used as a prognostic factor for early surgery in white children who have CD. Although this study is specific to pediatric-onset CD, the authors believe it also might serve as an example of how gene identification strategies can lead to new clinically important prognostic markers in pediatric disease [19].

RNA analysis

Because DNA variation influences diseases processes, it is obvious that RNA as the downstream product of genes similarly reflects the disease process. In some cases, such as cancer, changes in gene expression are fundamental characteristics of pathogenesis. The mechanisms for these changes can be complex. For example, mutations in coding regions can directly affect the gene product, mutations in splice sites can result in splice variants, mutations in 5′ regulatory regions can affect RNA levels, and 3′ mutations can influence RNA stability. Whatever mechanism of mutation ultimately is involved, the gene expression program of a cell reflects these changes at some point. Consequently, the quantitative analysis of gene expression evolved as a powerful tool for diagnosis and disease characterization. Most progress in this field has been made related to cancer and cancer diagnostics. For example, for adult patients who have acute myeloid leukemia, the current classification system

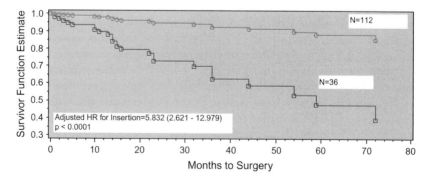

Fig. 1. Survival analysis in pediatric-onset Crohn disease in children stratified by CARD15 genotype. Squares denote children homozygous or heterozygous for 3020insC; circles denote children homozygous for wildtype. Children who have the 3020insC have a significant higher risk for surgery.

does not reflect fully the molecular heterogeneity of the disease, and treatment stratification is difficult. In a recent study by Bullinger and colleagues [20] expression profiling was used to identify patients at increased risk. Hierarchical clustering analysis to identify molecular subgroups with distinct gene-expression signatures identified a gene expression pattern grouped in a set of a 133-gene clinical-outcome predictor, which accurately predicted overall survival among these patients. Similar results have been described for other types of cancer, such as diffuse large B-cell lymphomas [21], ovarian cancer [22], or liver tumors [23]. Ultimately, the molecular classification of a disease on the RNA level in combination with the genetic analysis in the future should allow placing a patient in a specific molecular subgroup. The development of this genetic- and genomic-derived classification can direct the treatment toward genomic-tailored and more individualized treatment.

Protein analysis

Proteomics deals with the identification, characterization, and quantitative and functional analyses of proteins in cells. The systematic and comprehensive analysis of the protein remains a daunting task. This challenge is attributable in part to the substantial complexity of proteins, the great variability of their functional activity because of posttranslational modifications, and the functional importance of their localization. Furthermore, protein–protein interaction significantly influences the function of proteins. Significant technological progress has been made in protein sequencing. Various databases exist that systematically describe protein sequence and model the three-dimensional structure of proteins. Approaches exist to characterize functional classes linking protein families to predicted function. With the development of better and more sensitive methods determining protein concentrations by mass spectrometry, and the development of protein arrays, the technological basis has been established to increase the number of proteins that can be analyzed simultaneously. This technology will be important to link gene expression information with protein discovery to delineate posttranslational modifications. Significant technological challenges still remain, however. For example, sample preparation remains a critical component for a high-throughput analysis of biologic samples. Currently, protein analysis often is performed following indications from genetic and genomic studies. In the future, a comprehensive analysis of RNA expression patterns and protein levels and activity will be an important component to understand how genes and genetic factors determine disease phenotypes.

Moving functional genomics to clinical practice

Identifying disease-relevant genes will give us an unprecedented view of the molecular basis of disease. Developing specific knowledge about how a gene causes a disease, identifying detailed disease mechanisms, and systematically and comprehensively analyzing gene function in health and disease are daunting tasks. Bringing genetic knowledge to the clinic, however, might not depend on the final elucidation of the function of a gene because genetic markers, the expression profile, or a protein signature also can serve as a biomarker and disease correlate. In fact, it is perceivable that genetic biomarker information will be used in disease diagnosis and treatment before we fully understand exact genetic mechanisms. For example, measuring the prostate specific antigen is now a widely used test for early detection of hypertrophy and prostate cancer, whereas the exact role and function of this protein remains less clear [24].

Clinical correlates and functional genomics

As outlined above, the various technologies allow for a comprehensive analysis of molecular targets. Ultimately the information from these analyses will focus on a subset of novel molecular diagnostics that can be used as: (1) markers to identify patients at increased risk before onset of clinical disease manifests, (2) markers for earlier detection of disease because molecular changes may precede overt clinical disease manifestations, (3) markers to identify patients who have more severe disease progression requiring intensified treatment, and (4) markers to identify patients who may benefit from a specific treatment regimen because the drug affects specific disease mechanisms or drug metabolism or efficacy is influenced by genetic factors. Whatever technological platform is used—whether DNA, RNA, protein, or a combination of all these technologies—evaluation of clinical validity is fundamental to establish these molecular methods in clinical practice.

Molecular markers as clinical correlates

Prognostic markers correlate with clinical outcomes as either progression markers or risk markers. Markers related to the progression of a disease can be surrogates for other clinical criteria (clinical correlates) that are established predictors of the disease. Clinical correlates are good markers to evaluate and establish the response to treatment if the direct measurement of the disease is complex, invasive, or expensive. In many cases progression of disease determines prognosis. When the disease severity does not correlate closely with outcome, however, these clinical correlates have only a limited value to predict the overall outcome. Prognostic markers, conversely, are correlated with the progression of the disease or certain defined risks linked to the disease. Progression markers do not necessarily have to correlate with disease burden or disease mechanisms as long as these markers capture critical information related to the overall outcome. These markers have high potential as surrogate end-point markers in trials if the actual end-point is difficult to determine during a clinical trial. In some cases genetic and genomic information also might be used as risk markers to identify patients who have a severe disease prognosis. Risk markers do not necessarily have to respond to treatment, because these markers might only reflect the overall severity of a disease independent of treatment or clinical response. Finally, predictive markers are related to response, outcome, toxicity, or a combination of these factors. Ultimately, biologic markers might capture information as clinical correlates that determine the overall risk and severity of a disease, and correlate with the overall prognosis. Consequently, a critical validation of the proposed biomarkers for clinical benefit must be performed to be used in clinical practice. Most likely, the most promising leads will be identified from carefully designed clinical trials, which provide high-quality clinical data collected in a standardized environment combined with information on clinical outcome or therapeutic response. In addition, large-scale observational epidemiologic studies are necessary to provide baseline characteristics with regard to normal variation, such as gene mutation frequencies. The reanalysis of previous clinical trials or established study populations and information from disease registries with available biologic samples is a cost-efficient strategy to test these molecular markers. Finally, as the clinical importance of a test is always determined by its sensitivity, specificity, or positive predictive value, these characteristics have to be established in the relevant clinical populations. In that respect, it is important to perform adequately powered studies in the respective pediatric populations as a basis for clinical applications.

Summary

Technological development in genetics and genomics provides unprecedented possibilities to identify the underlying molecular basis of many common diseases. With the availability of the human genome sequence and growing information on the most frequent DNA variations combined with the molecular analysis on the RNA expression and protein level, diseases might be characterized in the future at the molecular level. Describing gene function and the specific role of DNA, RNA, and proteins in the disease process provides novel diagnostic tools and treatment. Ultimately, the goal is always to provide optimal therapy for each patient. Understanding how the unique genetic signature of an individual influences the risk and prognosis of disease is the basis for individualized medicine in the years to come.

References

[1] Lander ES, Linton LM, Birren B, et al. Initial sequencing and analysis of the human genome. Nature 2001;409:860–921.
[2] Stephens M, Sloan JS, Robertson PD, et al. Automating sequence-based detection and genotyping of SNPs from diploid samples. Nat Genet 2006;38:375–81.
[3] Service RF. Gene sequencing. The race for the $1000 genome. Science 2006;311:1544.
[4] Hannson J, Nelson-Williams C, Suzuki H, et al. Hypertension caused by a truncated epithelial sodium channel gamma subunit: genetic heterogeneity of Liddle syndrome. Nat Genet 1995;11:76–82.

[5] Risch N. Linkage strategies for genetically complex traits. I. Multilocus models. Am J Hum Genet 1990;46:222–8.

[6] Risch N, Merikangas K. The future of genetic studies of complex human diseases. Science 1996;273:1516–7.

[7] Pritchard JK. Are rare variants responsible for susceptibility to complex diseases? Am J Hum Genet 2001;69:124–37.

[8] Helgadottir A, Manolescu A, Thorleifsson G, et al. The gene encoding 5-lipoxygenase activating protein confers risk of myocardial infarction and stroke. Nat Genet 2004;36:233–9.

[9] Horikawa Y, Oda N, Cox NJ, et al. Genetic variation in the gene encoding calpain-10 is associated with type 2 diabetes mellitus. Nat Genet 2000;26:163–75.

[10] Hugot JP, Chamaillard M, Zouali H, et al. Association of NOD2 leucine-rich repeat variants with susceptibility to Crohn's disease. Nature 2001;411:599–603.

[11] Ogura Y, Bonen DK, Inohara N, et al. A frameshift mutation in NOD2 associated with susceptibility to Crohn's disease. Nature 2001;411:603–6.

[12] Ozaki K, Ohnishi Y, Iida A, et al. Functional SNPs in the lymphotoxin-alpha gene that are associated with susceptibility to myocardial infarction. Nat Genet 2002;32:650–4.

[13] Rioux JD, Daly MJ, Silverberg MS, et al. Genetic variation in the 5q31 cytokine gene cluster confers susceptibility to Crohn disease. Nat Genet 2001;29:223–8.

[14] Xu J, Zheng SL, Komiya A, et al. Germline mutations and sequence variants of the macrophage scavenger receptor 1 gene are associated with prostate cancer risk. Nat Genet 2002;32:321–5.

[15] Barrett JC, Cardon LR. Evaluating coverage of genome-wide association studies. Nat Genet 2006;38:659.

[16] Pe'er I, de Bakker PI, Maller J, et al. Evaluating and improving power in whole-genome association studies using fixed marker sets. Nat Genet 2006;38:663.

[17] Klein RJ, Zeiss C, Chew EY, et al. Complement factor H polymorphism in age-related macular degeneration. Science 2005;308:385–9.

[18] Herbert A, Gerry NP, McQueen MB, et al. A common genetic variant is associated with adult and childhood obesity. Science 2006;312:279–83.

[19] Kugathasan S, Collins N, Maresso K, et al. CARD15 gene mutations and risk for early surgery in pediatric-onset Crohn's disease. Clin Gastroenterol Hepatol 2004;2:1003–9.

[20] Bullinger L, Dohner K, Bair E, et al. Use of gene-expression profiling to identify prognostic subclasses in adult acute myeloid leukemia. N Engl J Med 2004;350:1605–16.

[21] Lossos IS, Czerwinski DK, Alizadeh AA, et al. Prediction of survival in diffuse large-B-cell lymphoma based on the expression of six genes. N Engl J Med 2004;350:1828–37.

[22] Heinzelmann-Schwarz VA, Gardiner-Garden M, Henshall SM, et al. A distinct molecular profile associated with mucinous epithelial ovarian cancer. Br J Cancer 2006;94:904–13.

[23] Lam SH, Wu YL, Vega VB, et al. Conservation of gene expression signatures between zebrafish and human liver tumors and tumor progression. Nat Biotechnol 2006;24:73–5.

[24] Vollmer RT. Predictive probability of serum prostate-specific antigen for prostate cancer: an approach using Bayes rule. Am J Clin Pathol 2006;125:336–42.

ELSEVIER
SAUNDERS

Pediatr Clin N Am
53 (2006) 817–842

PEDIATRIC CLINICS
OF NORTH AMERICA

Current Methods for the Rapid Diagnosis of Bioterrorism-Related Infectious Agents

Jiang Fan, MD[a], Andrea J. Kraft, MS[a], Kelly J. Henrickson, MD[b],*

[a]*Department of Pediatrics, Medical College of Wisconsin, 8701 Watertown Plank Road, Milwaukee, WI 53226, USA*
[b]*Pediatric Infectious Diseases, Children's Hospital of Wisconsin, Suite C450, P.O. Box 1997, Milwaukee, WI 53201-1997, USA*

Bioterrorism is the calculated use of violence against civilians to attain political, religious, or ideologic goals using weapons of biological warfare. Bioterrorism is particularly concerning because these weapons can be manufactured with ease and do not require highly sophisticated technology. Moreover, biologic agents can be delivered and spread easily and can affect a large population and geographic area. The terrorist attacks occurring around the world necessitate society's continued investment in adequate defense against these unpredictable and irrational events.

A bioterrorist attack, or even the threat of an attack, can have an enormous impact, with economic, political, and public health implications. The impact of a true bioterrorist attack depends on the specific agent or toxin used, the method and efficiency of dispersal, the population exposed, the level of immunity in the population, the availability of effective postexposure prophylaxis or therapeutic regimens, and the potential for secondary transmission [1]. Understanding and quantifying the impact of a bioterrorist attack are essential to developing an effective response.

Many events throughout history have involved the use of biological weapons. One of the first well-documented events was during the 14th century medieval siege of Kaffa [76]. The attacking Tartars catapulted dead and dying plague victims into the city to spread the plague among the enemy. This action hastened the ensuing plague pandemic in Europe, and hundreds

---

* Corresponding author.
E-mail address: khenrick@mcw.edu (K.J. Henrickson).

0031-3955/06/$ - see front matter © 2006 Elsevier Inc. All rights reserved.
doi:10.1016/j.pcl.2006.08.002
pediatric.theclinics.com

and thousands of people were killed by the disease. The biological and chemical weapons used during World War I resulted in many deaths. Modern technology significantly advanced biological weapons in the 20th century. The Geneva Protocol for the "Prohibition of the Use in War of Asphyxiating, Poisonous or Other Gases and of Bacteriological Methods of Warfare" was issued in 1925 and the Geneva Convention on the "Prohibition of the Development, Production, and Stockpiling of Bacteriological and Toxin Weapons and on Their Destruction" was developed and ratified in 1972 [126]. However, although many countries signed the convention, several continued offensive research and production of biological agents as recently as the mid-1990s. Additionally, increasingly more subnational terrorist and radical groups have independently worked on offensive use of biological weapons since the mid-1980s. A recent example was the *Bacillus anthrax* event in 2001, which resulted in few deaths but significant societal disruption and cost [2].

Because of its scientific leadership, talent, resources, and health systems, the United States has special responsibility for leading efforts to prepare for a bioterrorist attack. Such a crisis would also certainly have a grave impact on the global economy. Large corporations should be planning their own response to the absenteeism, travel restrictions, isolation, and quarantine policies a terrorist attack or threat might cause, including using their considerable resources to help communities handle an event. The measures taken in the United States and throughout the world will hopefully create systems that will control an outbreak caused by a deliberate release of bioterrorism agents [3]. Important tools in this planning are rapid, sensitive, and accurate diagnostic assays to help governments and public health organizations identify most infectious agents that might be used in bioterrorism attacks. This article discusses the current status of diagnostic assays for the most likely bioterrorism agents.

Organisms with the highest bioterrorism potential

Many virulent and pathogenic organisms can be used individually or together as weapons to harm a person or community. Infectious agents identified as posing the greatest threat are classified by the Centers for Disease Control and Prevention (CDC) as CDC category A, B, or C agents (Table 1).

Importance of laboratory diagnosis

Rapid, accurate detection and identification of bioterrorism agents are important not only for confirming that a bioterrorism event has occurred but also for treating individual patients and implementing suitable public health measures. Although diagnostic tests are available for most CDC category A, B, and C bioterrorism agents, many are time consuming, have less than optimal sensitivity and specificity, or cannot test for multiple agents

Table 1
List of the Centers for Disease Control and Prevention category A, B, and C agents

Category A	Category B	Category C
Variola major (smallpox)	*Brucella* spp. (brucellosis)	Influenza A and B viruses
Bacillus anthracis (anthrax)	*Burkholderia mallei* (glanders)	Nipah virus
Yersinia pestis (plague)	*Burkholderia pseudomallei*	Hantavirus
Clostridium botulinum toxin	(meliodosis)	Rabies
(botulism)	*Chlamydia psittaci*	Drug-resistant
Francisella tularensis	(psittacosis)	tuberculosis
(tularaemia)	*Coxiella burnetii* (Q fever)	Yellow fever
RNA viruses that cause	*Ricinus communis* (ricin)	*Rickettsia conorii*
hemorrhagic, fevers (viral	*Clostridium perfringens*	Tickborne encephalitis
hemorrhagic fevers)	(epsilon toxin)	Tickborne viral
	Rickettsia prowazekii	hemorrhagic fevers
	(typhus fever)	
	Staphylococcal enterotoxin B	
	Viral encephalitis (alphaviruses)	
	Food safety agents	
	(*Salmonella, Shigella,* and	
	Escherichia coli)	
	Water safety agents	
	(*Vibrio cholerae*)	

simultaneously. Diagnostic tests that can detect multiple pathogens simultaneously offer attractive advantages, including the ability to screen patients presenting with nonspecific symptoms (eg, rash, lower respiratory symptoms, sepsis, fever) or screening asymptomatic individuals who have possible exposure to an unknown agent.

The U.S. Food and Drug Administration (FDA) has not approved any diagnostic assays for CDC category A, B, and C bioterrorism agents. The Department of Defense (DOD) has assay design requirements and specifications for detecting virtually all agents in the CDC category A, B, and C lists, which include approximately 50 to 60 agents. Considering that the DOD requires multiple genes per agent to be analyzed for accurate evaluation of biological warfare agents, this number effectively doubles.

Routine assays for laboratory diagnosis of bioterrorism agents

The current gold standard for laboratory diagnosis of bioterrorism agents is standard culture, biochemical assays, or serologic assays. For bacterial agents, routine assays would include standard culture, modified staining with light microscopic analysis, motility testing, lysis by gamma phage, capsule production staining, hemolysis, wet mounts, staining for spores, slide agglutination, direct fluorescent antibody testing, rapid immunochromatography, and ELISAs to measure antibody titers. Biochemical assays are another method for diagnosing bacterial agents. Biochemical systems for recognizing biological agents include measuring products and enzymatic activity associated with microbial metabolism, but these methods generally are not as specific as antibody- or nucleic acid–based methods because the targeted product or enzyme may also be present in other organisms [4]. The routine assays for viral agents include virus isolation through tissue culture or growth in eggs, direct and indirect immunofluorescence assays (DFA/IFA), immunodiffusion in agar, electron microscopy, modified staining and light microscopic analysis, plaque reduction neutralization testing, hemagglutination inhibition assay, neuraminidase activity assays, complement fixation, enzyme and optical immunoassays, and ELISAs to measure antibody titers or antigen concentration [5,6]. Pathologic examination of tissues and immunohistochemistry staining can also play an important role in diagnosing bioterrorism-related agents, such as anthrax, plague, tularemia, botulism, smallpox, and viral hemorrhagic fevers [7].

Molecular methods for laboratory diagnosis of bioterrorism agents

Molecular assays are becoming the new gold standard for bioterrorism detection (Table 2). The published sensitivities and specificities are close to 100% when compared with culture or serologic assays [8–40]. In fact, studies comparing molecular assays with culture have shown significantly better sensitivity (10%–33%) if a method for determining true-positives is included. Examples of current molecular methods used in diagnosing bioterrorism agents are described later.

Molecular diagnostic assays to detect infectious agents in humans or other animals usually involve target isolation (usually nucleic acid [NA], either DNA or RNA), target amplification, and then specific pathogen identification or detection (amplification product detection). Efficient methods of target or signal amplification are needed because these assays must detect pathogens to less than 10 NA copies in a reaction starting with very little material. Target amplification has been favored over signal amplification methods because stoichiometry limits the amount of signal amplification possible without getting background amplification (signal-to-noise ratio). In identifying pathogens in the environment (eg, water, air), signal amplification may be adequate because the ability to concentrate the target out of large sample volumes lessens the need for target amplification. Proteomics may also offer diagnostic assay possibilities for these agents in the future. The following discussion identifies molecular assays by their method of amplification and detection.

Signal amplification

Branch-chained DNA assays

The branch-chained DNA (bDNA) assay uses centrifugation of clinical samples to concentrate pathogens, which releases their DNA. Special oligonucleotides are added to bind to the DNA and the wall of the vessel. Other oligonucleotides are added to bind to the previous oligonucleotides to begin creating a branching mechanism that will amplify the signal. Finally, a final oligonucleotide is added that binds to the previous oligonucleotide and also binds to an enzyme. The enzyme is added and a color change occurs that allows the DNA of the organism from the original sample to be quantified. This method shows high specificity but low sensitivity (25,000 copies/mL) [41]. However, in the second generation of bDNA assay, a pre-amplifier is used to increase the number of labeled probes that can be bound to the targets, and the sensitivity is increased by two logs. To reduce the background noise, in the third generation of bDNA the non-natural bases isocytidine and isoguanosine are incorporated into the amplification probes. For example, third-generation bDNA assays for HIV-1 detection report sensitivities to a detection limit of approximately 50 copies/mL [42].

Hybrid capture assay

Hybrid capture assays depend on the formation of DNA/RNA hybrids, and a DNA/RNA hybrid–specific antibody is used to capture and detect the hybrids. For DNA target detection, NA isolation occurs and an RNA probe that is complementary to the target DNA is added to the sample. The DNA/RNA hybrids are bound by the antibodies that have been coated on a solid support. Captured hybrids react with a second antibody conjugated with an enzyme. After this step, a chemiluminescent substrate is added and a color reaction occurs. This assay has been used to detect cytomegalovirus. Studies using signal amplification to detect CDC Category A through C agents could not be found.

Target amplification

Nucleic acid–based sequence amplification

Nucleic acid–based sequence amplification (NABSA) is a transcription-based isothermic amplification method that amplifies RNA from either an RNA or DNA target. Compared with polymerase chain reaction (PCR), NASBA assay needs three enzymes: avian myeloblastosis virus reverse transcriptase, RNase H, and T7 RNA polymerase. This assay involves three steps: (1) the formation of cDNA molecules from the target RNA by the oligonucleotide primers containing a T7 RNA polymerase binding site with reverse transcriptase, (2) RNase H degradation of the initial RNA target in the RNA-DNA hybrids, with the second primer binding to the cDNA and extending so that (3) the double-stranded DNA with T7 RNA polymerase binding site is formatted and serves as a substrate of T7 polymerase, resulting in transcription of multiple copies of antisense RNA that will be used as new targets to make more cDNA and double-stranded DNA. NASBA has been used to detect influenza viruses (including avian strains),

Table 2
Current molecular methods for diagnosis of bioterrorism agents

Molecular method	Specific amplification product detection methods	Organisms	Study
Nucleic acid sequence–based amplification		Influenza A, Flaviviruses, Escherichia coli, Salmonella	[43–48]
Polymerase chain reaction	Singleplex with gel detection	Orthopoxviruses, Burkholderia spp, Brucella spp, Francisella tularensis, Bacillus anthracis, Yersinia pestis	[16,19,37–39,70,71]
	Nested	Rickettsia conorii, R prowazekii, Y pestis, Coxiella burnetii, Chlamydia psittaci	[31,32,34,40]
	Multiplex with gel detection	F tularensis, Y pestis	[19,73]
	Multiplex with liquid bead array detection	Y pestis, Bacillus anthracis, F tularensis	[56]
	Multiplex with enzyme hybridization assay detection	F tularensis, Y pestis, Bacillus anthracis, Variola major	[55]
Polymerase chain reaction–based sequencing assay		Mycobacterium tuberculosis, Bacillus anthracis, Y pestis, F tularensis, Brucella spp, Burkholderia spp	[35,51]
Reverse-transcription polymerase chain reaction	Singleplex with gel detection	Dengue, hantavirus, Ebola, Lassa, Junin, arboviruses, influenza A and B	[8,24–28,30,86–88,94,106,108]
	Singleplex with enzyme hybridization assay detection	Influenza A and B	[9,106]
	Multiplex with gel detection	Dengue, influenza A and B	[10,24,58,118,105,107,115,125]
	Multiplex with enzyme hybridization assay detection	Influenza A and B	[9,111]

Quantitative competitive polymerase chain reaction	Singleplex	*Escherichia coli*	[50]
Real-time polymerase chain reaction	Singleplex	*Bacillus anthracis, Y pestis, F tularensis, Brucella* spp. *Burkholderia mallei, Burkholderia pseudomallei,* orthopoxviruses, dengue	[35,36,75,95]
	TaqMan-based	*Coxiella burnetii, F tularensis,* dengue, orthopoxviruses	[23,33,59,72]
	SYBR Green	*Y pestis, Bacillus anthracis,* dengue	[22,53]
	Multiplex	*Bacillus anthracis, Y pestis, Burkholderia mallei,* influenza A and B	[53,64,107,112,113,116,117,121]
DNA microarray		*Bacillus anthracis, Y pestis, F tularensis,* orthopoxviruses, hantavirus, *Clostridium botulinum, Brucella* spp. influenza A and **B**, *E coli*	[52,60–62,65,119,104,109,114, 120,124]

flaviviruses, and microbial pathogens that are concerns to food safety, such as *Salmonella* and *Escherichia coli* [43–48].

Polymerase chain reaction

Recent progress has been made in designing singleplex PCR assays for some of these agents, bringing the speed and accuracy of molecular biology to their diagnosis. This method amplifies specific DNA segments using cycles of template denaturation, primer annealing, and replication using thermostable DNA polymerase at varying temperatures [49]. Singleplex PCR with gel detection has been used for many bioterrorism agents, including orthopoxviruses, *Burkholderia* spp, and *Francisella tularensis* (see Table 2). Nested singleplex PCR reactions can also be used to detect *Rickettsia conorii*, *R prowazekii*, *Yersinia pestis*, *Coxiella burnetii*, and *Chlamydia psittaci* (see Table 2) [31,32,34,40].

Reverse transcription–polymerase chain reaction

To amplify an RNA target, the RNA must be reversely transcribed to cDNA by an RNA-dependent DNA polymerase using random hexamers or one of the PCR primers as the primer. MuLV and AvLV are two commonly used reverse transcriptases. Some reverse transcription–PCR (RT-PCR) assays use a single enzyme–a recombinant DNA polymerase from *Thermus thermophilus*–that has two functions: reversely transcribing the target RNA to cDNA and amplifying the cDNA to obtain the PCR product.

Quantitative competitive polymerase chain reaction

Quantitative competitive (QC) PCR is based on coamplifying a sequence that will be quantified with a known amount of competitor sequence resembling the target. Because both sequences amplify with the same primers, the two sequences should be from the same region of DNA for the primers to amplify each with equal efficiency, but should differ slightly in size so they can be distinguished by agarose gel electrophoresis. A dilution series of three to five PCR mixtures should be made, each with an unknown amount of target DNA and a known dilution series of competitor DNA. The target and competitor DNA compete for the same primers; when the concentration of each is equivalent, band intensities will be equivalent. The point of equivalence is determined by visually assessing band intensities or digitally analyzing the gel image and generating a regression line [50]. QC PCR has been used to detect and quantify *E coli* 0157 cells [50]. QC PCR is a useful tool for detecting and quantifying pathogens when real-time PCR equipment is not available.

Polymerase chain reaction–based sequencing assay

With the rapid development of sequencing equipment and reduced price, DNA sequencing has become a routine assay in many laboratories. The capillary-based electrophoresis instruments make the automatic sequencing reactions available. Although Sanger-based dideoxy sequencing method is used most, other methods, such as Pyrosequencing assay and mass spectrometry assay, are promising alternatives. Pyrosequencing is used mainly for analyzing single nucleotide polymorphisms and characterizing short sequences [51]. This method is based on an enzyme-cascade system with real-time monitoring, and the result is accurate and can be obtained in 1 hour [51]. A pyrosequencing assay was used to identify rifampin-resistant strains of *Mycobacterium tuberculosis* [51]. Other PCR-based DNA sequencing assays have been used to identify different strains of *Bacillus anthracis, Y pestis, F tularensis, Brucella* spp, and *Burkholderia* spp (see Table 2) [35].

Multiplex PCR

Multiplex PCR amplifies two or more DNA sequences in one reaction. The biochemical method is similar to singleplex PCR, with various methods used to improve amplification within the primer mixture or detection of the PCR product [52–54]. Several uses of this method have been reported for bioterrorism agents using different methods of PCR product detection (see later discussion and Table 2). Examples of PCR product detection other than gel electrophoresis include enzyme hybridization assay (EHA), which is similar to an ELISA assay and performed in 96 well plates [55]; Luminex beads, which allow amplification DNA targets with subsequent hybridization to fluorescent beads that pass through a flow cytometer for measurement [56]; and DNA microarray detection [52].

Multiplex reverse transcription–polymerase chain reaction

Multiplex RT-PCR detects multiple different RNA agents using RT-PCR. Examples of this method for detecting bioterrorism agents include assays for detecting flaviviruses (dengue) and influenza A and B viruses (see Table 2). One study developed a rapid and cost-effective multiplex RT-PCR–based diagnostic test for detecting and serotypically characterizing dengue viruses in the acute phase of illness in a single tube [24].

Real-time polymerase chain reaction

Real-time PCR allows simultaneous DNA quantification and amplification. In real-time PCR, the target amplification and PCR product detection occur in the same tube, at the same time. The real-time PCR machine uses precision optics that can monitor fluorescence emissions when target amplification occurs. A computer software program in the machine monitors and analyzes the data throughout the PCR cycles and generates amplification information in real time. Common quantification methods include using fluorescent dyes that intercalate with double-stranded DNA, and modified DNA oligonucleotides (called *probes*) that fluoresce when hybridized with a complementary DNA. The three main fluorescence-monitoring systems for DNA amplification are hydrolysis probes, hybridizing probes, and

DNA-binding agents [57]. Hydrolysis probes include TaqMan probes (Applied Biosystems, Foster City, California) [23], molecular beacons [53], and Scorpions (DxS Ltd, Manchester, United Kingdom) [57]. Hybridizing probes include LionProbes (Biotools, Madrid, Spain) [57], and DNA-binding agents include SYBR Green (Applied Biosystems, Foster City, California) and fluorescence resonance energy transfer (FRET) probes [22,53].

Although the CDC is currently developing several singleplex real-time PCR assays to be the new gold standard for detecting bioterrorism agents in the United States, no studies have been published on these tests, nor have they been clinically field tested. Real-time PCR has been shown to be an effective method of detection for small panels [58]. However, as the panels become larger, real-time PCR is limited by the number of fluorophores that can be detected in a single reaction (currently three or four). This method involves fewer steps and everything is added at the beginning, thus decreasing the risk for contamination seen in methods that require manipulation of the amplified DNA outside of the closed reaction tube. Additional advantages of this test over standard format PCR are that it is faster and slightly cheaper. However, disadvantages include higher start-up costs, higher reagent costs, more difficulty setting the low cutoff values, and less-stable commercial reagents. A TaqMan real-time PCR assay was developed for detecting orthopoxviruses, *F tularensis*, *Coxiella burnetii*, and dengue virus (see Table 2) [23,33,59,72]. Real-time PCR assays using SYBR Green probes were developed for *Y pestis*, *Bacillus anthracis*, and dengue virus [22,53]. As seen in Table 2, some multiplex real-time PCR assays are being used to detect *Bacillus anthracis*, *Y pestis*, *Burkholderia mallei*, and influenza A and B.

DNA microarray

DNA microarray is a collection of microscopic DNA spots attached to a solid surface, such as glass, plastic, or a silicon chip, to form an array. The affixed DNA segments are known as probes, thousands of which can be used in a single DNA microarray. Microarray technology evolved from Southern blotting. Measuring gene expression using microarrays is relevant to many areas of biology and medicine, such as studying treatments, disease, and developmental stages. Lapa and colleagues [60] described the use of microarrays (Micro Arrays of Gel Immobilized Compounds on a Chip [MAGIChip]) to detect and identify five different orthopoxviruses. However, because the clinical sample first had to be amplified using a singleplex PCR assay to detect a gene sequence common to all five species, the ultimate limit of detection (LOD) depended on the PCR, not the microarray. PCR linked with amplification product detection using electronic DNA microarrays have shown a tremendous amount of flexibility and control in detecting NA. Sites on the microarray can be easily configured and modified for a range of assay formats. Because nonactivated sites do not draw NA, multiple samples can be analyzed and multiple runs performed on the same microarray without cross-contamination [61,62].

Current laboratory diagnosis of selected important bioterrorism agents

Bacillus anthracis

Anthrax is a zoonotic disease that is transmissible to humans through handling or consumption of contaminated animal products. The etiologic agent of anthrax, *Bacillus anthracis*, is a spore-forming gram-positive bacillus. Human anthrax has three major clinical forms: cutaneous, inhalation, and gastrointestinal. The characteristics that make anthrax a potential bioterrorism weapon are its stability as a spore, its ease of culture and production, its ability to be aerosolized, and the serious disease it causes. If left untreated, all forms of anthrax can cause septicemia and death.

A standard culture on a 5% Sheep Blood agar plate and a Gram stain normally identifies *Bacillus* to the genus level through colony identification. Confirmatory identification of *Bacillus anthracis* performed by the CDC includes phage lysis, capsular staining, and direct fluorescent antibody (DFA) testing on capsule antigen and cell wall polysaccharide. Immunologic tests include specific ELISAs to measure antibody titers to particle agglutination or capsular components. Indirect microhemagglutination provides similar results to ELISA but has drawbacks, including short shelf life of reagents and longer preparation times [63]. All methods are labor intensive, lengthy, or lack sensitivity or specificity. In particular, rapid immunologic-based tests marketed for environmental testing in the United States lack sensitivity and specificity. More recent lateral flow immunoassay kits have shown improved specificity (100%) but still poor LOD and sensitivity [17]. Singleplex PCR tests have been developed to detect conserved regions common to all *Bacillus anthracis* strains and to try to detect specific subtypes of the organism. Higgins and colleagues [18] compared several PCR-based techniques for detecting pathogenic organisms. He was able to detect anthrax using the Taq-Man 5' nuclease assay (real-time PCR), but its clinical usefulness could not be assessed. PCR assays to the particle agglutination gene are available at national and some state reference laboratories. Moser and colleagues [64] used a real-time PCR platform called MultiCode-RTx to simultaneously analyze the presence of *Bacillus anthracis*–specific virulence plasmid-associated genes (three targets at one time) on a LightCycler-1 (Roche, Basel, Switzerland). The triplex showed high sensitivity and specificity (100%) and LODs nearing single copy levels [64].

Yersinia pestis

Yersinia are gram-negative bacilli and members of the family *Enterobacteriaceae*. The genus includes three species that are pathogens to humans and animals: *Y pestis*, *Y pseudotuberculosis*, and *Y enterocolitica* [66].

Y pestis is the most notorious species and causes bubonic plague, or "Black Death," which is usually fatal unless treated quickly with antibiotics. The fleas from rodents transmit the disease to humans and other animals. Past studies have shown that *Y pseudotuberculosis* and *Y pestis* are similar at the nucleotide level. According to Achtman and colleagues [67], *Y pestis* is a recently emerged clone of *Y pseudotuberculosis*. Despite this nucleotide similarity, the pathogenic mechanisms are different: *Y pseudotuberculosis* and *Y enterocolitica* cause gastrointestinal disease, whereas *Y pestis* causes plague. *Y pestis* is also known to disable the immune system in humans by injecting proteins into macrophages, one of the body's key defenders against bacterial attack. Inhaling a small number of *Y pestis* can lead to pneumonic plague, which is highly lethal and can spread from person to person. This bacterium can be grown and aerosolized easily and is available worldwide, making it a potent bioterrorism weapon.

Y pestis has been rapidly diagnosed using many traditional methods (eg, culture, microscopic observation, biochemical characteristics, anti–F1 antigen detection by slide agglutination, immunofluorescence, phage lytic assay). However, these methods are not very accurate in identifying or diagnosing different species of *Yersinia*. Chanteau and colleagues [68] compared F1 antigen capture ELISA assay with rapid immunogold dipstick for early diagnosis of bubonic plague (*Y pestis*) and concluded that bubo fluid rather than serum or urine specimens must be used to diagnose this agent. However, even these poor tests (F1 ELISA, dipstick assay) provided valuable tools for early diagnosis and the surveillance of plague. In their experiments to specifically detect plasmid-bearing *Yersinia* isolates with PCR, Neubauer and colleagues [19] concluded that all possible pathogenic *Yersinia* isolates could be identified based on PCR analysis with fewer false-positive reactions than the autoagglutination test. This PCR assay has not been evaluated for routine use.

Francisella tularensis

F tularensis is one of the two recognized species of the genus *Francisella*. It is a virulent, facultative, intracellular bacterium. According to Johansson and colleagues [69], the bacterium is widely distributed in nature and has been isolated from approximately 250 wildlife species, many of which can transmit disease to humans. Types A and B are the two major subtypes, with type A more virulent. Tularemia is acquired by direct contact with infected animals, through contaminated water or food, or from vectors such as biting insects or ticks. Airborne transmission can also occur during processing of agricultural products. This disease is epidemic in humans and animals, with clinical manifestation depending on the means of transmission. Tularemia is also known as *rabbit fever* and *deer fly fever*. In the natural setting, tularemia is a predominately rural disease with clinical presentations that include ulceroglandular, glandular, oculoglandular, oropharyngeal, pneumonic, typhoidal, and septic forms. Experts believe that of the various ways that *F tularensis* could be used as a weapon, an aerosol release would have the greatest adverse medical and public health consequences.

Rapid diagnostics for tularemia are not widely available. Culture is the definitive test for *F tularensis* but can take several days. In many clinical laboratories, the diagnosis of tularemia is usually confirmed by showing an antibody response to *F tularensis*. However, this method normally does not allow a definite diagnosis within the first 2 weeks, when antibiotic therapy would be most helpful [70]. Therefore, simple and reliable diagnostic tests that could be used to identify persons infected with *F tularensis* in the mass exposure setting must be developed. *F tularensis* has been detected from pus using PCR [71], and several PCR assays, including the TaqMan 5'-nuclease assay (real-time PCR), have been developed to identify *F tularensis* from bodily fluids of infected animals and vectors [72–75]. However, using rapid immunochromatography testing, ELISA, and PCR to analyze *F tularensis* bacterial cellular components, Berdal and colleagues [74] concluded that the rapid immunochromatography test was more handy and versatile, whereas Higgins and colleagues [18] showed that PCR had greater efficacy in identifying *F tularensis*. Rapid methods for identifying *F tularensis*, such as the immunofluorescence assay and ELISAs for detecting antigen and the RNA hybridization assay, have been tried but have not been included in routine diagnostics. These assays also lack the sensitivity and specificity of PCR. Singleplex PCR tests and multiplex PCR assays (see later discussion) are being studied for diagnosing tularemia. Overall, PCR has shown greater efficacy in identifying *F tularensis* compared with other methods [76].

Variola major

Smallpox caused by *Variola major* (family Orthopoxviruses) was a devastating disease and caused massive epidemics and fatalities. Although the disease was eradicated in 1977, the remaining stocks of smallpox virus constitute one of the most dangerous threats to humanity [77–79]. This agent is believed to be one of the most potentially deadly and effective biological weapons because it is easily transmitted, no effective therapy exists, and few people carry full immunity. Meltzer and colleagues [80,81] constructed a mathematical model to show the spread of smallpox once the virus is released after a bioterrorism attack. They assumed that if 100 people were initially infected with the virus, and every infected person transmitted the infection to 3 additional people, then stopping the outbreak would take up to 1 year if 9 million vaccine doses were used and effective quarantine implemented, and still 4200 people would become infected and approximately 1200 would die.

Smallpox is usually diagnosed by the presence of characteristic virus particles on electron microscopy of vesicular scrapings. Under a light microscope, aggregations of variola virus particles, called *Guarnieri bodies*, are found. Another rapid but insensitive method to detect Guarnieri bodies in vesicular scrapings is to use Gispen's modified silver stain, which stains cytoplasmic inclusions black. Neither of these laboratory tests is capable of discriminating variola from the other poxviruses, such as monkeypox and vaccinia (attenuated vaccine strain of smallpox). This differentiation classically requires isolation of the virus and characterization of its growth on specific media. Tarantola and colleagues [21] introduced a new and improved immunofluorescence staining technique to test scabs or vesicular or pustular impressions for smallpox, and compared it with the existing methods (immunodiffusion in agar and culture on chorioallantoic membranes of embryonated eggs). Although no false-negative results occurred, a high rate of false-positive results were found, and therefore immunofluorescence could not be recommended as a routine screening test for smallpox. The development of PCR and other molecular diagnostic techniques promises a more accurate and less cumbersome way to discriminate between variola and other orthopoxviruses [82]. Although MAGIChip detects and identifies five different orthopoxviruses (including smallpox), it does not allow multiple unrelated organisms to be detected without initial use of a multiplex PCR. A TaqMan real-time PCR assay was developed for single-organism diagnosis from pathology specimens [59].

Ebola and Lassa fever

Several enveloped RNA viruses that typically cause viral hemorrhagic fever (VHF) syndrome include the Filoviridae (Ebola, Marburg) and Arenaviridae (Junin, Lassa). These viruses are typically transmitted to humans through contact with infected animal reservoirs or arthropod vectors, and some may be highly infectious through aerosol [83]. However, the highest fatalities are caused by the filoviruses, whose genomic organization is well studied. The genus *Filovirus* contains four subtypes of Ebola (Zaire, Sudan, Ivory Coast, and Reston) and a single species of Marburg virus. Three of the Ebola species have caused death in humans, whereas the Ebola virus Reston has only caused disease in nonhuman primates. Arenaviruses belong to the family Arenaviridae, whose members are generally associated with rodent-transmitted disease. Based on their serologic properties, genetic composition, and geographic distribution, the arenaviruses are classified into two major groups: Old World and New World. Junin virus causes an endemoepidemic disease, acute hemorrhagic fever. The VHF agents may be used as weapons because no vaccines or treatments exist for the disease (except Lassa) and it is highly fatal.

Antigen capture ELISA testing, IgG ELISA, PCR, virus isolation, and real-time PCR can be used to diagnose VHF within a few days of the onset of symptoms [22–27,84–86]. Persons tested later in the disease course or after recovery can be tested for IgG and IgM antibodies The disease can also be diagnosed retrospectively in deceased patients through immunohisto-chemistry, virus isolation, or PCR. Leroy and colleagues [28] compared tra-ditional methods of ELISA antigen capture, Ebola-specific IgM and IgG antibody detection, and RT-PCR as diagnostic techniques. Compared with antigen or IgM detection, the sensitivity of RT-PCR in identifying acute infection was 100% and 91%, respectively, and specificity was 97%. Antigen capture detected only 83% of infections identified with PCR, whereas IgM identified only 67%. More significantly, RT-PCR detected Ebola RNA in blood even 1 to 3 weeks after symptoms disappeared, when the antigen was undetectable. RT-PCR was the most sensitive method and was able to detect virus over a broad time range during symptomatic disease.

Lozano and colleagues [29] designed an RT-PCR–based assay to detect Junin virus in whole blood samples. The RT-PCR–based assay was com-pared with traditional methodologies, including ELISA, plaque neutraliza-tion tests, and occasionally viral isolation. This assay showed a 98% sensitivity and 76% specificity. Using the consensus sequences of these re-gions, Lozano and colleagues [87] designed primers and used RT-PCR to perform restriction fragment length polymorphism analysis. They then com-pleted a phylogenetic analysis on Old World and New World arenaviruses and were able to show a clear relationship between these two groups. Using primers from a region of the small RNA segment of Lassa virus coding for the glycoprotein, Trappier and colleagues [30] evaluated PCR and hybrid-ization procedures for diagnosing Lassa fever. The study did not show a clear correlation between the results obtained with PCR and those using virus isolation methods. Of the results, 32% were false-positive. Bockstahler and colleagues [88] reported similar results with an RT-PCR–based assay. This problem is common with PCR assays when they "beat" the current gold standard, and these false-positives may have been true-positives.

Rift Valley fever, Hantavirus, and dengue

Other enveloped RNA viruses that typically cause VHF syndrome in-clude Bunyaviridae (*Nairovirus, Phlebovirus*, Rift Valley fever, *Hantavirus*), and Flaviviridae (yellow fever, dengue). Bunyaviridae and Flaviviridae are also known as Arboviruses (arthropod-borne). Flaviviridae contains the genera *flavivirus* (which includes the viruses causing Japanese encephalitis, dengue fever, yellow fever, and tickborne encephalitis). The hantaviruses (Bunyaviridae) have been implicated as the cause of two acute diseases: hemorrhagic fever with renal syndrome and hantavirus pulmonary syndrome.

Numerous methods are used to diagnose hantaviruses and flaviviruses, including indirect immunofluorescence, plaque reduction neutralization test, hemagglutination inhibition test, and complement fixation [89–92]. These tests are technically demanding and reproducibility of results is poor. A recent IgM antibody capture ELISA uses a defined set of antigens [93] for rapid screening of human samples for various arboviruses. However, it requires antigens that are tailored to the geographic origin of the specimen. In addition, ELISAs have decreased sensitivity and specificity compared with PCR assays. Kuno [94] used different PCR protocols to try to develop a universal diagnostic RT-PCR protocol for different arboviruses. However, several protocols would have been needed, with many optimizations regarding enzymes, reagents, and equipment, and would be generally cumbersome. Anwar and colleagues [95] described a method of detecting and quantifying dengue virus using a stem-loop mediated reverse transcription real-time PCR assay. Because of the use of a reverse transcription primer folded into the stem-loop structure and the use of primer sequences specific to this stem-loop structure, this assay has shown very high specificity and excellent sensitivities as low as 10 copies per reaction [95].

Influenza (avian, human, and other animals)

Influenza is an orthomyxovirus and can be separated morphologically from its cousin, the paramyxovirus, by its segmented genome. This characteristic also allows for the genetic reassortment, which leads to rapid shifts in antigenic characteristics within influenza and results in pandemic disease (ie, millions of deaths). The three major types of influenza (A, B, and C) are differentiated by stable type-specific RNA-associated nucleoprotein. Influenza A has 16 hemagglutinin (HA) and 9 neuraminidase (N) antigenic subtypes and influenza B has 1 major antigenic subtype with several different sublineages. Influenza is efficiently spread person to person through inhalation of aerosolized droplets produced by coughing and sneezing [96]. This efficient spread causes infection in up to 30% of school-aged children during a typical yearly epidemic, which can reach even higher levels ($>40\%$) during a pandemic or if a terrorist releases an engineered recombinant virus [97]. Until recently, influenza B was believed to only infect humans. However, the recent discovery in seals of strains genetically identical to those in humans has suggested that this virus may be able to reside in animal reservoirs and re-emerge, causing pandemic disease [98]. Influenza A viruses are well adapted to their natural hosts, causing only mild or subclinical forms of the disease; however, they are isolated in concentrations sufficient for effective transmission to other potential host species. All subtypes of influenza type A have been found in wild bird populations. HA and N have 144 possible combinations, but only a very small number have actually been found in nature. A much smaller range of subtypes has been found in other animals, such as pigs, horses, dogs, and marine mammals. The natural history of avian strains remains unclear, except that water birds like ducks and geese seem to have higher incidence rates then other species. Until the latest H5N1 epidemic, the wild avian hosts were believed to be immune to disease from these viruses. In 2005, influenza virus subtypes H5N1 became one of the most important zoonotic infections in Russia, Europe, and Asia.

Tissue culture and isolation in embryonated eggs (specific pathogen-free) was the gold standard for detecting influenza A and B in humans and influenza A in animals (eg, avian), respectively. However, these methods have been replaced with molecular methods over the past 10 years. Tissue culture and egg inoculation will (for the near future) remain regionally important to maintain a source for analyzing genetic and antigenic change in virus populations (eg, the yearly influenza vaccine). Serology is not usually helpful in acute diagnosis; 10% to 30% of patients who have documented influenza or other respiratory virus infections were found to be serologically negative [99,100].

Significant advancements in rapid diagnostic methods have occurred, with many more on the horizon. For influenza, antigen-based assays have been used for more than 30 years and, in order of their introduction, include IFA/DFA, enzyme immunoassay, optical immunoassay, and neuraminidase activity assays [12,99,101–103]. Although these methods are still used widely and have the advantage of being inexpensive and easy to use, they lack sensitivity and specificity, especially during times of low prevalence (off-season) or in special populations such as individuals who are immunocompromised or elderly. Some methods seem able to detect multiple avian and other animal strains, but few have been clinically tested against more then one or a few different influenza antigenic types. If they do not detect a specific antigenic subtype (eg, H7N2), they cannot be easily adapted to new agents or multiplexed.

PCR and microarrays have been used to study influenza antigenic subtypes [104–109], and large numbers of real-time PCR assays have been reported. Trani and colleagues [113] developed a highly sensitive one-step real-time PCR for detecting (but not subtyping) avian influenza viruses that used TaqMan MGB probes. They reported that this assay detected down to 0.001 median tissue culture infectious dose ($TCID_{50}$) or 5 to 50 RNA gene copies per reaction and detected 100% of H1–13 and N1–6, 8, 9 influenza A subtypes without any crossover with influenza B or other avian diseases [113]. However, the LOD was only determined in three runs with one antigenic type, and only a small number of clinical samples were tested. Individual real-time PCR assays to the N gene have been developed for five of the nine subtypes (Kathy Kurth, personal communication, 2006).

Multiplex detection of select bioterrorism agents

Several different technologies and methods have been used for multiplex detection of different bioterrorism agents, including standard oligonucleotide microarray with singleplex PCR [114]; real-time PCR assays [53, 115–117], which are currently limited to only one to four analytes; and multiplex immunoassay or PCR with detection by Luminex beads (MiraiBio, Alameda, California) read on a flow cytometer [56,115], which have decreased LOD and have only been tested for environmental samples. The autonomous pathogen detection system developed at Lawrence Livermore for environmental testing was only tested at higher target levels than needed for clinical testing.

Song and colleagues [65] developed a multiplex DNA fiberoptic microsphere–based microarray for detecting many different bioterrorism agents, including *Bacillus anthracis*. An optical fiber bundle was chemically etched to yield microwells. In these microwells, 18 different 50-mer single-stranded DNA probes that were covalently attached to 3.1-μm microspheres were distributed, forming a randomized multiplex high-density array. The microarray was able to detect target concentrations as low as 10 fM in a 50 μL volume [65]. Unfortunately, this LOD is equivalent to approximately $10^{5\text{-}6}$ DNA copies/mL, which would not be sensitive enough for clinical applications. This array was reported as highly specific [65]. A multiplex PCR assay for several different orthopoxviruses (including smallpox) with gel detection has been described [16] with good sensitivity.

Khanna and colleagues [55] reported a multiplex PCR assay, which includes *Bacillus anthracis, F tularensis, Y pestis, V zoster*, and smallpox using highly conserved regions of the PA genome, the *tul 4* protein gene, the virus-associated gene, the *ORF29* gene, and the *HA* gene to detect these agents. This multiplex PCR-EHA identified these bioterrorism agents using a simple 96-well plate format. The LOD for *F tularensis* was at 10^0 colony-forming units per mL, for *B anthracis* and *Y pestis* was at 10^{-8} dilution of the genomic DNA, and for *V zoster* was at 10^{-2} TCD_{50}/mL. Recombinant DNA controls for *F tularensis, Bacillus anthracis*, and *V major* were detected at 10^2 copies/mL, whereas *Y pestis* was detected at 10^1 copies/mL. The analytic specificity showed no cross-reactivity to 16 closely related organisms. *F philomiragia* obtained from the American Type Culture Collection showed some unexplained cross-reactivity in the assay. Further work on this assay has added an internal control without significant loss of analytic sensitivity, and a clinical trial is currently underway.

Previously, the only work reported on multiplex RT-PCR in bioterrorism viruses was within a specific virus family (eg, dengue [23,26,118], hantavirus [119]), but no attempts were made to detect different virus species. We developed a multiplex RT-PCR (RNA) assay to detect the Ebola virus (three types), Lassa virus, hantavirus (Sin Nombre strains), Rift Valley fever virus, and dengue virus (four strains). Preliminary analytic work has shown excellent LOD and specificity, and clinical testing will begin soon (Kelly J. Henrickson, Jiang Fan, Andrea J. Kraft, unpublished data, 2006). Considerable progress has been made in developing multiplexed amplification reactions suitable for diagnosing respiratory illness [110,111]. Although gel electrophoresis detection is still used by some laboratories, it requires considerable hands-on time and has limited resolution. Several laboratories have successfully used plate-based assays, such as the PCR-based EHA or enzyme-coupled probes. The oldest and most widely used commercial molecular assay for influenza A and B is the Hexaplex (Prodesse, Waukesha, Wisconsin), which uses multiplex RT-PCR–EHA to detect the seven most common respiratory viruses [112]. This assay was developed in our laboratory at the Medical College of Wisconsin and has recently been adapted to Nanogen's electronic microarray with excellent correlation between assays [120]. Spackman and colleagues [121] developed a multiplex real-time RT-PCR assay for detecting H5 and H7 subtypes of avian influenza, with the sensitivities determined to be 10^4 HA gene copies for H7 subtypes and 10^4 to 10^5 HA gene copies for H5 subtypes. When compared with hemagglutination inhibition assay results, the assays agreed on 95.2% of the samples tested [121].

Future

Continued research is critical to develop new detection strategies for bioterrorism agents, including NA isolation, amplification, and amplification product detection, each as separate stand-alone processes and as complete devices. Promising amplification product detection strategies for multiplex PCR include capillary electrophoresis, mass spectrometry, three-dimensional flow through microarray, and electronic microarrays [120,122–125]. Finally, whether NA-based or proteomic-based, more sensitive, specific, rapid, easy to use, and inexpensive techniques to identify most category A, B, and C agents must be developed, field tested, and made widely available. These methods must be adaptable to new agents and have the ability to detect multiple pathogens simultaneously.

Summary

The United States, European Union, and other countries have recently expended much time and funds to develop diagnostic assays to rapidly detect and identify bioterrorism agents. These efforts have resulted in great strides and the introduction of many detection technologies. Many of these technologies could ultimately be used to detect and identify all bioterrorism agents. However, challenges still remain, such as (1) false-positive PCR results, (2) positive samples unrelated to a bioterrorism event (ie, bioterrorism agents can be found naturally in human samples, such as respiratory secretions, blood, stool, and urine, or in powder, food, and water); (3) optimizing sample collection, storage, transportation, and target concentration for each method or assay; (4) isolating genomic material; (5) removing assay inhibitors; (6) keeping specific pathogens alive if using culture methods; (7) dealing with low sample volumes for clinical samples or high sample volumes for environmental samples; and (8) universal or multiplex pathogen detection.

Although several assays are available for detecting bioterrorism agents, only a few have been clinically evaluated. All assays must ultimately face the problem that many diseases caused by bioterrorism agents show similar symptoms, and exposed individuals must be tested for many potentially toxic or deadly pathogens. Therefore, multiplex assays seem to hold the key to solving this pressing global problem.

References

[1] Kaufmann AF, Meltzer MI, Schmid GP. The economic impact of a bioterrorist attack: are prevention and postattack intervention programs justifiable? Emerg Infect Dis 1997;3(2): 83–94.

[2] United States General Accounting Office. Capitol Hill Anthrax Incident: EPA's Cleanup was Successful; Opportunities Exist to Enhance Contract Oversight. Report to the Chairman, Committee on Finance, US Senate. Washington, DC: US Senate; 2003.

[3] Pennington H. Smallpox and bioterrorism. Bull World Health Organ 2003;81(10):762–7.

[4] Christensen JJ, Andresen K, Kemp M. New diagnostic methods for bacterial infections after the introduction of increased bioterrorism preparedness. Ugeskr Laeger 2005;167(36): 3416–7.

[5] Zhu Z, Dimitrov AS, Chakraborti S, et al. Development of human monoclonal antibodies against diseases caused by emerging and biodefense-related viruses. Expert Rev Anti Infect Ther 2006;4(1):57–66.

[6] Curry A, Appleton H, Dowsett B. Application of transmission electron microscopy to the clinical study of viral and bacterial infections: present and future. Micron 2006;37(2): 91–106.

[7] Guarner J, Zaki SR. Histopathology and immunohistochemistry in the diagnosis of bioterrorism agents. J Histochem Cytochem 2006;54(1):3–11.

[8] Atmar RL, Baxter BD, Dominguez EA, et al. Comparison of reverse transcription-PCR with tissue culture and other rapid diagnostic assays for detection of type A influenza virus. J Clin Microbiol 1996;34:2604–6.

[9] Fan J, Henrickson KJ, Savatski LL. Rapid simultaneous diagnosis of infections with respiratory syncytial viruses A and B, influenza viruses A and B, and human parainfluenza virus types 1, 2, and 3 by multiplex quantitative reverse transcription-polymerase chain reaction-enzyme hybridization assay (Hexaplex). Clin Infect Dis 1998;26:1397–402.

[10] Gilbert LL, Dakhama A, Bone BM, et al. Diagnosis of viral respiratory tract infections in children by using a reverse transcription-PCR panel. J Clin Microbiol 1996; 34:140–3.

[11] Henrickson KJ. Advances in the laboratory diagnosis of viral respiratory disease. Pediatr Infect Dis J 2004;23:S6–10.

[12] Covalciuc KA, Webb KH, Carlson CA. Comparison of four clinical specimen types for detection of influenza A and B viruses by optical immunoassay (FLU OIA test) and cell culture methods. J Clin Microbiol 1999;37(12):3971–4.

[13] Goff JL, Guerot E, Matta M, et al. Evaluation of the Hexaplex assay for the detection of respiratory viruses in Bronchoalveolar lavages from adults attending at a medical intensive care unit. Presented at the Infectious Disease and Microbiology Conference. Paris, France, December 4, 2003.

[14] Kehl S, Henrickson KJ. Cost effective utilization of a Multiplex RT-PCR assay (Hexaplex) for respiratory virus detection at a Children's Hospital. Presented at the 2nd International Symposium for Influenza and Other Respiratory Viruses, Cayman Islands, British West Indies. December 10–12, 1999.

[15] Weinberg A. Incidence and diagnosis of viral respiratory tract infections in a lung transplant population. Presented at Clinical Virology Symposium, Clearwater, Florida. April 29–May 2, 2001.

[16] Pulford D, Meyer H, Brightwell G, et al. Amplification refractory mutation system PCR assays for the detection of variola and Orthopoxvirus. J Virol Methods 2004;117(1): 81–90.

[17] King D, Luna V, Cannons A, et al. Performance assessment of three commercial assays for direct detection of Bacillus anthracis spores. J Clin Microbiol 2003;41(7):3454–5.

[18] Higgins JA, Ibrahim MS, Knauert FK, et al. Sensitive and rapid identification of biological threat agents. Ann N Y Acad Sci 1999;894:130–48.

[19] Neubauer H, Meyer H, Prior J, et al. A combination of different polymerase chain reaction (PCR) assays for the presumptive identification of Yersinia pestis. J Vet Med B Infect Dis Vet Public Health 2000;47(8):573–80.

[20] Johansson A, Berglund L, Errickson, et al. Comparative analysis of PCR versus culture for diagnosis of ulceroglandular tularemia. J Clin Microbiol 2000;38:22–6.

[21] Tarantola DJ, Huq F, Nakano JH, et al. Immunofluorescence staining for detection of variola virus. J Clin Microbiol 1981;13(4):723–5.

[22] Chutinimitkul S, Payungporn S, Theamboonlers A, et al. Dengue typing assay based on real-time PCR using SYBR Green I. J Virol Methods 2005;129(1):8–15.

[23] Ito M, Takasaki T, Yamada K, et al. Development and evaluation of fluorogenic TaqMan reverse transcriptase PCR assays for detection of dengue virus types 1 to 4. J Clin Microbiol 2004;42(12):5935–7.

[24] Kumaria R, Chakravarti A. Molecular detection and serotypic characterization of dengue viruses by single-tube multiplex reverse transcriptase-polymerase chain reaction. Diagn Microbiol Infect Dis 2005;52(4):311–6.

[25] Moreli ML, Sousa RL, Figueiredo LT. Detection of Brazilian hantavirus by reverse transcription polymerase chain reaction amplification of N gene in patients with hantavirus cardiopulmonary syndrome. Mem Inst Oswaldo Cruz 2004;99(6):633–8.

[26] Sanchez-Seco MP, Rosario D, Domingo C, et al. Generic RT-nested-PCR for detection of flaviviruses using degenerated primers and internal control followed by sequencing for specific identification. J Virol Methods 2005;126(1–2):101–9.

[27] Towner JS, Rollin PE, Bausch DG, et al. Rapid diagnosis of Ebola hemorrhagic fever by reverse transcription-PCR in an outbreak setting and assessment of patient viral load as a predictor of outcome. J Virol 2004;78(8):4330–41.

[28] Leroy EM, Baize S, Lu CY, et al. Diagnosis of Ebola hemorrhagic fever by RT-PCR in an epidemic setting. J Med Virol 2000;60(4):463–7.

[29] Lozano ME, Enria D, Maiztegui JI, et al. Rapid diagnosis of Argentine hemorrhagic fever by reverse transcriptase PCR-based assay. J Clin Microbiol 1995;33(5):1327–32.

[30] Trappier SG, Conaty AL, Farrar BB, et al. Evaluation of the polymerase chain reaction for diagnosis of Lassa virus infection. Am J Trop Med Hyg 1993;49(2):214–21.

[31] Choi YJ, Lee SH, Park KH, et al. Evaluation of PCR-based assay for diagnosis of spotted fever group rickettsiosis in human serum samples. Clin Diagn Lab Immunol 2005;12(6): 759–63.

[32] Fournier PE, Raoult D. Suicide PCR on skin biopsy specimens for diagnosis of rickettsioses. J Clin Microbiol 2004;42(8):3428–34.

[33] Klee SR, Tyczka J, Ellerbrok H, et al. Highly sensitive real-time PCR for specific detection and quantification of Coxiella burnetii. BMC Microbiol 2006;6(2):1–8.

[34] Fenollar F, Fournier PE, Raoult D. Molecular detection of Coxiella burnetii in the sera of patients with Q fever endocarditis or vascular infection. J Clin Microbiol 2004;42(11): 4919–24.

[35] Jones SW, Dobson ME, Francesconi SC, et al. DNA assays for detection, identification, and individualization of select agent microorganisms. Croat Med J 2005;46(4): 522–9.

[36] Niedrig M, Meyer H, Panning M, et al. Follow-up on diagnostic proficiency of laboratories equipped to perform orthopoxvirus detection and quantification by PCR: the second international external quality assurance study. J Clin Microbiol 2006;44(4):1283–7.

[37] Nalca A, Rimoin AW, Bavari S, et al. Reemergence of monkeypox: prevalence, diagnostics, and countermeasures. Clin Infect Dis 2005;41(21):1765–71.

[38] Inglis TJ, Merritt A, Chidlow G, et al. Comparison of diagnostic laboratory methods for identification of Burkholderia pseudomallei. J Clin Microbiol 2005;43(5):2201–6.

[39] Elfaki MG, Al-Hokail AA, Nakeeb SM, et al. Evaluation of culture, tube agglutination, and PCR methods for the diagnosis of brucellosis in humans. Med Sci Monit 2005; 11(11):MT69–74.

[40] Van Loock M, Verminnen K, Messmer TO, et al. Use of a nested PCR-enzyme immunoassay with an internal control to detect Chlamydophila psittaci in turkeys. BMC Infect Dis 2005;5(76):1–9.

[41] Kapke GE, Watson G, Sheffler S, et al. Comparison of the Chiron Quantiplex branched DNA (bDNA) assay and the Abbot Genostics solution hybridization assay for quantification of hepatitis B viral DNA. J Viral Hepat 1997;4(1):67–75.

[42] Collins ML, Irvine B, Tyner D, et al. A branched DNA signal amplification assay for quantification of nucleic acid targets below 100 molecules/mL. Nucleic Acids Res 1997;25: 2979–84.

[43] Lanciotti RS. Molecular amplification assays for the detection of flaviviruses. Adv Virus Res 2003;61:67–99.

[44] Lau LT, Banks J, Aherne R, et al. Nucleic acid sequence-based amplification methods to detect avian influenza virus. Biochem Biophys Res Commun 2004;313(2):336–42.

[45] D'Souza DH, Jaykus LA. Nucleic acid sequence based amplification for the rapid and sensitive detection of Salmonella enterica from foods. J Appl Microbiol 2003;95(6):1343–50.

[46] Collins RA, Ko LS, So KL, et al. A NASBA method to detect high- and low-pathogenicity H5 avian influenza viruses. Avian Dis 2003;47(3 Suppl):1069–74.

[47] Collins RA, Ko LS, Fung KY, et al. Rapid and sensitive detection of avian influenza virus subtype H7 using NASBA. Biochem Biophys Res Commun 2003;300(2):507–15.

[48] Collins RA, Ko LS, So KL, et al. Detection of highly pathogenic and low pathogenic avian influenza subtype H5 (Eurasian lineage) using NASBA. J Virol Methods 2002;103(2): 213–25.

[49] Higgins JA, Cooper M, Schroeder-Tucker L, et al. A field investigation of Bacillus anthracis contamination of US Department of Agriculture and other Washington, D.C., buildings during the anthrax attack of October 2001. Appl Environ Microbiol 2003;69:593–9.

[50] Li W, Drake MA. Development of a quantitative competitive PCR assay for detection and quantification of Escherichia coli O157:H7 Cells. Appl Environ Microbiol 2001;67(7): 3291–4.

[51] Jureen P, Engstrand L, Eriksson S, et al. Rapid detection of rifampin resistance in Mycobacterium tuberculosis by Pyrosequencing technology. J Clin Microbiol 2006;44(6):1925–9.

[52] Tomioka K, Peredelchuk M, Zhu X, et al. A multiplex polymerase chain reaction microarray assay to detect bioterror pathogens in blood. J Mol Diagn 2005;7(4):486–94.

[53] Varma-Basil M, El-Hajj H, Marras SA, et al. Molecular beacons for multiplex detection of four bacterial bioterrorism agents. Clin Chem 2004;50(6):1060–2.

[54] Elnifro EM, Ashshi AM, Cooper RJ, et al. Multiplex PCR: optimization and application in diagnostic virology. Clin Microbiol Rev 2000;13:559–70.

[55] Khanna M, Harrington KP, Gajewski A, et al. Simultaneous detection of CDC category "A" DNA bioterrorism agents and varicella in a single multiplex PCR-EHA assay. Presented at the ASM Biodefense Meeting. Baltimore, March 20–23, 2005.

[56] Wilson WJ, Erler AM, Nasarabadi SL, et al. A multiplexed PCR-coupled liquid bead array for the simultaneous detection of four biothreat agents. Mol Cell Probes 2005;19(2):137–44.

[57] Lay MJ, Wittwer CT. Real-time fluorescence genotyping of factor V Leiden during rapid-cycle PCR. Clin Chem 1997;43(12):2262–7.

[58] Syrmis MW, Whiley DM, Thomas M, et al. A sensitive, specific, and cost-effective multi-plex reverse transcriptase-PCR assay for the detection of seven common respiratory viruses in respiratory samples. J Mol Diagn 2004;6:125–31.

[59] Schoepp RJ, Morin MD, Martinez MJ, et al. Detection and identification of Variola virus in fixed human tissue after prolonged archival storage. Lab Invest 2004;84(1): 41–8.

[60] Lapa S, Mikheev M, Mikhailovich V, et al. Species-level identification of orthopoxviruses with an oligonucleotide microchip. J Clin Microbiol 2002;40(3):753–7.

[61] Gau JJ, Lan EH, Dunn B, et al. A MEMS based amperometric detector for *E. coli* bacteria using self-assembled monolayers. Biosens Bioelectron 2001;16:745–55.

[62] Westin L, Miller C, Vollmer D, et al. Antimicrobial resistance and bacterial identification utilizing a microelectronic chip array. J Clin Microbiol 2001;39:1097–104.

[63] Kolsto AB, Helgason E, Okstad AO. *Bacillus anthracis, Bacillus thuringiensis* and *Bacillus cereus*: Janus-faces in Microbiology. Abstract presented at the 4th International Conference on Anthrax. Annapolis, June 10–13, 2001.

[64] Moser MJ, Christensen DR, Norwood D, et al. Multiplexed detection of anthrax-related toxin genes. J Mol Diagn 2006;8(1):89–96.

[65] Song L, Ahn S, Walt DR. Fiber-optic microsphere-based arrays for multiplexed biological warfare agent detection. Anal Chem 2006;78:1023–33.

[66] Leclercq A, Guiyoule A, El Lioui M, et al. High homogeneity of the *Yersinia pestis* fatty acid composition. J Clin Microbiol 2000;38(4):1545–51.

[67] Achtman M, Zurth K, Morelli G, et al. *Yersinia pestis*, the cause of plague, is a recently emerged clone *Yersinia pseudotuberculosis*. Proc Natl Acad Sci U S A 1999;96:14043–8. Erratum in: Proc Natl Acad Sci U S A 2000;97(14):8192.

[68] Chanteau S, Ratsitorahina M, Rahalison L, et al. Current epidemiology of human plague in Madagascar. Microbes Infect 2000;(1):25–31.

[69] Johansson A, Goransson I, Larsson P, et al. Extensive allelic variation among *Francisella tularensis* strains in a short-sequence tandem repeat region. J Clin Microbiol 2001;39(9): 3140–6.

[70] Sjostedt A, Eriksson U, Berglund L, et al. Detection of *Francisella tularensis* in ulcers of patients with Tularemia by PCR. J Clin Microbiol 1997;35(5):1045–8.

[71] Karhukorpi EK, Karhukorpi J. Rapid laboratory diagnosis of ulceroglandular tularemia with polymerase chain reaction. Scand J Infect Dis 2001;33(5):383–5.

[72] Higgins JA, Hubalek Z, Halouzka J, et al. Detection of *Francisella tularensis* in infected mammals and vectors using a probe-based polymerase chain reaction. Am J Trop Med Hyg 2000;62(2):310–8.

[73] Johansson A, Ibrahim A, Goransson I, et al. Evaluation of PCR-based methods for dis-crimination of *Francisella* species and subspecies and development of a specific PCR that distinguishes the two major subspecies of *Francisella tularensis*. J Clin Microbiol 2000; 38(11):4180–5.

[74] Berdal BP, Mehl R, Haaheim H, et al. Field detection of *Francisella tularensis*. Scand J Infect Dis 2000;32(3):287–91.

[75] Fujita O, Tatsumi M, Tanabayashi K, et al. Development of a real time PCR assay for detection and quantification of *Francisella tularensis*. Jpn J Infect Dis 2006;59: 46–51.

[76] Christopher G, Cieslak T, Pavlin J, et al. Biological warfare: a historical perspective. JAMA 1997;278:412–7.

[77] Berche P. The threat of smallpox and bioterrorism. Trends Microbiol 2001;9(1):15–8.

[78] Henderson DA. Smallpox: clinical and epidemiologic features. Emerg Infect Dis 1999;5(4): 537–9.

[79] Henderson DA. The looming threat of bioterrorism. Science 1999;283(5406):1279–82.

[80] Meltzer MI, Damon I, LeDuc JW, et al. Modeling potential responses to smallpox as a bio-terrorist weapon. Emerg Infect Dis 2001;7(6):959–69.

[81] Jahrling PB, Fritz EA, Hensley LE. Countermeasures to the bioterrorist threat of smallpox. Curr Mol Med 2005;5(8):817–26.

[82] Ropp SL, Jin Q, Knight JC, ct al. PCR strategy for identification and differentiation of small pox and orthopoxviruses. J Clin Microbiol 1995;33(8):2069–76.

[83] Franz DR, Jahrling PB, Friedlander AM, et al. Clinical recognition and management of patients exposed to biological warfare agents. JAMA 1997;278:399–411.

[84] Teles FR, Prazeres DM, Lima-Filho JL. Trends in dengue diagnosis. Rev Med Virol 2005; 15(5):287–302.

[85] Weidmann M, Muhlberger E, Hufert FT. Rapid detection protocol for filoviruses. J Clin Virol 2004;30(1):94–9.

[86] Formenty P, Leroy EM, Epelboin A, et al. Detection of Ebola virus in oral fluid specimens during outbreaks of Ebola virus hemorrhagic fever in the Republic of Congo. Clin Infect Dis 2006;42:1521–6.

[87] Lozano ME, Posik DM, Albarino CG, et al. Characterization of arenaviruses using a family-specific primer set for RT-PCR amplification and RFLP analysis. Its potential use for detection of uncharacterized arenaviruses. Virus Res 1997;49(1):79–89.

[88] Bockstahler LE, Carney PG, Bushar G, et al. Detection of Junin virus by the polymerase chain reaction. J Virol Methods 1992;39(1–2):231–5.

[89] Beaty BJ, Calisher CH, Shope RE. Arboviruses. In: Lennette EH, Lennette ET, editors. Diagnostic procedures for viral, rickettsial and chlamydial infections, 7th edition. Washington (DC): American Public Health Association; 1995. p. 204–5.

[90] Casey HL. Standardized diagnostic complement fixation method and adaption to microtest. Public health monograph no. 74. Washington (DC): US Government Printing office; 1996.

[91] Clarke DH, Casals J. Techniques for hemagglutination-inhibition with arthropod-borne viruses. Am J Trop Med Hyg 1958;7:561–73.

[92] Lindsey HS, Calisher CH, Matthews JH. Serum dilution neutralization test for California group virus identification and serology. J Clin Microbiol 1976;4:503–10.

[93] Martin D, Muth DA, Brown T, et al. Standardization of immunoglobulin M capture enzyme-linked immunosorbent assays for routine diagnosis of arboviral infections. J Clin Microbiol 2000;38(5):1823–6.

[94] Kuno G. Universal diagnostic RT-PCR protocol for arboviruses. J Virol Methods 1998; 72(1):27–41.

[95] Anwar A, August JT, Too HP. A step-loop mediated reverse transcription real-time PCR for the selective detection and quantification of the replicative strand of an RNA virus. Anal Biochem 2006;352:120–8.

[96] Henrickson KJ. Viral pneumonia. Semin Pediatr Infect Dis 1998;9(3):217–33.

[97] Madjid M, Lillibridge S, Parsa M, et al. Influenza as a bioweapon. JR Soc Med 2003;96: 345–6.

[98] Osterhaus AD, Rimmelzwann GF, Martina BF, et al. Influenza B virus in seals. Science 2000;288:1051–3.

[99] Henrickson KJ. Parainfluenza viruses. Clin Microbiol Rev 2003;16(2):242–64.

[100] Kellner G, Popow-Kraupp T, Kundi M, et al. Clinical manifestations of respiratory tract infections due to respiratory syncytial virus and rhinoviruses in hospitalized children. Acta Paediatr Scand 1989;78:390–4.

[101] Peiris JS, Lai ST, Poon LL, et al. Coronavirus as a possible cause of severe acute respiratory syndrome. Lancet 2003;361:1319–25.

[102] Reimer LG, Carroll KC. Role of microbiology laboratory in the diagnosis of lower respiratory tract infections. Clin Infect Dis 1998;26:742–8.

[103] Uyeki TM. Influenza diagnosis and treatment in children: a review of studies on clinically useful tests and antiviral treatment for influenza. Pediatr Infect Dis J 2003;22(2): 164–77.

[104] Ivshina AV, Vodeiko GM, Kuznetsov VA, et al. Mapping of genomic segments of influenza B virus strains by an oligonucleotide microarray method. J Clin Microbiol 2004;42(12): 5793–801.

[105] Malik YS, Patnayak DP, Goyal SM. Detection of three avian respiratory viruses by single-tube multiplex reverse transcription-polymerase chain reaction assay. J Vet Diagn Invest 2004;16(3):244–8.

[106] Munch M, Nielsen LP, Handberg KJ, et al. Detection and subtyping (H5 and H7) of avian type A influenza virus by reverse transcription-PCR and PCR-ELISA. Arch Virol 2001; 146(1):87–97.

[107] Payungporn S, Phakdeewirot P, Chutinimitkul S, et al. Single-step multiplex reverse transcription-polymerase chain reaction (RT-PCR) for influenza A virus subtype H5N1 detection. Viral Immunol 2004;17(4):588–93.

[108] Ito M, Watanabe M, Nakagawa N, et al. Rapid detection and typing of influenza A and B by loop-mediated isothermal amplification: comparison with immunochromatography and virus isolation. J Virol Methods 2006;135:272–5.

[109] Lin B, Wang Z, Vora GJ, et al. Broad-spectrum respiratory tract pathogen identification using resequencing DNA microarrays. Genome Res 2006;16:527–35.

[110] Aguilar JC, Perez-Brena MP, Garcia ML, et al. Detection and identification of human parainfluenza viruses 1, 2, 3, and 4 in clinical samples of pediatric patients by multiplex reverse transcription-PCR. J Clin Microbiol 2000;38:1191–5.

[111] Puppe W, Weigl JA, Aron G, et al. Evaluation of a multiplex reverse transcriptase PCR ELISA for the detection of nine respiratory tract pathogens. J Clin Virol 2004;30:165–74.

[112] Templeton KE, Scheltinga SA, Beersma MF, et al. Rapid and sensitive method using multiplex real-time PCR for diagnosis of infections by influenza A and influenza B viruses, respiratory syncytial virus, and parainfluenza viruses 1, 2, 3, and 4. J Clin Microbiol 2004; 42(4):1564–9.

[113] Di Trani L, Bedini B, Donatelli I, et al. A sensitive one-step real-time PCR for detection of avian influenza viruses using a MGB probe and an internal positive control. BMC Infect Dis 2006;6:87–102.

[114] Burton JE, Oshota OJ, North E, et al. Development of a multi-pathogen oligonucleotide microarray for detection of Bacillus anthracis. Mol Cell Probes 2005;19(5):349–57.

[115] Hindson BJ, McBride MT, Makarewicz AJ, et al. Autonomous detection of aerosolized biological agents by multiplexed immunoassay with polymerase chain reaction confirmation. Anal Chem 2005;7(1):284–9.

[116] Kim K, Seo J, Wheeler K, et al. Rapid genotypic detection of Bacillus anthracis and the Bacillus cereus group by multiplex real-time PCR melting curve analysis. FEMS Immunol Med Microbiol 2005;43(2):301–10.

[117] Selvapandiyan A, Stabler K, Ansari NA, et al. A novel semiquantitative fluorescence-based multiplex polymerase chain reaction assay for rapid simultaneous detection of bacterial and parasitic pathogens from blood. J Mol Diagn 2005;7(2):268–75.

[118] Ayers M, Adachi D, Johnson G, et al. A single tube RT-PCR assay for the detection of mosquito-borne flaviviruses. J Virol Methods 2006;135:235–9.

[119] Nordstrom H, Johansson P, Li QG, et al. Microarray technology for identification and distinction of hantaviruses. J Med Virol 2004;72(4):646–55.

[120] Henrickson KJ, Kraft AJ, Canter D, et al. Comparison of electronic microarray to enzyme hybridization assay for multiplex RT-PCR detection of common respiratory viruses in children. Presented at the 22nd Annual Clinical Virology Symposium, Clearwater, Florida. April 30–May 3, 2005.

[121] Spackman E, Senne DA, Bulaga LL, et al. Development of multiplex real-time RT-PCR as a diagnostic tool for avian influenza. Avian Dis 2003;47(3 Suppl):1087–90.

[122] Briese T, Palacios G, Kokoris M, et al. Diagnostic system for rapid and sensitive differential detection of pathogens. Emerg Infect Dis 2005;11(2):310–3.

[123] Erdman DD, Weinberg GA, Edwards KM, et al. GeneScan reverse transcription-PCR Assay for detection of six common respiratory viruses in young children hospitalized with acute respiratory illness. J Clin Microbiol 2003;41:4298–303.

[124] Kessler N, Ferraris O, Palmer K, et al. Use of the DNA flow-thru chip, a three-dimensional biochip, for typing and subtyping of influenza viruses. J Clin Microbiol 2004;42:2173–85.

[125] Stockton J, Ellis JS, Saville M, et al. Multiplex PCR for typing and subtyping influenza and respiratory syncytial viruses. J Clin Microbiol 1998;36(10):2990–5.

[126] U.S. Department of State. Convention on the prohibition of the development, production, and stockpiling of bacteriological (biological) and toxin weapons and on their destruction. Available at http://www.state.gov/t/ac/trt/4718.htm#treaty. Accessed September 11, 2006.

ELSEVIER
SAUNDERS

Pediatr Clin N Am
53 (2006) 843–853

PEDIATRIC CLINICS

OF NORTH AMERICA

Human Artificial Chromosomes: Potential Applications and Clinical Considerations

Joydeep Basu, PhD*, Huntington F. Willard, PhD

Institute for Genome Sciences & Policy, Duke University, 101 Science Drive, Durham, NC 27708, USA

Gene therapy, defined as the introduction of an exogenous gene into a recipient cell to achieve a therapeutic benefit, is already a reality. Despite widespread negative publicity associated with vector-induced oncogenesis in several patients, sustained correction of an X-linked form of severe combined immunodeficiency as a result of retroviral-mediated gene therapy was achieved several years ago [1]. This success notwithstanding, these combined results effectively illustrate the very real possibility of insertional mutagenesis associated with any integrative modification of the human genome. In evaluating technology platforms with the potential to address this issue, a theoretical consideration of the broader properties of an ideal gene therapy vector system may be informative.

Such a vector should not be limited by any arbitrary constraints on the size of a desired gene imposed by the biology of the host virus but would instead be able to express that gene in a sustained, physiologically appropriate manner as determined by its endogenous regulatory elements, which may be spread over hundreds or even thousands of kilobases (kb) of genomic DNA. This vector should not express any foreign proteins that may trigger potentially fatal immunogenic reactions [2–4]. In addition, such a vector should be nonintegrative, thereby bypassing the potential for insertional oncogenesis, as well as being immune to gene silencing effects imposed by the local chromatin environment at the point of insertion [5]. Last, such a vector would be capable of replicating and segregating with high fidelity side by

The authors have an equity interest in Athersys, Inc.

* Corresponding author. Institute for Genome Sciences & Policy, Duke University, CIEMAS Room 2379, 101 Science Drive, Durham, NC 27708.

E-mail address: basu0005@mc.duke.edu (J. Basu).

side with the native chromosomes of the host cell, being faithfully transmitted through subsequent generations of daughter cells, while continuing to express its therapeutic protein payload. These properties are not consigned to a gedanken experiment; rather, they define the potential of the emerging technology of human artificial chromosomes (HACs).

The chromosome as vector

To appreciate fully the concept of using HACs as potential vectors and how HACs are designed and constructed, a brief synopsis of the salient features of naturally occurring human chromosomes may be useful. Stripped to its essentials, a typical chromosome is composed of genes, telomeres that are responsible for capping and protecting the linear ends of chromosomes from nucleolytic attack and degradation, and, perhaps most crucially from the standpoint of long-term stability, a centromere. The centromere is the cis-acting chromosomal locus responsible for mediating the establishment of the kinetochore, a trilaminar protein/DNA complex responsible for securing attachments to and movements of the chromosome along the mitotic spindle apparatus (Fig. 1) [6,7]. The kinetochore is composed of a number of constitutive proteins, including the centromere-specific histone variant CENtromere Protein (CENP)-A, as well as the centromeric chromatin-associated proteins CENP-B and -C. In addition, numerous other proteins associate dynamically with the kinetochore in a cell cycle–dependent manner, including microtubule motors such as CENP-E and components of the mitotic spindle checkpoint that control the onset of anaphase during cell division [6,7]. Notwithstanding the significant issues related to proper control of gene expression, the centromere represents the key structural and functional component of an autonomous, mitotically stable potential gene therapy vector [8].

The DNA component underlying the centromere of all normal human chromosomes is alpha-satellite. Alpha-satellite is a class of repetitive elements based on the hierarchical organization of a 171–base pair (bp) monomeric unit, tandemly multimerized into a higher-order repeat unit, itself tandemly repeated over several megabases within the centromeric region of all normal human chromosomes (see Fig. 1). Studies of both naturally occurring and experimentally derived human chromosome rearrangements have provided clear evidence that long arrays of tandemly repeated alpha-satellite DNA serve as the underlying genomic component of a functional centromere within human chromosomes [8–11].

A conclusive demonstration of the causal role of alpha-satellite in establishing the centromere was made possible by techniques permitting the systematic manipulation of synthetic alpha-satellite arrays capable of forming centromeres de novo [10]. Although the occurrence in rare abnormal chromosomes of neocentromeres at chromosomal locations not containing alpha-satellite suggests that alpha-satellite is not an absolute prerequisite for centromere function [7], only cloned alpha-satellite DNA can establish

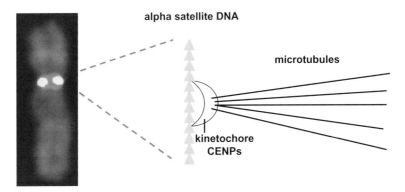

Fig. 1. The centromere is the locus at which the kinetochore, a protein/DNA complex mediating interactions with microtubules of the spindle apparatus, is assembled. As shown here, the centromere typically is located at the site of the cytogenetically visible primary constriction. The centromere is composed of tandemly organized repetitive arrays consisting of alpha-satellite DNA. The kinetochore, shown here as the typical "double dots" flanking the centromere as observed by immunostaining with an antibody against a kinetochore component, is assembled at the site of the centromere. CENPs, CENtromere Protein.

centromere function de novo [10,11]. How this is achieved mechanistically remains to be established. This point notwithstanding, alpha-satellite–based HACs as well as a number of classes of engineered natural chromosomes with functional centromeres are under active development as gene therapy vectors. The principles underlying the design, construction, and manipulation of these classes of vectors are outlined in more detail later.

Engineered and artificial chromosomes

Using the so-called "top-down" strategy, a variety of approaches have been applied to engineer native chromosomes to generate smaller chromosome derivatives, which in turn may be modified further by recombinogenic methodologies with a range of gene expression cassettes. For example, amplification, rearrangement, and truncation of native mouse chromosomes can result in the formation of huge (50–400 megabase) mega-amplicons, referred to by a variety of names including "sausage chromosomes" or "satellite-DNA–derived artificial chromosomes" (SATACs) [12,13]. These amplified mouse chromosomes have been manipulated through site-specific recombination and shown to express simple reporter constructs. Additionally, they may be transferred by microcell-mediated chromosome transfer (MMCT) into human primary cells as well as into mesenchymal and hematopoietic stem cells [13–15].

A more controlled and systematic engineering strategy involves the use of telomere-mediated truncation to pare down an existing human chromosome into a microchromosome derivative. Telomere-mediated chromosome fragmentation is based on the integration of cloned human telomeric DNA into

an existing chromosome arm, which occasionally may lead to de novo telomere seeding and consequent breakage of the chromosome arm at the integration site. The integration site of the cloned telomeric array then may be
targeted by homologous recombination. This method has been used to form
microderivatives of several normal human chromosomes as well as derivatives of rare, abnormal human chromosomes that contain neocentromeres
[16–19]. In all these cases, modification of the microchromosome with
recombinase recognition sites permits the subsequent introduction of gene
expression cassettes [20]. Additionally, these engineered human chromosomes can be transferred between cell lines, for example, between a host
cell line and a targeted recipient primary or stem cell line, by MMCT [21].

A fundamentally different strategy involves a "bottom-up" approach in
which cloned chromosomal elements, including alpha-satellite DNA, telomeric DNA, and genomic DNA, are preassembled into a defined artificial
chromosome vector or are assembled spontaneously by the host cell through
a combination of nonhomologous recombination and DNA repair mechanisms [10,11].

To facilitate the establishment of a clear and consistent nomenclature, the
authors reserve the term "human artificial chromosome" to describe a species
created entirely de novo from individual, structurally defined chromosomal
components, as first shown for the construction of yeast artificial chromosomes (YACs) [22]. Analogous to YAC vectors, HACs have clearly defined
centromeric, replication origin, and, where relevant, telomeric elements, all
of which typically are cloned into a bacterial artificial chromosome (BAC),
YAC, or P1 phage–based (PAC) vector backbone. BAC-based artificial chromosomes may be assembled as either linear or circular molecules requiring
only a mammalian selectable marker and a cloned alpha-satellite array, which
may be of natural origin or assembled synthetically (Fig. 2) [23]. The rapid
and reproducible assembly of unimolecular BAC-based vectors has been
assisted further by the development of specialized recombination-based
methodologies for the assembly of high-molecular-weight BAC vectors containing large, repetitive (>100-kb) arrays [23,24].

The essential elements required for assembly of an optimal HAC have
been under active investigation since the initial development of this technology [10]. Strategies for the establishment of de novo telomeres from
synthetic telomere seeds consisting of small tandem arrays of telomeric repetitive elements have greatly facilitated the construction of linear artificial
chromosomes [25,26]. Studies comparing circular BACs (which by definition
lack telomeres) and linear BAC vectors, however, have shown that they are
equally competent for the assembly of de novo human artificial chromosomes [27], suggesting that for most applications telomeres may be entirely
redundant.

The DNA sequence elements that demarcate mammalian replication
origins remain poorly defined. Nevertheless, because replication origins
may occur on average once in approximately every 100-kb of genomic

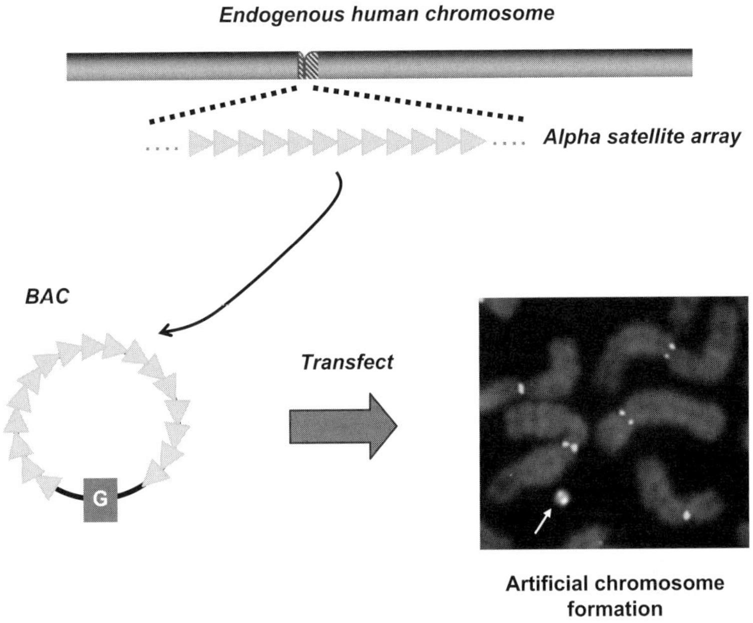

Fig. 2. One strategy for generating a de novo human artificial chromosome. A segment of alpha-satellite DNA is synthesized or cloned from an endogenous centromeric array into a bacterial artificial chromosome (BAC) vector containing a gene of interest (G). Alpha-satellite–containing BAC then is transfected into a recipient human cell, where it can be identified as an autonomously segregating human artificial chromosome (arrow) adjacent to the cohort of normal endogenous human chromosomes.

DNA [28,29], any sufficiently large genomic fragment may suffice to provide origin function in the context of an artificial chromosome. One of the few defined examples of a mammalian origin of replication lies within the well-characterized β-globin locus, which has been shown to have specific replicator function reproducible in *trans* to its native chromosomal location [30]. The entire β-globin locus control region has, in fact, been incorporated successfully into a HAC [24].

The demonstration of the unique ability of alpha-satellite to nucleate de novo centromere formation was the critical observation permitting the development of HAC technology [8,10,11]. Alpha-satellite derivatives of both natural and synthetic origin from a variety of human chromosomes have been shown to be capable of establishing de novo centromeres, with a frequency that seems to depend largely on the presence of certain key protein-binding elements known as CENP-B boxes [9–11,23,24,27,31–33]. In contrast, sequences other than alpha-satellite are unable to function in a de novo centromere formation assay [27,32,34]. Taken together, these results confirm the unique, albeit poorly understood, ability of alpha-satellite DNA to create artificial chromosomes, a property likely to underlie the continued development of artificial chromosome technology for the foreseeable future.

Toward physiologically relevant gene expression from engineered and artificial human chromosomes

Although the technology to generate mitotically stable HACs is now well established, from the standpoint of gene transfer studies related to eventual gene therapy, the ultimate aim of artificial chromosomes is to carry a genomic copy of a human gene of therapeutic interest and to express it in relevant recipient cells in a properly regulated manner. To this end, only limited progress with engineered chromosomes has thus far been reported. For example, a chromosome 21–derived minichromosome vector was created with a tetracycline-inducible expression cassette to generate DNA-dependent protein kinase (DNA-PKcs), a protein involved in nonhomologous end joining in a drug-responsive manner [35]. The same engineered vector also has been modified to express the human erythropoietin gene and has been transferred successfully to primary human fibroblasts by MMCT and shown to be functional [21]. Additionally, this chromosome derivative has been transferred into human mesenchymal stem cells [36] and engineered to express the precursor form of insulin at the RNA level, although no functional, secreted insulin was detected in this study [37].

Human gene expression also has been demonstrated from much larger genomic fragments engineered into human minichromosomes through an elaborate recombination scheme in the recombination-proficient chicken DT40 cell line [38]. This modified minichromosome then was transferred to mouse embryonic stem cells and used to make transgenic mice expressing human immunoglobulin genes. Additionally, minichromosome vectors containing the entire human immunoglobulin heavy chain and lambda light chain loci have been used to engineer transchromosomic cattle expressing human immunoglobulins [39,40]. In another experiment, a spontaneously arising linear minichromosome was co-opted as an expression vector for the human interleukin-2 (IL-2) cDNA [41]. Although IL-2 expression was demonstrated, the site of insertion of the cDNA into the minichromosome was not evaluated, so the chromosome context from which IL-2 is expressed is uncertain. This result underscores the potential advantage of cloning large genomic fragments, rather than small cDNAs, into vectors such as HACs that permit a more controlled environment.

Several studies have demonstrated, as a proof of principle, expression of a human gene from artificial chromosomes created de novo from individually cloned, defined chromosomal components. An approximately 150-kb *HPRT* genomic fragment has been shown to complement a *HPRT*-deficient cell line when expressed from the context of a unimolecular BAC-based artificial chromosome vector [42] or from a de novo microchromosome created by cotransfection of two different BACs, one containing the *HPRT* locus and the other an alpha-satellite array [43]. The cotransfection approach also has been used to generate artificial chromosomes expressing the guanosine triphosphate cyclohydrolase I locus [44]. Using a more systematic strategy, the authors demonstrated that prefabricated HACs containing the entire β-globin locus control region are capable of producing β-globin RNA in certain fibroblast cell lines [24]. Although these proof-of-principle experiments establish that large genes can indeed be expressed from HACs, no studies to date have rigorously demonstrated the regulated expression of a gene or examined the levels of expression relative to an endogenous gene copy.

One of the principal rate-limiting steps in the assembly of artificial chromosomes has been the technical difficulty associated with the manipulation of high-molecular-weight repetitive DNA. Progress in the development of HAC technology has been made possible, however, by the creation of novel recombinogenic methodologies for the rapid and reliable manipulation of BACs carrying defined, cloned chromosomal components. For example, any genomic BAC carrying any defined gene in its endogenous regulatory context may be converted into a BAC-based HAC vector by a single-step in vitro reaction based on the integration of a transposable element carrying a synthetic alpha-satellite array [23]. Other, more involved methodologies based on the Cre/lox recombination system also have been reported [24,45]. Taken together, these strategies permit any custom-built BAC-based HAC to be defined and constructed quickly and efficiently. Last, although preliminary studies indicate that engineered and artificial human chromosomes are capable of expressing custom-built gene cassettes in certain experimental cell lines, the successful expression of a therapeutic transgene in a physiologically relevant manner in a clinically relevant host cell (ie, a primary or stem cell line) remains an objective yet to be achieved.

In vitro and in vivo strategies for delivery of human artificial chromosomes

Certain classes of herpesvirus may be capable of delivering the large alpha-satellite arrays and genomic regulatory elements that typically constitute a HAC vector directly into the human body as an infectious particle [46]. Although delivery is technically feasible, it is difficult to imagine at the current stage of development how such particles may be targeted specifically within the body, and therefore this discussion is focused on in vitro strategies for HAC delivery. Such approaches typically revolve around the genetic modification of adult-derived hematopoietic or bone marrow stem cells with the vector carrying the therapeutic transgene, in this case an engineered or artificial chromosome vector. Engineered human chromosomes already have been transferred successfully into human mesenchymal and hematopoietic stem cells using the technique of MMCT [21], and expression of reporter transgenes has been observed. These initial results must be treated with caution, however; for technical reasons associated with the MMCT methodology, the engineered microchromosomes typically are maintained in a rodent cell line [14,15,36–39]. The effects of this alien epigenetic environment on the nature of chromatin or the functionality of the microchromosome have yet to be determined. Additionally, it remains to be rigorously demonstrated that the vector has not been subjected to rearrangements during the transfer. Although the sequence of human chromosome 21 is, of course, known, providing initial defined composition of matter for the microchromosome derivatives, detailed analysis of the structure of the microchromosome during and after transfer to a recipient cell may not be technically feasible. Some in vivo studies of the behavior of other engineered chromosomes, such as SATACs in transgenic mouse models, have been performed [47], and transgenic cattle have been created from engineered human chromosomes [39,40]. Again, however, detailed structural and stability analysis of the microchromosomes is required before their utility for human gene therapy can be contemplated seriously.

Unlike engineered human chromosomes, BAC-based HACs may be grown in massive scale in *Escherichia coli* using well-established good manufacturing practice (GMP) methodologies. A number of important technical obstacles remain to be overcome before such vectors achieve practical utility, however. Perhaps most importantly, such vectors have been shown to form de novo HACs only in certain immortalized human cell lines. Additionally, the de novo HACs reported to date typically are formed by the uncontrolled concatamerization of the starting vector, to form megabase-sized derivatives [9–11,23,24,31–33,42]. It will be crucial to demonstrate that de novo HACs can be formed in human primary or stem cell lines, that their composition of matter is fully definable, and that uncontrolled multimerization is not a necessary prerequisite for the assembly of a stable and functional HAC. Finally, reliable delivery of defined artificial chromosome vectors into human stem cells is a critical component of translating this technology into the clinic. Direct nuclear microinjection, erythrocyte-based "ghosts," invasive bacteria, and high-capacity viruses such as herpes simplex virus are all strategies under active development in various laboratories [46,48–50].

Future considerations

Regardless of whether the engineered or the artificial chromosome platform can be used eventually for clinical applications, reasonable extrapolations can be made based on the directions of current experimentation to advance this technology further. The authors have already described how, potentially, any gene may be delivered by an artificial chromosome in the context of its full complement of endogenous regulatory elements.

Pediatric genetic disorders involving haploinsufficiency of genes whose open reading frames and regulatory regions span hundreds of kilobases may be especially attractive candidates for the use of artificial chromosome vectors capable of delivering large amounts of genomic DNA. Duchenne's muscular dystrophy, polycystic kidney disease, lysosomal storage disorders such as Hurler's disease, and cystic fibrosis are disorders that fall into this category.

In the most direct demonstration of the potential of engineered chromosome vectors, functional cystic fibrosis transmembrane conductance regulator (CTFR, the protein affected in cystic fibrosis) has been shown to be expressed from minichromosome vectors engineered to incorporate a 320-kb genomic region encompassing the entire *CFTR* locus and its upstream regulatory regions [51]. Additionally, the authors have created *HAC* vectors based around a 208-kb genomic region containing the *PKD1* gene [24], mutations in which are responsible for polycystic kidney disease.

Disorders of the hematopoietic system, including the thalassemias, hemophilias, and anemias, are another class of pediatric genetic diseases potentially suitable for correction with gene therapy vectors. Toward this end, considerable effort has been spent on the design, construction, and evaluation of retroviral vectors containing globin minigene cassettes that must be capable of reproducing physiologically relevant patterns of globin gene expression, a technically demanding undertaking given the strict 12-kb upper packaging limit associated with retroviral vectors and the distribution of the genomic regulatory sequences associated with globin gene regulation over some 150-kb [52,53]. An alternative approach would take advantage of the substantially larger payload capacity of HAC vectors; in initial studies, the authors have constructed such vectors using a 200-kb genomic fragment containing the β-globin gene locus, including its native locus control region elements. Although preliminary, these and other artificial chromosomes illustrate the foundational principles for artificial chromosome vector design, assembly, and evaluation that will form the basis of future generations of artificial chromosome vector systems [24,50].

References

[1] Hacein-Bey-Abina S, Von Calle C, Schmidt M, et al. LMO2-associated clonal T cell proliferation in two patients after gene therapy for SCID-X1. Science 2003;302(5644):415–9.

[2] Somia N, Verma IM. Gene therapy: trials and tribulations. Nat Rev Genet 2000;1(2):91–9.

[3] Williams DA, Baum C. Gene therapy—new challenges ahead. Science 2003;302(5644): 400–1.

[4] Rosenberg LE, Schechter AN. Gene therapist, heal thyself. Science 2000;287(5459):1751.

[5] Recillas-Targa F, Valvadez-Graham V, Farrell CM. Prospects and implications of using chromatin insulators in gene therapy and transgenesis. Bioessays 2004;26(7):796–807.

[6] Cleveland DW, Mao Y, Sullivan KF. Centromeres and kinetochores: from epigenetics to mitotic checkpoint signaling. Cell 2003;112(4):407–21.

[7] Sullivan BA, Blower MD, Karpen GH. Determining centromere identity: cyclical stories and forking paths. Nat Rev Genet 2001;2(8):584–96.

[8] Willard HF. Centromeres: the missing link in the development of human artificial chromosomes. Curr Opin Genet Dev 1998;8(2):219–25.

[9] Schueler MG, Higgins AW, Rudd MK, et al. Genomic and genetic definition of a functional human centromere. Science 2001;294(5540):109–15.

[10] Harrington JJ, Van Bokkelen G, Mays RW, et al. Formation of de novo centromeres and construction of first-generation human artificial microchromosomes. Nat Genet 1997; 15(4):345–55.

[11] Ikeno M, Grimes B, Okazaki T, et al. Construction of YAC-based mammalian artificial chromosomes. Nat Biotechnol 1998;16(5):431–9.

[12] Kereso J, Praznovsky T, Cserpan I, et al. De novo chromosome formations by large scale amplification of the centromeric region of mouse chromosomes. Chromosome Res 1996; 4(3):226–39.

[13] Hadlackzky G. Satellite DNA-based artificial chromosomes for use in gene therapy. Curr Opin Mol Ther 2001;3(2):125–32.

[14] Vanderbyl S, MacDonald GN, Sidhu S, et al. Transfer and stable transgene expression of a mammalian artificial chromosome into bone marrow-derived human mesenchymal stem cells. Stem Cells 2004;22(3):324–33.

[15] Vanderbyl SL, Sullenbarger B, White N, et al. Transgene expression after stable transfer of a mammalian artificial chromosome into human hematopoietic cells. Exp Hematol 2005; 33(12):1470–6.

[16] Itzhaki JE, Barnett MA, MacCarthy AB, et al. Targeted breakage of a human chromosome mediated by cloned, telomeric DNA. Nat Genet 1992;2(4):283–7.

[17] Yang JW, Pendon C, Yang J, et al. Human mini-chromosomes with minimal centromeres. Hum Mol Genet 2000;9(12):1891–902.

[18] Mills W, Critcher R, Lee C, et al. Generation of an ~2.4-Mb human X centromere-based minichromosome by targeted telomere-associated chromosome fragmentation in DT40. Hum Mol Genet 1999;8(5):751–61.

[19] Wong LH, Saffery R, Choo KH. Construction of neocentromere-based human minichromosomes for gene delivery and centromere studies. Gene Ther 2002;9(11):724–6.

[20] Moralli D, Vagnarelli P, Bensi M, et al. Insertion of a loxP site in a size-reduced human accessory chromosome. Cytogenet Cell Genet 2001;94(3–4):113–20.

[21] Kakeda M, Hiratsuka M, Nagata K, et al. Human artificial chromosome (HAC) vector provides long-term therapeutic transgene expression in normal human primary fibroblasts. Gene Ther 2005;12(10):852–6.

[22] Murray AW, Szostak JW. Construction of artificial chromosomes in yeast. Nature 1983; 305(5931):189–93.

[23] Basu J, Stromberg G, Compitello G, et al. Rapid creation of BAC-based human artificial chromosome vectors by transposition with synthetic alpha-satellite arrays. Nucleic Acids Res 2005;33(2):587–96.

[24] Basu J, Compitello G, Stromberg G, et al. Efficient assembly of de novo human artificial chromosomes from large genomic loci. BMC Biotechnol 2005;5:21.

[25] Shampay J, Szostak JW, Blackburn EH. DNA sequences of telomeres maintained in yeast. Nature 1984;310(5973):154–7.

[26] Barnett MA, Buckle VJ, Evans EP, et al. Telomere directed fragmentation of mammalian chromosomes. Nucleic Acids Res 1993;21(1):27–36.

[27] Ebersole TA, Ross A, Clark E, et al. Mammalian artificial chromosome formation from circular alphoid input DNA does not require telomere repeats. Hum Mol Genet 2000;9(11): 1623–31.

[28] Hamlin JL. Mammalian origins of replication. Bioessays 1992;14(10):651–9.

[29] Todorovic V, Falaschi A, Giacca M. Replication origins of mammalian chromosomes: the happy few. Front Biosci 1999;4:D859–68.

[30] Aladjem MI, Rodewald LW, Kolman JK, et al. Genetic dissection of a mammalian replicator in the human beta-globin locus. Science 1998;281(5379):1005–9.

[31] Rudd MK, Mays RW, Schwartz S, et al. Human artificial chromosomes with alpha satellite-based de novo centromeres show increased frequency of nondisjunction and anaphase lag. Mol Cell Biol 2003;23(21):7689–97.

[32] Grimes BR, Rhoades AA, Willard HF. Alpha-satellite DNA and vector composition influence rates of human artificial chromosome formation. Mol Ther 2002;5(6):798–805.

[33] Ohzeki J, Nakano M, Okada T, et al. CENP-B box is required for de novo centromere chromatin assembly on human alphoid DNA. J Cell Biol 2002;159(5):765–75.

[34] Saffery R, Wong LH, Irvine DV, et al. Construction of neocentromere-based human minichromosomes by telomere-associated chromosomal truncation. Proc Natl Acad Sci U S A 2001;98(10):5705–10.

[35] Otsuki A, Tahimic CG, Tomimatsu N, et al. Construction of a novel expression system on a human artificial chromosome. Biochem Biophys Res Commun 2005;329(3):1018–25.

[36] Ren X, Katoh M, Hoshiya H, et al. A novel human artificial chromosome vector provides effective cell lineage-specific transgene expression in human mesenchymal stem cells. Stem Cells 2005;23(10):1608–16.

[37] Suda T, Katoh M, Hiratsuka M, et al. Heat regulated production and secretion of insulin from a human artificial chromosome vector. Biochem Biophys Res Commun 2006;340(4): 1053–61.

[38] Kuroiwa Y, Tomizuka K, Shinohara T, et al. Manipulation of human minichromosomes to carry greater than megabase-sized chromosome inserts. Nat Biotechnol 2000;18(10):1086–90.

[39] Kuroiwa Y, Kasinathan P, Choi YJ, et al. Cloned transchromosomic calves producing human immunoglobulin. Nat Biotechnol 2002;20(9):889–94.

[40] Robl JM, Kasinathan P, Sullivan E, et al. Artificial chromosome vectors and expression of complex proteins in transgenic animals. Theriogenology 2003;59(1):107–13.

[41] Guiducci C, Ascenzioni F, Auriche C, et al. Use of a human minichromosome as a cloning and expression vector for mammalian cells. Hum Mol Genet 1999;8(8):1417–24.

[42] Mejia JE, Willmott A, Levy E, et al. Functional complementation of a genetic deficiency with human artificial chromosomes. Am J Hum Genet 2001;69(2):315–26.

[43] Grimes BR, Schindelhauer D, McGill NI, et al. Stable gene expression from a mammalian artificial chromosome. EMBO Rep 2001;2(10):910–4.

[44] Ikeno M, Inagaki H, Nagata K, et al. Generation of human artificial chromosomes expressing naturally controlled guanosine triphosphate cyclohydrolase I gene. Genes Cells 2002; 7(10):1021–32.

[45] Kotzamanis G, Cheung W, Abdulrazzak H, et al. Construction of human artificial chromosome vectors by recombineering. Gene 2005;351:29–38.

[46] Moralli D, Simpson KM, Wade-Martins R, et al. A novel human artificial chromosome gene expression system using herpes simplex virus type 1 vectors. EMBO Rep 2006;(Aug):11.

[47] Co DO, Borowoski AH, Leung JD, et al. Generation of transgenic mice and germline transmission of a mammalian artificial chromosome introduced into embryos by pronuclear microinjection. Chromosome Res 2000;8(3):183–91.

[48] Byun HM, Suh D, Yoon H, et al. Erythrocyte ghost-mediated gene delivery for prolonged and blood targeted expression. Gene Ther 2004;11(5):492–6.

[49] Laner A, Goussard S, Ramalho AS, et al. Bacterial transfer of large functional genomic DNA into human cells. Gene Ther 2005;12(21):1559–72.

[50] Basu J, Willard HF. Artificial and engineered chromosomes: non-integrating vectors for gene therapy. Trends Mol Med 2005;11(5):251–8.

[51] Auriche C, Carpani D, Conese M, et al. Functional human CFTR produced by a stable minichromosome. EMBO Rep 2002;3(9):862–8.

[52] Li Q, Peterson KR, Fang X, et al. Locus control regions. Blood 2002;100(9):3077–86.

[53] Pannell D, Ellis J. Silencing of gene expression: implications for design of retrovirus vectors. Rev Med Virol 2001;11(4):205–17.

ELSEVIER
SAUNDERS

Pediatr Clin N Am
53 (2006) 855–871

PEDIATRIC CLINICS
OF NORTH AMERICA

Inborn Errors of Development: Disruption of Pathways Critical for Normal Development

Anthony Wynshaw-Boris, MD, PhD

Department of Pediatrics, Center for Human Genetics and Genomics, University of California San Diego School of Medicine, 9500 Gilman Drive, La Jolla, CA 92093-0627, USA

The development of the single cell of a fertilized egg into a fully formed human with a highly ordered and stereotypic body form requires the precise choreography of events controlling numerous cellular processes, including proliferation, cell fate determination, and cell migration. Although development generally proceeds normally, there is an approximately 2% to 3% risk that an individual child will have a recognizable malformation or malformations at birth [1]. In about half the cases, a single isolated malformation is found, whereas the other half display multiple malformations [2]. Looking at this a slightly different way, although the vast majority of newborns have no recognizable abnormalities, 1 in 40 have a recognizable defect, and thus are seen by pediatricians and pediatric subspecialists.

How should a pediatrician think about children who have birth defects or other genetic defects? Traditionally, congenital birth defects have been classified descriptively [3]. Is there a single defect or are there multiple anomalies? Are the malformations caused by intrinsic or extrinsic forces? Single primary defects can be classified by the nature of the presumed cause of the defect as a malformation, dysplasia, deformation, or disruption [3]. Malformations and dysplasias are primary structural defects arising from a localized error in morphogenesis that results in the abnormal formation of a tissue or organ or an abnormal organization of cells into tissues, respectively. Deformations and disruptions, on the other hand, are secondary effects that result from forces generated extrinsic to the affected tissue or organ, by alteration or destruction in the shape of a structure or organ that has differentiated normally.

E-mail address: awynshawboris@ucsd.edu

0031-3955/06/$ - see front matter © 2006 Elsevier Inc. All rights reserved.
doi:10.1016/j.pcl.2006.08.008

Malformations affecting intrinsic structures are attributable to genetic defects 20% to 30% of the time, and as those genes are identified our understanding of congenital anomalies is advancing rapidly. Approximately 7% to 8% of developmental abnormalities are caused by mutations in a single gene and display characteristic Mendelian patterns of inheritance [1]. The genes for more than 100 of these single-gene disorders have been identified. The molecular understanding of the pathogenesis of these disorders is useful for improving our understanding of mammalian development and for improving patient care.

The development of genetic approaches in various model organisms from yeast to worm to fly to mouse and even in the human has contributed greatly to our understanding of mechanisms that control embryologic development. In the post-genome era, the sequence of the entire human genome and the genomes of various model organisms are completed and immediately accessible by way of public web browsers. It is becoming increasingly clear that developmental processes in all eukaryotic organisms, including humans, are controlled by evolutionarily conserved signal transduction pathways, transcription factors, or regulatory proteins required for key developmental events. In humans, several of the genes identified that are mutated in malformation syndromes, along with genes whose expression is disrupted by environmental agents or teratogens, are part of these conserved signal transduction pathways important for controlling development throughout evolution. These studies have increased our understanding to the point that we can consider malformations to be inborn errors of development [2,4–6], much as metabolic disorders are considered inborn errors of metabolism, a term coined by Sir Archibald Garrod more than a century ago.

The goal of this article is to provide a framework that allows pediatricians to relate the phenotype in humans who have birth defects to the function of a gene or genes signal transduction pathway that regulates development. In its broadest sense, a signal transduction pathway "transduces" an external signal in the form of a ligand into changes in gene transcription by binding of the ligand to specific cellular receptors (Fig. 1). There may be a few or several intracellular events that come between the ligand–receptor interaction and changes in gene transcription. Although there are several conserved developmental signal transduction pathways important for organogenesis that can be described, this article focuses on three highly conserved pathways: the sonic hedgehog (SHH) pathway; the wingless-int1 (WNT) pathway, and a recently described branch of this pathway called the planar cell polarity (PCP) pathway; and the fibroblast growth factor (FGF) pathway. Each of these pathways or gene families is conserved in invertebrates, such as worms (*Caenorhabditis elegans*) and flies (*Drosophila melanogaster*), where the outline of each pathway and its importance during development was first described. A brief description of each pathway is followed by the developmental processes regulated by that pathway as defined in model organisms, particularly in mouse models, in which the genes and

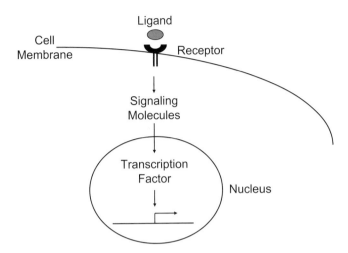

Fig. 1. An idealized signal transduction pathway in which an extracellular ligand binds to a surface receptor, resulting in the activation of intracellular signaling molecules to modify transcription factor activity in the nucleus and alter transcription of specific genes.

developmental phenotypes are highly conserved. The human diseases with known mutations in each pathway are described. Finally, a brief discussion of how the coordination and integration of the activity of these pathways during development is presented, to underscore the complexity that is layered on top of developmental pathways.

Sonic hedgehog pathway

The SHH pathway (Fig. 2) is developmentally important during embryogenesis to induce controlled proliferation in a tissue-specific manner, and disruption of this pathway results in various related developmental disorders and malformations [7,8,9]. By contrast, activation of this pathway in the adult leads to abnormal proliferation and cancer.

SHH is a ligand expressed in the embryo in various regions important for development of the brain, face, limbs, and gut. SHH is processed by proteolytic cleavage to an active N-terminal form, which is then further modified by the addition of cholesterol. The modified and active form of SHH binds to its transmembrane receptor Patched (PTCH), and there are two family members (PTCH-1 and PTCH-2) in mammals. SHH binding to PTCH inhibits the activity of the transmembrane protein Smoothened (SMOH). SMOH acts to suppress downstream targets of the SHH pathway, the GLI family of transcription factors, so inhibition of SMOH by PTCH results in activation of GLI1, GLI2, and GLI3, resulting in alteration of transcription of GLI targets.

Studies in vertebrate model organisms revealed that the SHH pathway is important for early development and for regulating proliferation. SHH itself

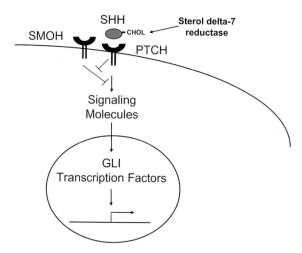

Fig. 2. A simplified version of the SHH pathway.

regulates several vertebrate developmental processes, including the definition of the posterior region of the limb and the ventral region of the central
nervous system. In the limb, SHH is expressed in a posterior structure of the
developing limb bud known as the zone of polarizing activity (ZPA). The
ZPA was identified as an area of the developing vertebrate limb that defines
the posterior side of the limb bud (see Fig. 5 below). Transplants of an embryonic chicken ZPA to the anterior side of a developing chick limb bud resulted in mirror image posterior duplications of the limb, suggesting that the
ZPA produces a morphogen, a diffusible substance that can change the fate
of an embryonic structure. SHH was identified as the morphogen in the
ZPA that defines the posterior region of the developing limb bud. Similarly,
SHH was found to be a morphogen in the developing central nervous system. It is expressed first in the notochord, a structure just below the future
ventral portion of the neural plate and neural tube. SHH is expressed later in
the ventral-most portion of the neural tube, the floor plate, where a gradient
of SHH expression specifies the types of neurons generated from the ventral
half of the neural tube. PTCH, on the other hand, acts as a tumor suppres-
sor. Mice heterozygous for null mutations of PTCH display skeletal defects
and tumors, whereas homozygous mutants die in midgestation with an open
and overgrown neural tube.

Human diseases

Several human diseases are associated with defects in the SHH pathway
(Table 1). Most of the diseases result in defects in the central nervous system
and limbs or result in cancer, phenotypes expected based on the developmental role of this pathway. Sporadic and inherited loss-of-function mutations in SHH are found to cause holoprosencephaly, a variably severe

Table 1
Human genetic diseases caused by mutations in the SHH pathway

Gene mutated	Disease	Inheritance	Manifestations
SHH	Holoprosencephaly	AD	Variable midline defects (single maxillary incisor, hypotelorism, holoprosencephaly, cyclopia)
sterol delta-7-reductase	Smith-Lemli-Opitz	AR	Syndactyly, polydactyly, upturned nose, ptosis, cryptorchidism, CNS hypoplasia, holoprosencephaly
PTCH-1	Gorlin syndrome	AD	Dysmorphic features (short metacarpals, rib defects, broad face, dental abnormalities), cancer predisposition (rhabdomyosarcoma, medulloblastoma)
PTCH-1 or -2	Tumor suppressors	Somatic	Basal cell carcinomas, medulloblastomas
SMOH	Oncogene	Somatic	Basal cell carcinomas, medulloblastomas
GLI1	Oncogene	Somatic	Glioblastoma, osteosarcoma, rhabdomyosarcoma, B cell lymphomas
GLI3	Greig syndrome	AD	Hypertelorism, syndactyly, preaxial polydactyly, broad thumbs and great toes
	Pallister-Hall syndrome	AD	Postaxial polydactyly, syndactyly, hypothalamic hamartomas, imperforate anus
	Postaxial polydactyly A	AD	
	Preaxial polydactyly IV	AD	

Abbreviations: AD, autosomal dominant; AR, autosomal recessive.

midline defect with phenotypes ranging from a single maxillary incisor with hypotelorism to cyclopia [10]. Smith-Lemli-Opitz syndrome (SLOS) results from mutations in the sterol delta-7-reductase gene, an enzyme important in cholesterol biosynthesis. Patients who have SLOS display syndactyly (fusion of the fingers and toes) often with polydactyly, upturned nose, ptosis, crypt-orchidism, central nervous system hypoplasia, and holoprosencephaly. These mutations link cholesterol biosynthesis to the SHH pathway, because many of the features of this disorder are related to defects in sonic hedge-hog, which is posttranslationally modified by cholesterol [11]. Somatic inac-tivating mutations in PTCH-1 and PTCH-2 act as tumor suppressors, whereas activating mutations in SMOH function as oncogenes, particularly in basal cell carcinomas and medulloblastomas [12]. Germline inactivating mutations in PTCH-1 result in Gorlin syndrome, an autosomal dominant disorder characterized by dysmorphic features (short metacarpals, rib defects, broad face, and dental abnormalities), basal cell nevi that undergo malignant transformation, and an increased risk for cancers, such as rhabdomyosarcoma and medulloblastoma. The phenotypes produced by mutations in the PTCH and SMO receptors are consistent with the function of these coreceptors in the pathway, as described above. GLI1 amplification has been found in several human tumors, including glioblastoma, osteosarcoma, rhabdomyosarcoma, and B cell lymphomas. By contrast, mutations or alterations in GLI3 have been found in Greig cephalopolysyndactyly syndrome (GCPS), Pallister-Hall syndrome (PHS), postaxial polydactyly type A (and A/B), and preaxial polydactyly type IV [13]. GCPS consists of hypertelorism, syndactyly, preaxial polydactyly, and broad thumbs and great toes. PHS is an autosomal dominant disorder characterized by postaxial polydactyly, syndactyly, hypothalamic hamartomas, imperforate anus, and occasionally holoprosencephaly. GLI3 binds to CBP, the protein coded for by the gene for a broadly acting transcriptional coactivator called CBP, or CREB-binding protein. Humans who have 50% reduction in CBP, by virtue of heterozygous loss-of-function mutations of this gene, display Rubinstein-Taybi syndrome (RTS). The CBP coactivator regulates the transcription of several genes, which helps to explain why patients who have mutations in CBP have a wide-ranging phenotype that includes mental retardation, broad thumbs and toes, and congenital heart disease [14]. One of the transcription factors that binds to CBP is GLI3, a transcription factor that is part of the SHH pathway.

Mutations in genes that function together in the SHH pathway commonly have overlapping clinical manifestations. Brain defects are found in holoprosencephaly, SLOS, and PHS. Facial abnormalities are found in holoprosencephaly, Gorlin syndrome, GCPS, and PHS. Limb defects are found in SLOS, Gorlin syndrome, GCPS, PHS, and the polydactyly syndromes. Overexpression or activating mutations of the SHH pathway result in cancer. An understanding of the SHH developmental pathway therefore allows us to place mutant genes into these pathways to consider birth defects as inborn errors of development, and provides insight into the pathogenesis of these related syndromes.

WNT pathway and planar cell polarity pathways

The WNT pathway is known to play many important roles in development, with particularly important effects in proliferation, cell fate specification, cellular polarity, and cell migration. Inactivation of members of the WNT pathway results in several specific developmental defects that span all of development and occur in all organs and tissues. The first member identified in this pathway was *Wnt1*, which was the site of mouse mammary tumor virus integration. This integration event resulted in the constitutive activation of *Wnt1* in the mammary gland, an event that resulted in mouse mammary gland cancer. Dysregulation of this pathway also can result in cancer. Importantly, when *wingless*, the *Drosophila* homolog of *Wnt1*, was cloned, the critical role of the Wnt pathway in cell fate determination also was revealed.

WNT pathway

Genome sequencing has revealed that the mammalian genome encodes at least 19 WNT ligands; 10 Frizzled (FZ) receptors; two coreceptors, lipoprotein receptor-related protein (LRP) 5 and 6; and a large number of additional proteins related to the WNT pathways. Depending on whether the pathways result in β-catenin–mediated gene transcription, one can divide the multiple WNT pathways into canonical (β-catenin–dependent, Fig. 3) and noncanonical (β-catenin–independent) WNT pathways. These two pathways share some common components but also use distinct members. Through phenotypic characterization of genetically engineered, radiation-induced, or spontaneous mutations in many of the components in the mouse, we have now gained a basic understanding of both pathways in mammalian patterning and morphogenesis. The role of the canonical WNT pathway in implantation, gastrulation, and organogenesis and the role of the PCP pathway, a primary branch of the noncanonical WNT pathway, in mammalian polarity determination and morphogenesis are discussed.

The WNT pathway was first discovered in *Drosophila*, where several segment polarity genes were identified that were required for the wingless signal

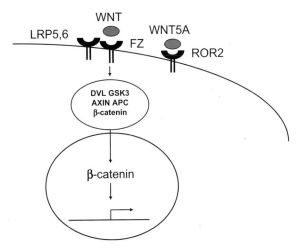

Fig. 3. A simplified version of the canonical WNT pathway.

transduction pathway [15,16]. In the canonical WNT pathway (Fig. 3), when the WNT signal is absent, glycogen synthase kinase-3 (GSK3) is active and phosphorylates armadillo/β-catenin. This activity results in the ubiquitination and degradation of β-catenin through the proteosome pathway. Transcription factors of the TCF/LEF family are associated with corepressors in the nucleus, and act to repress transcription of genes containing response elements for these transcription factors. In the presence of the WNT signal, WNT, a secreted protein associated with the extracellular matrix, binds to its cellular coreceptors, FZ and LRP/arrow. In an unknown fashion, Dishevelled (DVL) activation leads to the inactivation of GSK3. This activation of DVL and inactivation of GSK3 probably occurs in a large multiprotein complex in association with other members of the pathway, including axin, β-catenin, and APC, the product of the gene mutated in the human disorder adenomatous polyposis coli. As a result, β-catenin is stabilized and binds to transcription factors of the TCF/LEF families in the nucleus to modulate transcription. β-catenin binding dismisses the associated corepressors from TCF and LEF and activates transcription of genes containing response elements for these transcription factors. The result of WNT signaling thus is to convert extracellular signals into changes in transcriptional activity.

Given that there are so many broadly expressed genes in this pathway, it is not surprising that mutations in this pathway affect the development of virtually all stages of development and all organ systems. Members of this pathway are expressed at many developmental stages, in unique but often overlapping patterns with other members of the pathway. Phenotypes of loss-of-function mutations in the WNT pathway are revealing. For example, loss of WNT1 results in defects of the midbrain and cerebellum, loss of WNT2 or WNT7B result in placental defects, loss of WNT3 results in severe gastrulation defects, loss of WNT4 or WNT11 results in kidney and urogenital defects, and loss of WNT5A and WNT7A result in limb defects. Loss of function of APC results in human and mouse colorectal cancer. Finally, mutations in the DVL homologs in the mouse display defects in social behavior (DVL1), conotruncal development (DVL2 and DVL3), and neural tube closure (double mutants of DVL1 and DVL2). A complete and up-to-date listing of the genes in this pathway and the phenotypes of mice and humans with defects resulting from mutations in members of this pathway can be found at the Wnt Homepage, maintained by Roel Nusse at Stanford University (http://www.stanford.edu/~rnusse/wntwindow.html).

Planar cell polarity pathway

In addition to their critical roles in the Wnt/wg pathway, some members of the Wnt/wingless pathway, such as *Dishevelled*, and several other genes from *D. melanogaster* participate in the planar cell polarity (PCP) pathway [17,18]. The PCP pathway regulates the polarity of a cell within the plane of the epithelium, perpendicular to the apical–basilar axis of the cell. Activation of this pathway results in membrane localization of DVL and activation of the small GTPase RHO. In some instances, the PCP pathway activates JNK (c-Jun N-terminal kinase) signaling, whereas in others the RHO-associated kinase ROK becomes membrane localized. *Fz* and *Dishevelled* are required for the PCP/convergent extension pathway.

The major manifestation of the PCP pathway in *Drosophila* is in orienting cellular extensions called trichomes from the epithelial cells of the wing into parallel arrays, and in the oriented parallel arrays of photoreceptors in the compound eye. In *Drosophila*, several genes are required for the PCP pathway, including *Fz*, *Dsh*, and *Strabismus/Van Gogh* (*Stbm*). These genes are conserved in vertebrates, where they appear to be involved in a common pathway to generate traction and move these cells against one another to drive the elongation of the A–P axis with simultaneous shortening of the medial–lateral axis in a process called convergent extension. Recent evidence suggests that the PCP pathway in *Drosophila* and convergent extension in vertebrates are regulated by the same genetic pathway [17,18]. A third developmental process regulated by the PCP pathway seems to be the orientation of cell division in zebrafish [19].

A homologous PCP pathway also exists in mammals and regulates planar cell polarity in the development of the inner ear and convergent extension movements to regulate neurulation, or neural tube closure. When any of the mammalian homologs of the fly PCP pathway are disrupted in the mouse, the uniform orientation of stereocilia on the sensory hair cells is disrupted. In addition to the inner ear polarity defects, disruption of mammalian PCP pathway members results in a unique and severe neural tube closure defect in which the entire neural tube from mid-brain to tail fails to close, a severe congenital neural tube defect termed craniorachischisis in humans. More recently, roles for PCP noncanonical Wnt signaling in mammalian heart development and axonal tract development have been identified, suggesting that this pathway has surprisingly broad effects during development.

Human diseases

Several human genetic diseases result from defects in the Wnt pathway (Table 2). The diseases identified to date involve the skeleton, eye, and reproductive tract. Wnt-1–induced signaling protein 3 (WISP3), initially identified by increased expression in WNT1-transformed cells, was found to be associated with the autosomal recessive skeletal disorder progressive pseudorheumatoid dysplasia, a disorder often misdiagnosed as juvenile rheumatoid arthritis [20]. Patients display cartilage loss and destructive bone changes with age. AXIN2 is one of the essential intracellular proteins required to negatively control WNT signaling. Mutations in human AXIN2 result in familial tooth agenesis and a predisposition to colorectal cancer

Table 2

Human genetic diseases caused by mutations in the Wnt/PCP pathway

Gene mutated	Disease	Inheritance	Manifestations
WISP3	Progressive pseudorheumatoid dysplasia	AR	Cartilage loss, bone destruction
AXIN2	Tooth agenesis	AD	Tooth agenesis, cancer predisposition
LRP5	Juvenile osteoporosis	AR	Osteoporosis
	Osteoporosis-pseudoglioma syndrome	AR	Osteoporosis, blindness
Norrin	Norrie disease	X-linked	Retinal dysplasia, hearing loss, mental retardation
FZD4	Familial exudative vitreoretinopathy	AR	Retinal vascular disorder
ROR2	Brachydactyly type B	AD	Terminal deficiencies of fingers, toes
	Robinow syndrome	AR	Bone shortening, spine defects, brachydactyly, dysmorphic facies
WNT3	Tetra-amelia	AR	Absent limbs
WNT4	Rokitansky-Kuster-Hauser syndrome	AR	Absent vagina, uterus

Abbreviations: AD, autosomal dominant; AR, autosomal recessive.

[21]. Several of the known members of the WNT coreceptor complex result in inherited diseases. A specific activating mutation in the coreceptor LRP5 was found in a single family with autosomal dominant high bone mass [22]. By contrast, several familial cases of juvenile osteoporosis result from loss-of-function mutations in LRP5, including osteoporosis-pseudoglioma syndrome, an autosomal recessive disorder manifested by severe juvenile osteoporosis and juvenile-onset blindness. Frizzled-4 (FZ4) was found to be mutated in familial exudative vitreoretinopathy, and the gene for Norrie disease (X-linked congenital retinal dysplasia accompanied by hearing loss and mental retardation) seems to code for a novel ligand for FZ4 [23]. ROR2 is an orphan tyrosine kinase receptor that seems to mediate the signal of WNT5A (Fig. 3). Mutations in ROR2 result in brachydactyly type B, an autosomal dominant disorder characterized by terminal deficiencies in the fingers and toes [24] and the autosomal recessive form of Robinow syndrome, a severe skeletal dysplasia with limb bone shortening, spine defects, brachydactyly, and dysmorphic facial features [25]. Mutations in two WNT ligands have been found in two genetic disorders. One of the ligands, WNT3, was found to be mutated in an autosomal recessive form of tetra-amelia, a rare disorder consisting of complete absence of all four limbs and other disorders [26]. These WNT3 mutations were truncations and likely loss-of-function mutations. The other ligand, WNT4, was found to be mutated in Rokitansky-Kuster-Hauser syndrome, which consists of absence of the vagina and uterus, among other defects [27]. In the latter two cases, these

mutations were found in few individuals, so one should view these findings with some degree of caution until they are replicated.

Although the WNT pathway has broad known functions in development, mutations in genes that function together in the WNT pathway have overlapping clinical manifestations. Retinal defects are found in osteoporosis-pseudoglioma syndrome, Norrie disease, and familial exudative vitreoretinopathy. Limb abnormalities are found in brachydactyly type B, Robinow syndrome, and tetra-amelia. Skeletal defects are found in progressive pseudorheumatoid dysplasia, osteoporosis syndromes, and Robinow syndrome. AXIN2 and APC mutations result in cancer predisposition. An understanding of the WNT developmental pathway is another example in which birth defects can be classified as inborn errors of development.

Fibroblast growth factor pathway

The fibroblast growth factor (FGF) pathway is known to play many important roles in development, with particularly important effects in proliferation, cell fate specification, cellular polarity, and cell migration. Like the Wnt pathway, inactivation of members of the FGF pathway results in several specific developmental defects that span all of development and occur in the development of all organs and tissues.

The mammalian genome encodes at least 23 FGF ligands, 4 FGF receptors (FGFR), and many additional proteins related to downstream pathways activated by the tyrosine kinase activity of the activated FGFR [28–30]. Three downstream pathways have been identified: the Ras mitogen-activated protein kinase (MAPK) pathway, the phosphoinositol pathway, and the signal transducer and activator of transcription (STAT) pathway (Fig. 4). These three pathways share some common components, mainly the ligand–receptor combination, but also use distinct members to transduce the signal to the nucleus.

FGF binding to the FGFR results in dimerization of the receptor and stimulation of the intracellular tyrosine kinase domain of the dimerized receptor, resulting in autophosphorylation of the FGFR dimer at intracellular tyrosine residues. The activated receptor either binds directly to signaling molecules or recruits adapter molecules to link the activated receptor to downstream targets at the cell membrane. The cellular context determines which of the downstream pathways are activated after FGFR activation.

Two of the pathways activated by FGF signaling are classic growth factor signal transduction pathways: the Ras-MAPK and the phosphoinositol pathways. Activation of the classic Ras-MAPK pathway results in the stimulation of the protooncogene Ras by recruitment of scaffolding proteins, such as Grb2 and Sos, to the membrane. Activated Ras binds to Raf and stimulates a MAPK cascade that ultimately leads to transcription factor activation and the transcription of genes activated by FGF signaling. The

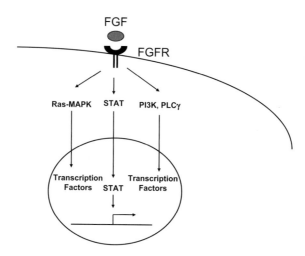

Fig. 4. A simplified version of the FGF pathway.

phosphoinositol pathway also is activated by FGF signaling by way of the activation of phosphoinositol-3 kinase (PI3K). The result of this activation is that potent lipid messengers, such as diacylglycerol (DAG) and inositol triphosphate (PIP3), activate phospholipase Cγ (PKCγ), which results in the phosphorylation of various transcription factors. Finally, STAT proteins are inactive in the cytosol, but when phosphorylated by activated FGFR (and other receptors) STATs are translocated to the nucleus where they regulate transcription. As in the Wnt pathway, there are multiple branch points downstream of the ligand–receptor interaction, providing several potential readouts from receptor activation that depend on the precise ligand and receptor and the cellular context.

The phenotypes of model organisms with both loss-of-function and gain-of-function mutations of many of the FGFs and FGFRs have been determined from genetically engineered, radiation-induced, or spontaneous mutations, so that we have now gained a basic understanding of the role of the FGF pathway in mammalian patterning and morphogenesis. For example, loss-of-function mutations in FGFs in the mouse demonstrate critical roles for these proteins in early development (FGF4, FGF8), inner ear development (FGF3), limb development (FGF10), neurologic development and function (FGF2, FGF8, FGF14, FGF17), cardiac development (FGF8), hair length (FGF5, FGF7), skin and wound healing (FGF2), branching morphogenesis in lung or kidney (FGF7, FGF9, FGF10), skeletal development (FGF2, FGF18), and in male sexual development (FGF9). The FGFR mutants display similarly broad but distinct phenotypes: early gastrulation defects (FGFR1, FGFR2), limb defects (FGFR2), skeletal defects (FGFR3), and growth retardation (FGFR4).

Human diseases

Several human genetic diseases result from defects in the FGF pathway (Table 3), most of which can be classified as either craniosynostosis or short-limbed skeletal dysplasias. All of the known diseases of the FGF pathway are inherited in an autosomal dominant fashion, and many represent gain-of-function or activating mutations in which the receptors are active in the absence of ligand.

Craniosynostosis is the abnormal shape of the skull because of the premature fusion of sutures of the skull during development. Several craniosynostosis syndromes have been defined based on the sutures involved (causing a particular type of shape of the skull) and whether or not there is distal limb involvement. Several of these syndromes are caused by heterozygous point mutations in the FGFRs, including Apert (FGFR2), Crouzon (FGFR2), Pfeiffer (FGFR1, FGFR2), Jackson-Weiss (FGFR2), and Beare-Stevenson (FGFR2, FGFR3) syndromes. The phenotypic details that differentiate each of these syndromes are beyond the scope of this article, but further details can be found elsewhere [3]. When these mutations have been studied, they have been found to result in various degrees of activation of the receptors.

The short-limbed skeletal dysplasias resulting from disruptions in the FGF pathway are caused by point mutations in FGFR3. As noted above, when these mutations have been studied they have been found to result in various degrees of activation of the receptors, and the degree of activation correlates somewhat with the severity of the phenotype. The most common disorder is achondroplasia. Most cases of achondroplasia are the result of a new mutation, and most patients have a single point mutation resulting

Table 3
Human genetic diseases caused by mutations in the FGF pathway

Disease	Gene mutated	Inheritance
Craniosynostosis syndromes		
Apert	FGFR2	AD
Crouzon	FGFR2	AD
Pfeiffer	FGFR1, FGFR2	AD
Jackson-Weiss	FGFR2	AD
Beare-Stevenson	FGFR2, FGFR3	AD
Short-limbed skeletal dysplasias		
Achondroplasia	FGFR3	AD
Hypochondroplasia	FGFR3	AD
Thanatophoric dysplasia	FGFR3	AD
SADDAN	FGFR3	AD
Other		
Cerebellar ataxia	FGF14	AD
Hypophosphatemic rickets	FGF23	AD

Abbreviations: AD, autosomal dominant; SADDAN, severe achondroplasia with developmental delay and acanthosis nigricans.

in a specific amino acid change in FGFR3 (Gly346Glu) that results in constitutive activation of the receptor. Hypochondroplasia is a less severe form of achondroplasia that also results from point mutations in FGFR3, and when these mutations were studied the mutant FGFR3s were less active than achondroplasia FGFR3 mutations. Thanatophoric dysplasia is a severe neonatal lethal form of achondroplasia that results from point mutations in FGFR3 that display greater activity than achondroplasia FGFR3 mutations.

Two other types of genetic disorders have been described in humans who have mutations in this pathway: AD cerebellar ataxia caused by a point mutation in FGF14 (Phe145Ser), and AD hypophosphatemic rickets caused by point mutations in a small region of FGF23.

Disorders caused by mutations in the FGF pathway have clear phenotypic overlap in their clinical manifestations. Most of the phenotypes cluster into craniosynostosis and short-limbed dwarfism syndromes. Of the two other genetic disorders, hypophosphatemic rickets also affects the skeleton, as predicted from mouse and human disorders, and the cerebellar ataxia phenotype is similar to some of the phenotypes seen in mouse mutants of FGFs. Similar to the SHH and FGF pathways, therefore, an understanding of the FGF developmental pathway allows us to place mutant genes into these pathways and consider birth defects as inborn errors of development, providing further insight into the pathogenesis of these related syndromes.

Integration and coordinate regulation of developmental pathways

Severe mutations in single genes result in severe and recognizable inborn errors of development because of the disruption of individual developmental pathways. We also know that several pathways simultaneously regulate the development of a given structure or organ. The complexity of form of mammalian organisms requires that these pathways are coordinately regulated and integrated. As an example of this integration, the coordinate regulation of the three pathways discussed in this article during the formation of the limbs is described.

Limb bud formation is localized in specific sites along the body wall of the developing embryo by a combination of FGF and WNT signaling. There are three axes in limb development: proximal–distal, anterior–posterior (AP), and dorsal–ventral (Fig. 5). Before limb bud initiation, *Fgf10* expression in the mesenchyme is localized precisely by the expression of *Wnt3* produced from the surface ectoderm. The initiation of limb bud formation thus is accomplished by coordinate regulation by the WNT and FGF pathways. As the limb bud grows and protrudes away from the body wall, the most distal part of the limb bud contains a thickened apical ectodermal ridge (AER). FGF expression, especially FGF4 and FGF8, is required to maintain the AER and to mediate the growth and elongation of the limb

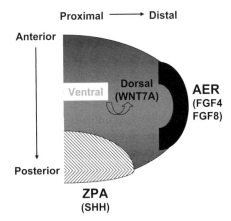

Fig. 5. The major axes of the developing limb bud and the location of SHH, WNT, and FGF in the developing limb bud. The axes are proximal–distal, anterior–posterior, and dorsal–ventral.

bud in a proximal-to-distal direction. As noted above, SHH is expressed in the ZPA to regulate the formation of the AP axis in the limb (in the hand the anterior is the thumb side, whereas the posterior is the little finger side). WNT signaling, primarily WNT7A, is responsible for the development of the dorsal–ventral axis of the limb (in the hand, the dorsal surface is the back of the hand, whereas the ventral surface is the palm). WNT7A is required to maintain the AER and the expression of FGF4 and FGF8, and also participates in regulatory feedback signaling with the ZPA to affect AP axis formation indirectly. FGF4 in the AER is required to maintain expression of SHH in the ZPA, whereas SHH also is able to modulate FGF4 levels in the AER, thereby creating a positive feedback loop that links the two signaling centers. WNT7A is also important for regulating SHH expression and consequently patterning along the limb AP axis. These three pathways are coordinately regulated to integrate signaling during the formation of the limb.

Summary

The mammalian SHH, WNT, and FGF pathways are large signaling networks that often display intricate interactions to determine, ultimately, the course of development. For example, WNTs can act either as morphogens to specify different cell lineages along the anterior–posterior axis or as mitogens to promote cell proliferation of a defined population. Some pathways may affect either cell fate or proliferation but other pathways may impact morphogenesis through remodeling cell arrangements along different axes. Understanding how the individual pathways are coordinately regulated and orchestrated to achieve the desired pattern and morphology will be one of the greatest challenges in developmental biology in the future. For human dysmorphology, the challenge will be to understand further the pathophysiology and cause of inborn errors of development.

There are several reasons that pediatricians should recognize that birth defects are inborn errors of development. Consideration of malformations as alterations of important developmental pathways provides a molecular framework to understand normal human development and the causes of human birth defects and disorders of organogenesis. In addition to providing an improved understanding of the pathophysiology of these defects, it will allow the distinction of similarities and differences among related disorders. Finally, a more complete understanding of how a pathway is disrupted in individuals who have severe birth defects may reveal treatment options for otherwise difficult-to-treat disorders [31].

References

[1] Winter R. Analysing human developmental abnormalities. Bioessays 1996;18:965–71.
[2] Epstein CJ. Human malformations and their genetic basis. In: Epstein CJ, Erickson RP, Wynshaw-Boris A, editors. Inborn errors of development: the molecular basis of clinical disorders of morphogenesis. Oxford: Oxford University Press; 2004. p. 3–9.
[3] Jones KL. Smith's recognizable patterns of human malformation. Philadelphia: WB Saunders; 1997.
[4] Holmes LB. Inborn errors of morphogenesis. A review of localized hereditary malformations. N Engl J Med 1974;291:763–73.
[5] Epstein CJ. The new dysmorphology: application of insights from basic developmental biology to the understanding of human birth defects. Proc Natl Acad Sci USA 1995;92:8566–73.
[6] Epstein CJ, Erickson RP, Wynshaw-Boris A, editors. Inborn errors of development: the molecular basis of clinical disorders of morphogenesis. Oxford: Oxford University Press; 2004.
[7] Villavicencio EH, Walterhouse DO, Iannaccone PM. The sonic hedgehog-patched-Gli pathway in human development and disease. Am J Hum Genet 2000;67:1047–54.
[8] Ho KS, Scott MP. Sonic hedgehog in the nervous system: functions, modifications and mechanisms. Curr Opin Neurobiol 2002;12:57–63.
[9] Cohen MM Jr. An introduction to sonic hedgehog signaling. In: Epstein CJ, Erickson RP, Wynshaw-Boris A, editors. Inborn errors of development: the molecular basis of clinical disorders of morphogenesis. Oxford: Oxford University Press; 2004. p. 210–28.
[10] Roessler E, Belloni E, Gaudenz K, et al. Mutations in the human Sonic Hedgehog gene cause holoprosencephaly. Nat Genet 1996;14:357–60.
[11] Irons M. DHCR7 and the Smith-Lemli-Opitz (RSH) syndrome. In: Epstein CJ, Erickson RP, Wynshaw-Boris A, editors. Inborn errors of development: the molecular basis of clinical disorders of morphogenesis. Oxford: Oxford University Press; 2004. p. 229–39.
[12] Wechsler-Reya R, Scott MP. The developmental biology of brain tumors. Annu Rev Neurosci 2001;24:385–428.
[13] Biesecker LG. Polydactyly: how many disorders and how many genes? Am J Med Genet 2002;112:279–83.
[14] Petrij F, Breuning MH, Hennekam RCM, et al. CBP and the Rubinstein-Taybi syndrome. In: Epstein CJ, Erickson RP, Wynshaw-Boris A, editors. Inborn errors of development: the molecular basis of clinical disorders of morphogenesis. Oxford: Oxford University Press; 2004. p. 11–2.

[15] Cadigan KM, Nusse R. Wnt signaling: a common theme in animal development. Genes Dev 1997;11:3286–305.

[16] Bienz M, Clevers H. Linking colorectal cancer to Wnt signaling. Cell 2000;103:311–20.

[17] Axelrod JD. Strabismus comes into focus. Nat Cell Biol 2002;4:6–10.

[18] Wallingford JB. Closing in on vertebrate planar polarity. Nat Cell Biol 2004;6:687–9.

[19] Gong Y, Mo C, Fraser SE. Planar cell polarity signalling controls cell division orientation during zebrafish gastrulation. Nature 2004;430:689–93.

[20] Hurvitz JR, Suwairi WM, Hul WV, et al. Mutations in the CCN gene family member WISP3 cause progressive pseudorheumatoid dysplasia. Nat Genet 1999;23:94–8.

[21] Lammi L, Arte S, Somer M, et al. Mutations in AXIN2 cause familial tooth agenesis and predispose to colorectal cancer. Am J Hum Genet 2004;74:1043–50.

[22] Levasseur R, Lacombe D, de Vernejoul MC. LRP5 mutations in osteoporosis-pseudoglioma syndrome and high-bone-mass disorders. Joint Bone Spine 2005;72:207–14.

[23] Xu Q, Wang Y, Dabdoub A, et al. Vascular development in the retina and inner ear: control by Norrin and Frizzled-4, a high-affinity ligand-receptor pair. Cell 2004;116:883–95.

[24] Oldridge M, Fortuna AM, Maringa M, et al. Dominant mutations in ROR2, encoding an orphan receptor tyrosine kinase, cause brachydactyly type B. Nat Genet 2000;24:275–8.

[25] Afzal AR, Rajab A, Fenske CD, et al. Recessive Robinow syndrome, allelic to dominant brachydactyly type B, is caused by mutation of ROR2. Nat Genet 2000;25:419–22.

[26] Niemann S, Zhao C, Pascu F, et al. Homozygous WNT3 mutation causes tetra-amelia in a large consanguineous family. Am J Hum Genet 2004;74:558–63.

[27] Biason-Lauber A, Konrad D, Navratil F, et al. WNT4 mutation associated with Mullerian-duct regression and virilization in a 46,XX woman. N Engl J Med 2004;351:792–8.

[28] Givol D, Eswarakumar VP, Lonai P. Molecular and cellular biology of FGF signaling. In: Epstein CJ, Erickson RP, Wynshaw-Boris A, editors. Inborn errors of development: the molecular basis of clinical disorders of morphogenesis. Oxford: Oxford University Press; 2004. p. 367–79.

[29] Cohen MM. FGFs/FGFRs and Associated disorders. In: Epstein CJ, Erickson RP, Wynshaw-Boris A, editors. Inborn errors of development: the molecular basis of clinical disorders of morphogenesis. Oxford: Oxford University Press; 2004. p. 380–400.

[30] Eswarakumar VP, Lax I, Schlessinger J. Cellular signaling by fibroblast growth factor receptors. Cytokine Growth Factor Rev 2005;16:139–49.

[31] Cassidy SB, Allanson JE. Management of genetic syndromes. Hoboken, NJ: Wiley-Liss; 2005.

PEDIATRIC CLINICS
OF NORTH AMERICA

Pediatr Clin N Am
53 (2006) 873–887

Transcriptional Regulation of Perinatal Lung Maturation

Jeffrey A. Whitsett, MD[a],*, Yohei Matsuzaki, MD[a,b]

[a]*Department of Pediatrics, Division of Pulmonary Biology, Cincinnati Children's Hospital Medical Center and the University of Cincinnati College of Medicine, 3333 Burnet Avenue Cincinnati, OH 45229-3039, USA*
[b]*Department of Pediatrics, School of Medicine, Keio University, 35 Shinanomachi Shinjuku, Tokyo 160-8582, Japan*

The respiratory tract undergoes remarkable structural, biochemical, and functional changes during the transition from fluid- to gas-filled status that occurs immediately following birth. The timing of lung maturation is mediated by genetic, hormonal, and autocrine/paracrine signaling, which in turn instructs transcriptional processes that regulate the expression of genes required for perinatal adaptation to breathing. The importance of pulmonary maturation to postnatal adaptation is evidenced by the severity of lung disease occurring in respiratory distress syndrome (RDS) and bronchopulmonary dysplasia (BPD), common sequelae of preterm birth that contribute to morbidity and mortality in premature infants. It is perhaps not surprising that perinatal lung maturation is accompanied by the induction of a complex genetic program designed to enhance surfactant function, establish postnatal alveolar fluid balance, and host defense, all processes that are required for lung function after birth. There is increasing evidence that the process of epithelial cell maturation is controlled by a network of nuclear transcription factors that interact to influence gene expression in the lung.

In this article, the role of several transcription factors mediating perinatal respiratory adaptation is discussed. Lung maturation depends on a carefully balanced interaction between the alveolar epithelial cells (Type I and Type II cells) and mesenchymal cells, including those of the pulmonary vasculature, smooth muscle, and stroma, that results in the production of signaling molecules that, in turn, regulate gene expression. A complex and interacting

---

* Corresponding author.
E-mail address: jeff.whitsett@cchmc.org (J.A. Whitsett).

doi:10.1016/j.pcl.2006.08.009
pediatric.theclinics.com

transcriptional network, mediated in mesenchyme via the glucocorticoid receptor (GR) and several transcription factors determining cell differentiation in the respiratory epithelium, influence lung maturation before birth. In addition to the important role of the GR, transcription factors in the respiratory epithelium, including thyroid transcription factor-1 (TTF-1), forkhead homolog a2 (FOXA2), and CCAT enhancer binding protein α (C/EBPα), regulate groups of genes that are required for the architectural and functional maturation of the lung.

Epithelial-mesenchymal interactions during lung morphogenesis

Formation of the lung during the embryonic period is dependent upon the balanced interactions between epithelial cells of the lung tubules and the underlying mesenchymal cells that ultimately differentiate into vascular, smooth muscle, and fibroblastic cells characteristic of the mature lung [1–3]. As in other organs undergoing branching morphogenesis, proliferation and differentiation of pulmonary cells are dependent upon reciprocal interactions between these epithelial and mesenchymal cellular compartments [4]. Removal of the underlying mesenchyme abrogates branching morphogenesis and growth of respiratory tubules [5]. Branching morphogenesis is regulated by fibroblast growth factor FGF) receptor-mediated signaling that influences epithelial cell migration and proliferation [6–9]. Deletion of FGF-10 or FGF-R2IIIb blocks branching morphogenesis during formation of the embryonic lung [7,9]. FGF-10 is synthesized by the lung mesenchyme, activating receptors on endodermally derived tubules via the FGF-R2IIIb receptor. Growth and differentiation of the peripheral lung saccules are highly dependent upon these interactions until late gestation. FGF signaling is required for the migration, differentiation, and proliferation of respiratory tubules, and plays a role later in lung development, when it influences sacculation and alveolarization [10]. Formation of respiratory tubules in the embryonic lung also requires the expression of TTF-1, a member of the Nkx family of homeodomain-containing transcription factors. TTF-1 plays a critical role in lung formation during the embryonic period of lung development, and is required for normal maturation of the respiratory epithelium before birth [11,12]. Thus reciprocal interactions mediated by autocrine and paracrine signaling between epithelial cells and mesenchymal cells control transcriptional events required for proliferation, migration, and differentiation of the cells that make up the mammalian lung.

Glucocorticoids and the glucocorticoid receptor

Liggins and Howie [13] demonstrated the clinical utility of glucocorticoids (GCs) for the enhancement of lung function in the preterm infant, a finding that has served as an important therapy for the reduction of morbidity and mortality in preterm infants at risk for RDS. Prenatal exposure of the preterm neonate to pharmacological doses of GCs, including betamethasone or dexamethasone, reduces the incidence and severity of RDS, resulting in increased perinatal survival [13–15]. GCs have important effects on lung architecture and function. Structurally, GCs enhance many aspects of the so-called "maturation," resulting in thinning of the pulmonary mesenchyme and alveolar walls. Dilatation of peripheral lung saccules occurs in late gestation, as pulmonary capillary endothelial cells come into close apposition to alveolar Type I epithelial cells, creating an efficient gas exchange region, a process that continues after birth with the formation of the alveoli [1,16]. During the process of sacculation and alveolarization, the respiratory epithelium thins and the lining of peripheral lung saccules is increasingly composed of squamous Type I epithelial cells. Type I cells arise from differentiation of Type II epithelial cells, the latter a cuboidal cell type that synthesizes and secretes surfactants, proteins, and lipids. Type II cells, although composing a relatively small fraction of the surface of peripheral lung saccules, synthesize surfactant proteins and lipids that are required for reduction of surface tension at the air-liquid interface after birth [17]. The increased synthesis of surfactant by Type II cells is associated with the maturation of lung structure, a process also stimulated by GCs [18]. Surfactant prevents atelectasis, thereby maintaining lung volumes and function. Pulmonary surfactant is a complex mixture of lipids (primarily phospholipids), including dipalmityl phosphatidylcholine (DPPC), phosphatidylglycerol, and associated proteins, the most abundant of which are surfactant proteins A, B, C, and D (SP-A, SP-B, SP-C, and SP-D) that regulate surfactant structure, function, and metabolism [17,19,20]. Surfactant proteins also play important protective roles during lung injury and infection. SP-A and SP-D, the pulmonary collectins, bind and inactivate various microbial pathogens, enhancing their uptake and clearance by alveolar macrophages [21]. Pulmonary adaptation to air breathing also requires the rapid removal of lung liquid at birth, a process dependent upon the regulation of electrolyte and water transport that is also influenced by GCs.

Mechanism of action of glucocorticoids on lung maturation

GCs, including cortisol, hydrocortisone, betamethasone, dexamethasone, and others, complex with a specific cytoplasmic receptor, the GR in pulmonary cells (Fig. 1) [22]. GR is a 94 Kd polypeptide, consisting of steroid and DNA-binding domains, encoded by a single gene located on human chromosome 5 [23,24]. There are two GR isoforms, GRα and GRβ. GRα is thought to mediate most of GC activity in endocrine target tissues, whereas GRβ may serve as a negative inhibitor of GRα [25]. GR complexes with several heat shock proteins that bind GR and prevent its nuclear transport in the absence of GC. Binding of GC to the cytoplasmic

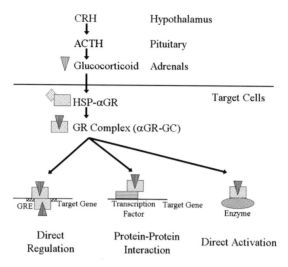

Fig. 1. GC regulation of perinatal lung maturation. Corticotrophin-releasing hormone produced by the hypothalamus, induces adrenocorticotropic hormone (ACTH) release from the pituitary, which stimulates GC production from the adrenal cortex. GCs enter target cells and bind to GRα, causing its dissociation from heat shock protein, causing the translocation of GR/GC complex to the nucleus of the target cells. GR often dimerizes, binds into glucocorticoid regulatory elements (GREs) located in regulatory regions of target genes, which in turn controls gene transcription (direct regulation). GR/GC can also regulate transcription by binding to other transcriptional factors (eg, AP1) to regulate gene expression via protein-protein interactions. Lastly, GR can bind directly to some cellular proteins to influence cell function by direct activation. ACTH, ; CRH corticotrophin-releasing hormone.

GRα causes dissociation of the Hsp-GR complex, causing translocation of GRα into the nucleus of target cells, where it binds to glucocorticoid-responsive elements (GREs) located on regulatory regions of GC target genes [26]. GRα binding to regulatory elements in target genes activates or inhibits transcription. GR also forms complexes with other transcription factors. Thus, GRα regulates gene expression primarily through its interactions with other transcription factors by binding to *cis*-active elements, shared by both GR and other nuclear transcription factors [27].

Deletion of GRα causes respiratory distress at birth

GRα$^{-/-}$ mice develop respiratory distress and die following birth [28,29]. Deficient GR signaling caused by mutation of the corticotrophin-releasing hormone (CRH) causes similar changes in lung architecture and function, resulting in thickened alveolar septae, atelectasis, and impaired lung function at birth [30]. Although lung function was severely impaired, minimal changes in the expression of surfactant proteins A, B, and surfactant lipids were observed in the lungs of GR$^{-/-}$ or CRH$^{-/-}$ mice. In contrast, exposure of fetal lung explant tissue to pharmacologic doses of GC markedly induces surfactant lipid and surfactant protein expression [31,32].

Cellular effects of glucocorticoids during lung development

GRα and GRß are expressed in relative abundance in both epithelial and nonepithelial cells of the fetal lung [25]. Although fetal lung growth and branching morphogenesis are not substantially altered by deletion of GRα or CRH, delayed sacculation and respiratory distress indicate its important role in pulmonary maturation before birth. This finding is consistent with the stimulatory effects of GCs on lung maturation in the preterm lung. Effects of GCs on lung maturation are likely associated with effects on both epithelial and mesenchymal cells of the lung. Stimulatory effects of GCs on surfactant lipid and protein synthesis have been observed in fetal lung explant culture and in vivo models of lung development in various species [31,32]. In isolated cells, stimulatory effects of GCs on lung maturation are dependent upon paracrine effects between epithelial cells and mesenchymal cells of the fetal lung. Stimulatory effects of GCs on surfactant lipid synthesis are mediated by the induction of cytidylytransferase, fatty acid synthase, and other enzymes mediating lipid synthesis. In isolated cells, the induction by GCs requires co-culture with lung fibroblasts, findings that led to a proposed "fibroblast pneumocyte factor," although the proposed "factor" has neither been isolated nor identified [33]. A number of polypeptides, for example FGF-7, are produced by the lung mesenchyme that can activate FGF receptors in the respiratory epithelium to enhance surfactant lipid and protein expression [34,35]. Although GR elements are found in the promoters of surfactant-related genes encoding SP-A, SP-D, and ABCA3 [36–38], it is unclear whether these genes are direct transcriptional or indirect targets of the glucocorticoids signaling in respiratory epithelial cells in vivo.

Glucocorticoids influence alveolar vasculogenesis and lung liquid clearance

The transition from intrauterine to extrauterine respiration requires the rapid removal of lung liquid at birth, a process also influenced by GCs. GREs and GC responsivity are observed in several genes critical for sodium transport across the respiratory epithelium, including the α-epithelial sodium channel subunit (αENaC) or α1 and β1 subunits of sodium-potassium adenosinetriphosphatases (ATPases) [39–41]. Deletion of αENaC, the apical amiloride-sensitive sodium channel in the respiratory epithelium, resulted in the failure to absorb lung liquid at birth [42]. Sodium-potassium ATPase, the basolateral sodium pump, is required for the generation of intracellular/extracellular sodium-potassium gradients. The finding that the promoters of both αENaC and sodium-potassium ATPase subunits contain GRE and are activated by GC in vitro supports the concept that GR mediates their expression in respiratory epithelial cells before birth. GCs influence lung formation during the saccular to alveolar phase of lung development. Prolonged or repetitive exposure to pharmacologic levels of GC in the prenatal or postnatal period inhibits somatic and lung growth, increasing the size of lung saccules, causing abnormal air space enlargement with features typical of emphysema [43,44]. Although GC therapy for the prevention of respiratory distress syndrome before birth was shown to be of therapeutic benefit, the potential for GC-related toxicity following multiple doses in the prenatal and postnatal period merits further study [45].

Mechanisms underlying the inhibiting effects of GCs on alveolarization are poorly understood; however, GC influences both vasculogenesis and angiogenesis in various organs, including the lung. Influence of GC on alveolar development is likely to be mediated in part by its role in the regulation of vascular endothelial growth factor (VEGF) expression [44,46,47]. Developmental and dose-dependent effects of GC on the regulation of polypeptides and receptors mediating pulmonary vasculogenesis may influence lung sacculation, growth, and alveolarization.

Clinical importance of glucocorticoids for prevention of lung disease in preterm infants

GC therapy for prevention and treatment of RDS and BPD has been extensively studied for more than 30 years. The therapeutic benefit of fetal GCs has been repeatedly documented in clinical studies. The National Institutes of Health Consensus Development Panel on the Effect of Corticosteroids for Fetal Maturation on Perinatal Outcomes strongly recommended the use of prenatal GC for women at high risk for preterm delivery, a practice now regarded as standard of care [14]. Because GCs have both beneficial and harmful effects on various organs, further refinement of the indications, dose, duration, and timing of GC for prevention and treatment of lung disease in the prenatal and postnatal period is indicated [48].

Transcriptional controls in the respiratory epithelium: thyroid transcription factor-1

TTF-1 is a 43 kDa phosphorylated transcription factor of the Nkx family of nuclear proteins that is expressed in the developing forebrain, thyroid, and lung [49]. Deletion of TTF-1 in the mouse results in central nervous system malformations and causes deficits in the formation of forebrain, thyroid gland, and lung [11]. Although TTF-1 is not required for formation of the trachea and bronchi, morphogenesis of the peripheral lung tubules is dependent upon TTF-1. The airway and lungs of TTF-1$^{-/-}$ mice consist of a tracheal-esophageal fistula, tracheal and bronchial tubes, and a peripheral lung consisting of saclike cysts, indicating the absence of peripheral lung tubules [11,50]. TTF-1 is expressed at high levels in the endodermally derived cells composing the respiratory epithelium from the onset of lung morphogenesis. TTF-1 is readily detected in the nucleus of subsets of respiratory epithelial cells, including those of the conducting airway and the peripheral lung throughout development, where it regulates the expression of genes controlling surfactant homeostasis and innate host defense [51]. TTF-1 binds to the promoters of a number of genes expressed selectively in the lung, including the surfactant proteins A, B, C, and D, and Scgb1a1 (CCSP [Clara cell secretory protein]). Genes encoding SP-B,SP-C, and ABCA3 play important roles in perinatal pulmonary adaptation [52]. TTF-1 interacts with numerous other transcription factors, forming direct partners with other transcription factors and other coactivators to influence target gene expression. Both the levels of TTF-1, selectivity for regulation of specific target genes, and its interactions with other transcription factors influence gene expression in respiratory epithelial cells, in both conducting airways and peripheral lung saccules/alveoli, during development and after birth.

TTF-1 regulates genes influencing perinatal lung adaptation and host defense

Deletion of TTF-1 in the mouse severely impaired the formation of the peripheral lung, thereby limiting the use of the TTF-1$^{-/-}$ mouse in the identification of TTF-1 target genes. Substitution of the mouse TTF-1 gene with a gene in which phosphorylation sites were mutated substantially rescued lung formation (compared with TTF-1$^{-/-}$ mice), but resulted in perinatal death related to respiratory insufficiency (Fig. 2) [12]. RNA microarray analysis of lungs from transgenic mice in which TTF-1 was replaced with a phosphorylation mutant (TTF-1^{PM}) was used to identify genes influenced by TTF-1 genes that are critical for perinatal lung adaptation. Expression of genes encoding proteins regulating surfactant homeostasis (surfactant proteins and lipids), fluid and electrolyte transport, alveolarization/vasculogenesis, and host defense (SP-A, SP-B, CCSP, lysozyme, and others) were decreased [12]. Binding sites for TTF-1 are present in promoter-enhancer regions of many of these genes [51], indicating that they are likely direct transcriptional targets of TTF-1 in vitro. Thus, TTF-1 plays distinct roles at various stages of development, being required for differentiation and proliferation of the primordial lung during the embryonic period, for maturation of the respiratory epithelium before birth, and for synthesis of pulmonary surfactant after birth. It is of clinical interest that mutations in TTF-1 cause CNS malformations, hypothyroidism, and pulmonary malformation/dysplasia in infants [53].

Forkhead family members FOXA1 and FOXA2

FOXA1 and FOXA2 are closely related members of a large, highly conserved family of forkhead/winged helix domain containing transcription factors that play important roles in many developmental processes in diverse organisms. FOXA2 is expressed in the foregut endoderm in the early

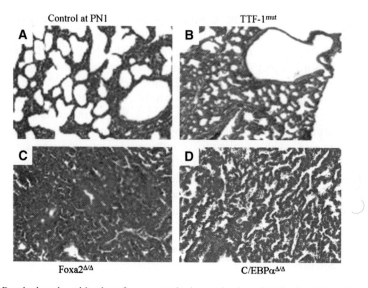

Fig. 2. Panels show lung histology from control mice on the day of birth (A), TTF-1 phosphorylation mutant mice (B), FOXA2$^{\Delta/\Delta}$ mice in which FOXA2 has been specifically deleted in respiratory epithelial cells of the developing lung (C), and C/EBPα$^{\Delta/\Delta}$ mice (D) in which C/EBPα has been conditionally deleted from respiratory epithelial cells. Mutant mice share defects in peripheral lung maturation and differentiation, resulting in respiratory distress following birth.

embryo, and is required for formation of anterior-posterior axis and specification of endoderm in the early mouse embryo [54]. During lung morphogenesis, both FOXA1 and FOXA2 are present in nuclei of the early lung buds. Later in development, nuclear staining for FOXA1 and FOXA2 is observed in respiratory epithelial cells of the conducting and peripheral respiratory tubules, where they are co-expressed with TTF-1 [55]. FOXA2 binds and activates a number of genes expressed selectively in the lung, including the gene encoding surfactant protein B, a protein required for surfactant function at birth [51,52,56]. Because deletion of FOXA2 causes death of the early embryo, FOXA2 was conditionally removed using a doxycycline inducible, lung-specific promoter system, to selectively delete FOXA2 [57] during pulmonary organogenesis. Although branching morphogenesis proceeded relatively normally, newborn mice in which the FOXA2 gene was deleted from peripheral respiratory epithelial cells developed atelectasis and respiratory distress, with the pathological and biochemical features associated with RDS in preterm infants (see Fig. 2) [57]. Differentiation of Type II alveolar cells was delayed and the alveoli remained immature in the absence of FOXA2. Surfactant proteins and lipids and the expression of SP-A, B, C, and ABCA3 were decreased, consistent with delayed pulmonary differentiation. RNA microarray analysis indicated that the deletion of FOXA2 resulted in the decreased expression of a number of genes that overlapped with those genes identified in the

TTF-1 phosphorylation mutant studies (Figs. 3, 4) [12,57]. These findings are consistent with the interacting or shared roles of TTF-1 and FOXA2 in maturation of the respiratory epithelium in late gestation. Expression of genes involved in surfactant synthesis, including ABCA3, SP-B, sterol Co-A desaturase, and SP-A are regulated by both TTF-1 and FOXA2. In contrast to the lethal effects of deletion of FOXA2 in the respiratory epithelium, mice in which FOXA1 was targeted survive at birth, but exhibit stage specific defects in perinatal lung maturation that do not cause respiratory distress [58].

Complementary roles of FOXA1 and FOXA2 during lung morphogenesis in the embryonic period

FOXA1 and FOXA2 are closely related FOXA family members that are expressed in an overlapping manner during lung morphogenesis and in the postnatal lung [58]. FOXA1 mRNA was increased after deletion of FOXA2 in respiratory epithelial cells, indicating a potentially compensatory role for FOXA1 in formation of the lung. To assess the role of FOXA activity during lung morphogenesis, mice were produced in which expression of both genes was absent in the lung [59]. Branching morphogenesis of the lung was arrested at an early stage of development, demonstrating that FOXA1 and FOXA2 play partially overlapping roles, and that FOXA activity is required for early lung formation. RNA analysis of embryonic lung tissue demonstrated a marked decrease in the expression of sonic

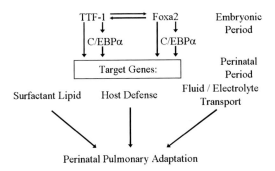

Fig. 3. Transcriptional control of perinatal maturation of the respiratory epithelium. FOXA2 is required for formation of the foregut endoderm in the developing mammalian embryo. TTF-1 is required for specification and differentiation of respiratory epithelial cells during early lung morphogenesis. Both TTF-1 and FOXA2 are required for regulation of C/EBPα expression in the respiratory epithelium. Mutation or targeted deletion of any of these factors results in respiratory failure at birth that is associated with the lack of expression of genes regulating surfactant lipid, host defense, fluid, and electrolyte transport. Many of the target genes share regulatory elements for TTF-1, FOXA2 and C/EBPα. Thus, these transcription factors regulate a shared group of target genes, and also regulate one another, functioning in a complex transcriptional network that controls perinatal lung adaptation.

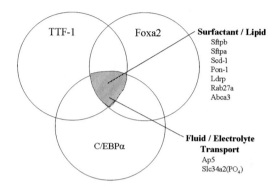

Fig. 4. TTF-1, FOXA2, and C/EBPα share regulatory targets in the respiratory epithelium of the developing lung. Represented are diagrams generated from microarray analysis of mice bearing TTF-1, FOXA2, and C/EBPα mutation/deletions, demonstrating the overlapping effects of these transcription factors on a subset of genes. Genes regulating surfactant lipid synthesis, fluid, and electrolyte transport are direct transcriptional targets of TTF-1, FOXA2, and C/EBPα. Target genes, including Sftpb (encodes SP-B) and Abca3, play critical roles in lung function at birth.

hedgehog (SHH) and a number of genes that participate in the SHH pathway required for smooth muscle differentiation after deletion of both FOXA1 and FOXA2. Because SHH is required for pulmonary smooth muscle development, the branching morphogenesis defects seen in the FOXA1/FOXA2 mutant mice are likely mediated by the absence of SHH production. Morphological and gene expression abnormalities observed after FOXA1 and FOXA2 deletion were similar to those seen after deletion of SHH in early lung morphogenesis [60]. Thus, FOXA controls SHH expression in the respiratory epithelium that is required for paracrine signaling, regulating smooth muscle differentiation necessary for branching morphogenesis of the peripheral lung [59].

Role of C/EBPα in lung maturation

C/EBPα is a member of the bZiP domain-containing transcription factor family that is expressed in epithelial cells of the developing lung [61]. C/EBPα regulates gene expression in numerous tissues, including adipocytes and hepatocytes, where it plays an important role in energy and substrate use, and the regulation of genes involved in lipid synthesis. C/EBPα$^{-/-}$ mice die early in the perinatal period, a finding initially thought to be linked to hypoglycemia; however, pulmonary abnormalities were also observed after deletion of C/EBPα [62,63]. Selected deletion of C/EBPα in epithelial cells of the fetal lung did not result in hypoglycemia, but caused respiratory failure following birth, with findings similar to those observed in TTF-1 mutant and FOXA2 deleted mice [64,65]. Morphologic maturation of the lung was markedly delayed, surfactant lipid and protein synthesis was decreased, and the expression of a group of mRNAs was decreased after deletion of C/EBPα (see Fig. 2). Many of the genes regulated by C/EBPα were also decreased in the TTF-1^{PM} and FOXA2$^{\Delta/\Delta}$ mice (see Fig. 4). These findings indicated that C/EBPα participates in a transcriptional network with TTF-1 and FOXA2. Deletion of either of TTF-1 or FOXA2 resulted in the absence of C/EBPα expression in the early respiratory epithelium [64]. C/EBPα directly binds to and regulates a number of genes critical for perinatal lung maturation itself, and is also regulated by TTF-1 and FOXA2 (see Fig. 3). Taken together, transcription factors of three distinct families, TTF-1, FOXA2, and C/EBPα, interact directly or indirectly to regulate expression of shared transcriptional targets that are required for lung maturation and function at birth (see Fig. 4).

Functional importance of transcriptional targets of the TTF-1, FOXA2, and C/EBPα

Analysis of potential transcriptional targets regulated by TTF-1, FOXA2, and C/EBPα in the developing lung identified a cluster of genes that are critical for perinatal lung maturation and function, including other transcription factors, growth factors, and their receptors. The TTF-1, FOXA2, C/EBPα "network" regulates: (1) fluid and electrolyte transport, including the aquaporins, several solute carriers, and the endothelial sodium channel (ENaC); (2) lipid homeostasis; and (3) proteins required for surfactant lipid synthesis and packaging, including SP-A, SP-B, SP-C, SP-D, and ABCA3. Genes regulating vasculogenesis and alveolarization, critical for the morphogenetic and structural transition of the lung from the saccular to the alveolar stage, were also identified. Several of these target genes are known to cause respiratory failure or chronic lung disease in newborns and infants, including *SFTPB*, *SFTPC*, and *ABCA3*. Mutations in these genes cause hereditary respiratory diseases typified by full-term infants who develop respiratory failure with clinical features that are usually associated with surfactant deficiency in preterm infants [19,52]. This group of genes associated with perinatal lung maturation, and the transcription factors controlling their expression, have evolved to control the unique characteristics of lung organogenesis and function, including formation of gas exchange area, surfactant homeostasis, mucociliary clearance, fluid and electrolyte homeostasis, and innate host defenses. It will be of interest to discern whether genes in this cluster represent novel genes causing hereditary lung disease or are modifiers of lung disease after birth.

Summary

The process of perinatal lung maturation includes remarkable changes in lung tissue architecture, cell differentiation, and gene expression, upon which respiration at birth depends. At the transcriptional level, pulmonary maturation is controlled by the concerted actions of a group of transcription factors mediating gene expression in the lung. An interacting network of transcription factors that includes TTF-1, FOXA2, and C/EBPα is an important regulator of gene expression in the respiratory epithelium that, in turn, influence maturational events in cells throughout the lung. Likewise, glucocorticoids (via the GR) acting primarily in the pulmonary mesenchyme, influence maturational processes in the respiratory epithelium. Elucidation of the intersecting pathways that control perinatal lung function may provide opportunities to induce pulmonary maturation in preterm infants at risk for RDS before birth, and will help identify genes and processes important for various aspects of lung function.

References

[1] Burri PH. Structural aspects of prenatal and postnatal development and growth of the lung. In: McDonald JA, editor. Lung growth and development. New York: Marcel Dekker; 1997. p. 1–35.

[2] Cardoso WV. Molecular regulation of lung development. Annu Rev Physiol 2001;63: 471–94.

[3] Shannon JM, Hyatt BA. Epithelial-mesenchymal interactions in the developing lung. Annu Rev Physiol 2004;66:625–45.

[4] Hogan LM. Morphogenesis. Cell 1999;96:225–33.

[5] Spooner BS, Wessells NK. Mammalian lung development: interactions in primordium formation and bronchial morphogenesis. J Exp Zool 1970;175:445–54.

[6] Peters K, Werner S, Liao X, et al. Targeted expression of a dominant negative FGF receptor blocks branching morphogenesis and epithelial differentiation of the mouse lung. EMBO J 1994;13:3296–301.

[7] Min H, Danilenko DM, Scully SA, et al. *Fgf-10* is required for both limb and lung development and exhibits striking functional similarity to *Drosophila branchless*. Genes Dev 1998;12: 3156–61.

[8] Bellusci S, Grindley J, Emoto H, et al. Fibroblast growth factor 10 (FGF10) and branching morphogenesis in the embryonic mouse lung. Development 1997;124: 4867–78.

[9] De Moerlooze L, Spencer-Dene B, Revest J, et al. An important role for the IIIb isoform of fibroblast growth factor receptor 2 (FGFR2) in mesenchymal-epithelial signalling during mouse organogenesis. Development 2000;127:483–92.

[10] Weinstein M, Xu X, Ohyama K, et al. FGFR-3 and FGFR-4 function cooperatively to direct alveogenesis in the murine lung. Development 1998;125:3615–23.

[11] Kimura S, Hara Y, Pineau T, et al. The T/ebp null mouse: thyroid-specific enhancer-binding protein is essential for the organogenesis of the thyroid, lung, ventral forebrain, and pituitary. Genes Dev 1996;10:60–9.

[12] deFelice M, Silberschmidt D, DiLauro R, et al. TTF-1 phosphorylation is required for peripheral lung morphogenesis, perinatal survival, and tissue-specific gene expression. J Biol Chem 2003;278:35574–83.

[13] Liggins GC, Howie RN. A controlled trial of antepartum glucocorticoid treatment for prevention of the respiratory distress syndrome in premature infants. Pediatrics 1972;50: 515–25.

[14] Effect of corticosteroids for fetal maturation on perinatal outcomes. NIH Consensus Development Panel on the Effect of Corticosteroids for Fetal Maturation on Perinatal Outcomes. JAMA 1995;273:413–8.

[15] Sinclair JC. Meta-analysis of randomized controlled trials of antenatal corticosteroid for the prevention of respiratory distress syndrome: discussion. Am J Obstet Gynecol 1995;173: 335–44.

[16] Ten Have-Opbroek AA. The development of the lung in mammals: an analysis of concepts and findings. Am J Anat 1981;162:201–19.

[17] Rooney SA, Young SL, Mendelson CR. Molecular and cellular processing of lung surfactant. FASEB J 1994;8:957–67.

[18] Ballard PL. Hormonal regulation of pulmonary surfactant. Endocr Rev 1989;10:165–81.

[19] Whitsett JA, Weaver TE. Hydrophobic surfactant proteins in lung function and disease. N Engl J Med 2002;347:2141–8.

[20] Whitsett JA. Composition of pulmonary surfactant lipids and proteins. In: Polin RA, Fox WW, S Abman S, editors. Fetal & neonatal physiology. 3rd edition. Philadelphia: WB Saunders Co.; 2004. p. 1005–13.

[21] McCormack FX, Whitsett JA. The pulmonary collectins, SP-A and SP-D, orchestrate innate immunity in the lung. J Clin Invest 2002;109:707–12.

[22] Bolt RJ, van Weissenbruch MM, Lafeber HN, et al. Glucocorticoids and lung development in the fetus and preterm infant. Pediatr Pulmonol 2001;32:76–91.

[23] Francke U, Foellmer BE. The glucocorticoid receptor gene is in 5q31-q32. Genomics 1989;4: 610–2.

[24] Hollenberg SM, Weinberger C, Ong ES, et al. Primary structure and expression of a functional human glucocorticoid receptor cDNA. Nature 1985;318:635–41.

[25] Oakley RH, Sar M, Cidlowski JA. The human glucocorticoid receptor beta isoform. Expression, biochemical properties, and putative function. J Biol Chem 1996;271: 9550–9.

[26] Sanchez ER, Toft DO, Schlesinger MJ, et al. Evidence that the 90-kDa phosphoprotein associated with the untransformed L-cell glucocorticoid receptor is a murine heat shock protein. J Biol Chem 1985;260:12398–401.

[27] Beato M, Arnemann J, Chalepakis G, et al. Gene regulation by steroid hormones. J Steroid Biochem 1987;27:9–14.

[28] Cole TJ, Blendy JA, Monaghan AP, et al. Targeted disruption of the glucocorticoid receptor gene blocks adrenergic chromaffin cell development and severely retards lung maturation. Genes Dev 1995;9:1608–21.

[29] Berger S, Cole TJ, Schmid W, et al. Analysis of glucocorticoid and mineralocorticoid signalling by gene targeting. Endocr Res 1995;22:641–52.

[30] Muglia L, Jacobson L, Dikkes P, et al. Corticotropin-releasing hormone deficiency reveals major fetal but not adult glucocorticoid need. Nature 1995;373:427–32.

[31] Gross I, Ballard PL, Ballard RA, et al. Corticosteroid stimulation of phosphatidylcholine synthesis in cultured fetal rabbit lung: evidence for de novo protein synthesis mediated by glucocorticoid receptors. Endocrinology 1983;112:829–37.

[32] Whitsett JA, Weaver TE, Clark JC, et al. Glucocorticoid enhances surfactant proteolipid Phe and pVal synthesis and RNA in fetal lung. J Biol Chem 1987;262:15618–23.

[33] Smith BT. Lung maturation in the fetal rat: acceleration by injection of fibroblast-pneumonocyte factor. Science 1979;204:1094–5.

[34] Tichelaar JW, Lu W, Whitsett JA. Conditional expression of fibroblast growth factor-7 in the developing and mature lung. J Biol Chem 2000;275:11858–64.

[35] Yano T, Mason RJ, Pan T, et al. KGF regulates pulmonary epithelial proliferation and surfactant protein gene expression in adult rat lung. Am J Physiol 2000;279: L1146–58.

[36] Chen Q, Boggaram V, Mendelson CR. Rabbit lung surfactant protein A gene: identification of a lung-specific DNase I hypersensitive site. Am J Physiol 1992;262:L662–71.

[37] Rust K, Bingle L, Mariencheck W, et al. Characterization of the human surfactant protein D promoter: transcriptional regulation of SP-D gene expression by glucocorticoids. Am J Respir Cell Mol Biol 1992;14:121–30.

[38] Yoshida I, Ban N, Inagaki N. Expression of ABCA3, a causative gene for fatal surfactant deficiency, is up-regulated by glucocorticoids in lung alveolar type II cells. Biochem Biophys Res Commun 2004;323:547–55.

[39] Champigny G, Voilley N, Lingueglia E, et al. Regulation of expression of the lung amiloride-sensitive Na + channel by steroid hormones. EMBO J 1994;13:2177–81.

[40] Tchepichev S, Ueda J, Canessa C, et al. Lung epithelial Na channel subunits are differentially regulated during development and by steroids. Am J Physiol 1995;269:C805–12.

[41] Barquin N, Ciccolella DE, Ridge KM, et al. Dexamethasone upregulates the Na-K-ATPase in rat alveolar epithelial cells. Am J Physiol 1997;273:L825–30.

[42] Hummler E, Barker P, Gatzy J, et al. Early death due to defective neonatal lung liquid clearance in alpha-ENaC-deficient mice. Nat Genet 1996;12:325–8.

[43] Luyet C, Burri PH, Schittny JC. Suppression of cell proliferation and programmed cell death by dexamethasone during postnatal lung development. Am J Physiol 2002;282: L477–83.

[44] Clerch LB, Baras AS, Massaro GD, et al. DNA microarray analysis of neonatal mouse lung connects regulation of KDR with dexamethasone-induced inhibition of alveolar formation. Am J Physiol 2004;286:L411–9.

[45] Jobe AH, Newnham J, Willet K, et al. Fetal versus maternal and gestational age effects of repetitive antenatal glucocorticoids. Pediatrics 1998;102:1116–25.

[46] Folkman J, Langer R, Linhardt RJ, et al. Angiogenesis inhibition and tumor regression caused by heparin or a heparin fragment in the presence of cortisone. Science 1983;221: 719–25.

[47] Nauck M, Karakiulakis G, Perruchoud AP, et al. Corticosteroids inhibit the expression of the vascular endothelial growth factor gene in human vascular smooth muscle cells. Eur J Pharmacol 1998;341:309–15.

[48] Jobe AH, Soll RF. Choice and dose of corticosteroid for antenatal treatments. Am J Obstet Gynecol 2004;190:878–81.

[49] Lazzaro D, Price M, de Felice M, et al. The transcription factor TTF-1 is expressed at the onset of thyroid and lung morphogenesis and in restricted regions of the foetal brain. Development 1991;113:1093–104.

[50] Minoo P, Su G, Drum H, et al. Defects in tracheoesophageal and lung morphogenesis in Nkx2.1 (−/−) mouse embryos. Dev Biol 1999;209:60–71.

[51] Bohinski RJ, DiLauro R, Whitsett JA. Lung-specific surfactant protein B gene promoter is a target for thyroid transcription factor 1 and hepatocyte nuclear factor 3 indicating common factors for organ-specific gene expression along the foregut axis. Mol Cell Biol 1994;14: 5671–81.

[52] Whitsett JA, Wert SE, Trapnell BC. Genetic disorders influencing lung formation and function at birth. Hum Mol Genet 2004;13:R207–15.

[53] Devriendt K, Vanhole C, Matthijs G, et al. Deletion of thyroid transcription factor-1 gene in an infant with neonatal thyroid dysfunction and respiratory failure. N Engl J Med 1998;338: 1317–8.

[54] Ang SL, Wierda A, Wong D, et al. The formation and maintenance of the definitive endoderm lineage in the mouse: involvement of HNF3/forkhead proteins. Development 1993; 119:1301–15.

[55] Zhou L, Lim L, Costa RH, et al. Thyroid transcription factor-1, hepatocyte nuclear factor-3β, surfactant protein B, C, and Clara cell secretory protein in developing mouse lung. J Histochem Cytochem 1996;44:1183–93.

[56] Clark JC, Wert SE, Bachurski CJ, et al. Targeted disruption of the surfactant protein B gene disrupts surfactant homeostasis, causing respiratory failure in newborn mice. Proc Natl Acad Sci U S A 1995;92:7794–8.

[57] Wan H, Xu Y, Ikegami M, et al. Foxa2 is required for transition to air breathing at birth. Proc Natl Acad Sci U S A 2004;101:14449–54.

[58] Besnard V, Wert SE, Kaestner KH, et al. Stage specific regulation of respiratory epithelial cell differentiation by Foxa1. Am J Physiol 2005;289:L750–9.

[59] Wan H, Dingle S, Xu Y, et al. Compensatory roles of Foxa1 and Foxa2 during lung morphogenesis. J Biol Chem 2005;280:13809–16.

[60] Pepicelli CV, Lewis PM, McMahon AP. Sonic hedgehog regulates branching morphogenesis in the mammalian lung. Curr Biol 1998;8:1083–6.

[61] Cassel TN, Nord M. C/EBP transcription factors in the lung epithelium. Am J Physiol 2003; 285:L773–81.

[62] Flodby P, Barlow C, Kylefjord H, et al. Increased hepatic cell proliferation and lung abnormalities in mice deficient in CCAAT/enhancer binding protein α. J Biol Chem 1996;271: 24753–60.

[63] Wang ND, Finegold MJ, Bradley A, et al. Impaired energy homeostasis in C/EBP alpha knockout mice. Science 1995;269:1108–12.

[64] Martis PC, Whitsett JA, Xu Y, et al. C/EBPα is required for lung maturation at birth. Development 2006;133:1155–64.

[65] Bassères DS, Levantini E, Ji H, et al. Respiratory failure due to differentiation arrest and expansion of alveolar cells following lung-specific loss of the transcription factor C/EBP in mice. Mol Cell Biol 2006;26:1109–23.

ELSEVIER
SAUNDERS

Pediatr Clin N Am
53 (2006) 889–909

PEDIATRIC CLINICS
OF NORTH AMERICA

Renal Cystic Disease: New Insights for the Clinician

Ellis D. Avner, MD[a,b,*], William E. Sweeney, Jr[a,b]

[a]*Children's Research Institute, Children's Hospital & Health System of Wisconsin,
999 North 92nd Street, Suite 730, Milwaukee 53226, USA*
[b]*Medical College of Wisconsin, Department of Pediatrics, Division of Pediatrics,
8701 Watertown Plank Road, Milwaukee 53225, USA*

Until recently, inherited renal diseases such as renal cystic disease (RCD) were characterized solely by a description of disease symptoms and the natural progression of the disease. One of the greatest recent advances in medicine has been the emergence of genomic techniques that facilitate the rapid identification of disease-causing genes. Modern molecular genetics has allowed what was once a descriptive clinical phenotype to now be classified as a unique disease entity, confirmed at the molecular level. Molecular genetics, through the identification and cloning of disease-causing genes, has enhanced our understanding of the pathophysiology of many diseases. Molecular techniques have allowed the generation or identification of animal models with mutations in the same gene affected in a human disease (an orthologous model), so that the pathophysiology can be studied at the cellular level. The molecular characterization of diseases has revolutionized our understanding of disease processes, and in many cases can direct clinical treatment. The cloning of defective genes can permit the prenatal diagnosis of many diseases and establish a definitive diagnosis to guide disease-specific, directed therapeutic intervention. Genetic diagnosis provides confidence for clinicians that they are treating a defined disease, particularly in the setting in which two or more diseases may have similar clinical presentations.

This article cannot comprehensively cover the enormous strides made in defining the molecular and cellular basis of RCDs over the last decade.

Supported by 1-P50-DK57306 from the National Institutes of Health; the PKD Foundation, Grant # 76a2r; Medical College of Wisconsin: Advancing A Healthier WI; and Children's Research Institute, Children's Hospital of Wisconsin.

* Corresponding author. Children's Corporate Center, Suite C-730, 999 North 92nd Street, Wauwatosa, WI 53226.

E-mail address: eavner@mcw.edu (E.D. Avner).

doi:10.1016/j.pcl.2006.08.012

Therefore, it includes a brief overview and categorization of inherited, developmental, and acquired RCDs, providing a relevant, up-to-date bibliography as well as a useful list of informative Internet Web sites. It's major focus is "translational." It also demonstrates how emerging molecular and cellular knowledge of the pathophysiology of particular diseases such as autosomal dominant polycystic kidney disease (ADPKD) and autosomal recessive polycystic kidney disease (ARPKD) can translate into innovative therapeutic insights.

RCD encompasses a broad spectrum of hereditary, nonhereditary, and acquired conditions that cause significant morbidity and mortality. A renal cyst is an abnormal fluid-filled, epithelial-lined, dilated sac that arises within the renal parenchyma from an existing tubule or collecting duct. A cystic kidney is arbitrarily defined as a kidney with three or more cysts [1].

RCD can be acquired or inherited, and when associated with extra-renal manifestations, often occurs as part of a well-defined syndrome. Autosomal dominant forms of RCD, such as ADPKD, are generally characterized by development of end-stage renal disease (ESRD) in adulthood. Autosomal recessive forms of RCD, such as nephronophthisis (NPHP) and ARPKD, generally produce ESRD in childhood or adolescence. When RCD appears as part of complex clinical syndromes, disease manifestations are usually dictated by the other involved organ systems.

In 1964, Osathanondh and Potter [2] developed a classification system based on microdissection of cystic kidneys and hypothesized that cyst formation was mechanistically related to specific segments of affected nephrons. Inclusion of clinically diverse cystic conditions/diseases within the same "anatomical" category limited the clinical usefulness of such classifications, however. Improvements in genetic and pathologic classifications over the years have provided more precise clinicopathologic correlations. The interested reader is referred to recent comprehensive overviews [3–6], and useful online resources, listed in Appendix 1.

Despite the large number of identified "cystic" genes, the differential diagnosis of the infant or child with enlarged cystic kidneys is readily limited to four diseases following initial clinical and laboratory evaluation: ARPKD, ADPKD, glomerulocystic kidney disease (GCKD), and tuberous sclerosis complex (TSC). After a brief description of the latter two entities, the remainder of this article focuses on the renal polycystic kidney diseases, ARPKD and ADPKD. These serve as excellent examples of how twenty-first century molecular and cellular pathophysiology has led to exciting and innovative disease-specific therapies.

Glomerulocystic kidney disease

Glomerular cysts may be an early manifestation of ADPKD, or can occur in multiple syndromes. Isolated GCKD also occurs as a defined genetic entity, and hypoplastic GCKD, an autosomal dominant disease, appears to be a clinically distinct subgroup.

GCKD cysts are characterized by dilated Bowman's spaces, lined with cuboidal or columnar cells containing primitive or immature glomeruli scattered within normal cortical parenchyma. Ultrasonographically, minute cysts are seen in an echogenic renal cortex. No cysts are observed in the renal medulla. The lack of tubular involvement distinguishes GCKD from other renal cyst diseases that generally involve tubular dilatation.

Most GCKD patients suffer some degree of renal failure and many present with hypertension. The typical presentation is that of an infant with abdominal masses and varying degrees of renal insufficiency. Sonography reveals enlarged kidneys with an echogenic cortex [7]. GCKD can present in adulthood with flank pain, hematuria, and hypertension [7]. Hepatic cysts have also been reported in patients with GCKD [8].

Although usually bilateral, asymmetric manifestations of this condition have been reported [8]. Most GCKD cases are transmitted in an autosomal dominant fashion, but the responsible gene has yet to be mapped to a specific locus.

GCKD is usually discovered in infants within the context of a familial history of ADPKD. Although a higher incidence of GCKD has been noted among patients with ADPKD, GCKD is not linked to *PKD1* or *PKD2* loci. Information regarding the molecular basis of ADPKD and reported familial associations of GCKD, TS, and ADPKD raises the possibility that autosomal dominant GCKD, TS, and ADPKD are genetically linked in some kindreds [7].

Patients with familial hypoplastic GCKD present with small kidneys, abnormal collecting systems, and abnormal or completely absent papillae [9]. Family pedigree studies demonstrate an autosomal dominant inheritance pattern [9].

In summary, GCKD is a heterogeneous collection of clinical entities with variable clinical courses. Prognosis often is dependent on associated disorders [7].

Tuberous sclerosis complex

TSC (OMIM 191100) is an autosomal dominantly inherited systemic malformation syndrome, linked to *TSC1* and *TSC2*-suppressor genes, mapped on chromosome 9q and chromosome 16p, respectively, with the former encoding hamartin [10] and the latter, which accounts for the two thirds of mutations, encoding tuberin [11]. TSC causes tumors to form in many different organs, primarily in the brain, eyes, heart, kidney, skin, and lungs.

TSC involves abnormalities of the skin (hypomelanotic macules, facial angiofibromas, shagreen patches, fibrous facial plaques, ungual fibromas), brain (cortical tubers, subependymal nodules, seizures, mental retardation/developmental delay), kidney (angiomyolipomas, cysts), and heart (rhabdomyomas, arrhythmias). Central nervous system (CNS) tumors are the leading cause of morbidity and mortality, and renal disease is the second leading cause of early death.

The diagnosis of TSC is based on clinical findings that have recently been refined [12]. Two causative genes, *TSC1* and *TSC2*, have been identified, and molecular testing for both genetic subtypes is available on a clinical basis (www.genetests.org). Prenatal testing is available if the disease-causing allele has been identified in an affected family member (www.genetests.org).

Renal manifestations such as cysts and angiomyolipomas occur in 40% to 80% of TSC patients. TSC renal cysts occur bilaterally. They are the second most frequently occurring renal manifestation of TSC. The cystic kidney in TSC usually presents with numerous medullary and cortical cysts, imparting a spongelike appearance to the kidneys. Sometimes the classic cystic kidney pattern of TSC may appear in association with the GCKD pattern.

Modern molecular genetics led to the discovery that the *TSC2* gene was located in close proximity to the disease gene for ADPKD-1 (*PKD1*) on chromosome 16 (see below). This led to the recognition that individuals with large deletions in segments of chromosome 16 may have mutations in both *TSC2* and *PKD1* genes. These individuals most often will have polycystic kidneys from birth, and will require close monitoring and treatment throughout the childhood years.

Individuals with TSC and ADPKD will generally be hypertensive. Hypertensive control, especially early in the disease process, is important. Dialysis, and sometimes even renal transplantation, may eventually be necessary. Renal transplantation has successfully been performed in individuals with TSC, and recurrence of angiomyolipomas in transplanted kidneys does not appear to occur [13].

Polycystic kidney disease: autosomal dominant polycystic kidney disease and autosomal recessive polycystic kidney disease

Current convention restricts the use of the term polycystic kidney disease (PKD) to two genetically distinct conditions: ADPKD, previously known as adult polycystic kidney disease, and ARPKD, previously referred to as infantile polycystic kidney disease.

PKD is one of the most common human genetic disorders, and is a major cause of ESRD in children and adults [14]. ADPKD (OMIM 173900; 173910) occurs in 1:1000 individuals and is caused by mutations in one of two genes, *PKD1* or *PKD2* [14]. ARPKD (OMIM 263200) is less frequent (1:20,000 live births) and occurs as a result of mutations in a single gene, polycystic kidney and hepatic disease 1 (*PKHD1*) [15–17].

Clinical spectrum and pathology of autosomal dominant polycystic kidney disease

ADPKD is generally a late-onset, multisystem disorder characterized by bilateral renal cysts with sporadic presentation of cystic lesions in seminal vesicles, pancreas, and liver. Other extra-renal presentations may include vascular abnormalities, including intracranial aneurysms, dilatation of the aortic root, dissection of the thoracic aorta, and mitral valve prolapse; and abdominal wall hernias [18].

The renal manifestations of ADPKD include renal function abnormalities, hypertension, renal pain, and renal insufficiency. The mean age of ESRD in PKD1 patients is 57 years, and it is 69 years in PKD2 patients [19]. Polycystic liver disease is the most common extra-renal manifestation of ADPKD. The prevalence of liver cysts in individuals with ADPKD increases from 20% in the third decade to approximately 75% after the sixth decade [19]. Intracranial aneurysms occur in approximately 10% of individuals with ADPKD. The prevalence is higher in those with a positive family history of aneurysms or subarachnoid hemorrhage (22%) than in those with a negative history (6%) [20]. Mitral valve prolapse is the most common valvular abnormality, and has been demonstrated in up to 25% of affected individuals. Substantial variability in the severity of renal disease and other extra-renal manifestations occurs within the same family, implying a major role for modifying genes and environmental factors. The site of the mutation in either gene (germline and somatic) is also known to affect the phenotype. Thus ADPKD disease shows both locus and allelic heterogeneity [19].

The *PKD1* gene mutated in the majority of ADPKD cases encodes the 450,000 to 460,000 MW (molecular weight, in kilodaltons) transmembrane protein polycystin-1 [21]. Polycystin-1 is predicted to be a membrane receptor, with a large extracellular domain mediating cell-cell and cell-extracellular matrix binding, and a multifunctional carboxy-terminal region capable of binding and interacting with many proteins and eliciting intracellular responses [22]. The *PKD2* gene product, polycystin-2, is thought to act as a calcium-permeable channel and play an integral role in polycystin-1 localization and function [23]. ADPKD is usually asymptomatic until the middle decades; however, 2% to 5% of ADPKD patients present with a severe neonatal course, with consequent significant morbidity and mortality.

Although ADPKD is usually a disease of adults, about 2% to 5% of patients manifest an early clinical course and may die perinatally. Such early manifestations of ADPKD may be identical to ARPKD, and can be differentiated only by histological or genetic analysis. The absence of a family history in such cases maybe misleading, because 5% to 8% of all ADPKD cases appear to represent new mutations [24,25].

Clinical spectrum and pathology of autosomal recessive polycystic kidney disease

ARPKD is a significant cause of renal and liver-related morbidity and mortality in childhood. Estimates of disease prevalence vary widely, but an overall frequency of 1 in 20,000 live births and a carrier level up to 1:70 have been recently proposed [26].

The majority of ARPKD patients present clinically as newborn or young children. Despite dramatic improvements in neonatal and intensive care over the past decade, neonatal mortality remains as high as 25% to 35%. The clinical spectrum of surviving patients is considerably more variable. Principal manifestations of the disease involve the fusiform dilation of renal collecting tubules or ducts (CT) and dysgenesis of the hepatic portal triad caused by a primary ductal plate abnormality.

ARPKD is a renal and hepatic developmental disorder caused by mutations in the PKHD1 gene located on chromosome 6p21.1-p12 [16,17]. PKHD1 is a large gene, with a minimum of 86 exons that are assembled into a variety of alternatively spliced transcripts that may be organ-specific, or temporally and spatially regulated.

ARPKD was first recognized as a distinct morphologic form of cystic disease in 1902, although its histologic characteristics were not well-described until later. In a landmark study, Blyth and Ockenden [27] classified ARPKD into four distinct phenotypes: perinatal, neonatal, infantile, and juvenile, on the basis of clinical manifestations and the age at presentation.

Before the identification of PKHD1, these phenotypes were thought to be distinct disease entities caused by different mutant genes. Though clinically useful as a guide, the Blyth and Ockenden classification has many exceptions because phenotypic variations extend across the four groups, even in isolated families with the same disease mutation.

ARPKD belongs to a group of congenital hepatorenal fibrocystic syndromes characterized by dual renal and hepatic involvement of varying severity. Renal manifestations include both ectasia and cystic dilatation of renal CT. The fusiform dilated CT are lined by undifferentiated epithelium and enclosed with thick layers of connective tissue. Unlike ADPKD cysts, ARPKD cysts retain both their afferent and efferent tubular connections [28,29]. The kidney appears spongy, and there is no clear division between the cortex and medulla.

A wide variability of phenotype and degree of renal dysfunction occurs, depending on the number of affected CT involved.

Liver disease is invariably present in all ARPKD patients. The manifestations generally vary according to the patient's age at presentation [7]. The chief pathologic hallmarks of ARPKD liver disease are hepatic lesions of biliary dysgenesis caused by a primary ductal plate malformation with associated periportal fibrosis, resulting in congenital hepatic fibrosis (CHF) and dilatation of intrahepatic bile ducts (Caroli's disease). Liver manifestations can be the major disease complication in older patients [18,27,30–32]. In these patients, particularly in those following treatment of ESRD with dialysis or transplantation, complications of CHF and Caroli's disease can result in portal hypertension (requiring a portocaval shunt) with consequent gastroesophageal varices, hypersplenism, and recurrent attacks of bacterial ascending cholangitis [33,34]. Generally, there is a reciprocal relationship between the degree of renal and hepatic involvement in individual patients. Those with more severe renal involvement often have less severe hepatic disease [27] although this varies [35].

Despite medical advances in neonatal care, the short-term and long-term morbidity and mortality of ARPKD remain substantial. Notwithstanding the variable clinical spectrum of ARPKD [35], the majority of patients are identified either in utero or at birth [7,34]. The most severely affected fetuses have enlarged echogenic kidneys and oligohydramnios caused by poor fetal urine output. These signs are potentially detectable in utero, but may not appear until late in the third trimester [26]. Improved neonatal intensive care and disease recognition have increased survival of the newborns, but death still occurs in the neonatal period in approximately 25% to 30% of affected individuals, primarily caused by respiratory insufficiency [33,36,37]. ARPKD patients surviving the neonatal period have a more optimistic prognosis [33].

Approximately 50% of affected individuals surviving the neonatal period progress to ESRD within the first decade of life [33,38]. Modern neonatal respiratory support and renal replacement therapies have improved the 10-year survival of patients who survive the first year to 82% [32]. For infants who survive the perinatal period, a wide range of associated morbidities can develop, including systemic hypertension, renal failure, portal hypertension, and renal and hepatic fibrosis [7,39,40]. The 15-year survival for infants who survive the perinatal period, is estimated to be 67% to 79% [32].

A minority of individuals present as older children, usually with hepatosplenomegaly as the presenting feature. Later childhood presentation is usually associated with less renal enlargement and more variability in cyst size [27]. As described above, these patients are more likely to develop complications of CHF and Caroli's disease, and may require porto-systemic shunting. In rare cases sequential or simultaneous liver-kidney transplants can be considered a viable therapeutic option [40]. The clinical spectrum of ARPKD has been expanded by a recent study using molecular characterization [35]. Almost one third of the patients presenting with classical hepatic phenotype and documented mutations in the *PKHD1* gene were over 20 years old at the time of diagnosis.

Hypertension may occur in up to 80% of children with ARPKD, is frequently severe, and may be correlated with decreased renal function. The mechanisms of hypertension are unknown, although increased intravascular volume secondary to dysregulation of renal sodium transport or activation of the renin-angiotension axis have been implicated [37].

Angiotension-converting enzyme inhibitors or angiotensin II (ATII) receptor inhibitors are particularly effective therapies [34,37,41]. Additional clinical complications include nephrogenic diabetes insipidus, failure to thrive, and hyponatremia [7,34,42].

Despite the variable clinical spectrum of ARPKD, genetic linkage studies indicate that mutations at a single locus, PKHD1, mapped to human chromosome region 6p21.1-p12, are responsible for all phenotypes of ARPKD, including seemingly isolated CHF [15,26].

Characterization of the polycystic kidney disease mutational spectrum

Molecular genetic testing for both ADPKD (PKD1 and PKD2) and ARPKD (PKHD1) are currently available (www.genetests.org). Molecular genetic testing in ADPKD is rarely used to confirm or establish the diagnosis. The diagnosis of ADPKD is primarily established by clinical evaluation and renal imaging studies. Molecular testing is primarily used when presymptomatic diagnosis is required.

In ARPKD, newly developed methodologies have yielded detection rates of 85% for the entire clinical spectrum of ARPKD patients [24,25,43,44]. Denaturing high performance liquid chromatography (DHPLC) and polymerase chain reaction (PCR)-based strategies have been successfully used for mutation screening. In general, sequence analysis, combined with haplotype analysis in multiply affected families, has proven to provide the most reliable and comprehensive results [18,45].

Molecular genetic studies in both ADPKD and ARPKD demonstrated that mutations are scattered throughout the genes without evidence of clustering at specific sites, and that neutral polymorphisms are common. Most mutations were unique to single families ("private mutations"), and most affected patients represent compound heterozygotes.

An ARPKD database that catalogs published mutations in the PKHD1 gene can be found at http://www.humgen.rwth-aachen.de. As of August 1, 2006, 296 different PKHD1 micromutations (point mutations and small deletions/duplications/insertions) on 670 mutated alleles are listed in the locus-specific database.

Molecular diagnosis and prenatal diagnosis

An anticipated benefit from genomic analysis is the ability to understand the molecular basis of clinical variations in disease presentation, progression, and outcome. Genotype-phenotype correlations should enhance understanding of the molecular pathogenesis of the disease and provide improved patient care by predicting disease progression; however, the combination of the large size of PKD1 and PKHD1, allelic heterogeneity, high level of missense mutations, and the complicated pattern of splicing pose significant challenges to DNA-based diagnostic testing for both ADPKD and ARPKD.

Autosomal dominant polycystic kidney disease

Molecular genetic testing for ADPKD can be used for presymptomatic diagnosis when imaging results are equivocal or when a definite diagnosis is required in a younger individual, such as a potential living related kidney donor.

Molecular testing for prenatal diagnosis or preimplantation diagnosis is generally not feasible for ADPKD because the disease is usually diagnosed in adults beyond their childbearing years. A possible exception is rare families in which severe, early onset disease in one child suggests a significant risk of recurrence of severe disease in a sibling. As noted, diagnosis of ADPKD is established primarily by clinical evaluation and renal imaging studies; however, molecular genetic testing can be used to confirm or establish the diagnosis when necessary [14].

Autosomal recessive polycystic kidney disease

Although the improved methodologies provide high detection rates, the ability to definitively assess the likelihood of micromutations being pathogenic is still lacking. To predict whether a variant is likely to be disease-causing, several factors are taken into account: evolutionary conservation of the amino acids, class of amino acid, no other mutations in "cis," cosegregation with the disease, or published previously pathogenic variant. Obviously, the correct classification of missense variants as pathogenic mutations or harmless polymorphisms is crucial for a correct diagnosis.

The bulk of mutational data currently available permit broad categorization of missense mutations into severe, moderate, or mild changes. Therefore, genotype-phenotype correlations can be drawn for the type of mutation rather than for the site of individual mutations. All patients carrying two truncating mutations have displayed a severe phenotype with peri- or neonatal demise [46], whereas patients surviving the neonatal period have had, on average, at least one missense mutation [47]. This indicates that some missense changes may not entirely inactivate the gene, but generate a hypomorphic allele. Additionally, some missense mutations may only disrupt specific splice forms of PKHD1 without affecting other functional variants [45].

In addition, the roles of the various splice forms in determining disease severity have yet to be determined. A potential biological function of the alterations identified in alternatively spliced exons must await the confirmation and definition of transcripts containing these alternative spliced exons and their predicted reading frames. Continued cataloging of mutations, especially pathogenic missense variants and the resulting disease phenotypes, are required to fully define genotype-phenotype correlations.

Because of the significant morbidity and mortality of ARPKD, many parents of ARPKD children seek prenatal diagnosis to guide future family planning. Before the identification of the *PKHD1* gene, prenatal diagnosis was only feasible by indirect genotyping (haplotype based analysis); however, interpretation of haplotype based analysis is difficult in cases without an unambiguous clinicopathologic diagnosis. If parental renal, hepatic, or pancreatic ultrasound reveals cyst formation, severe, early-onset ADPKD must be considered. Thus, in families with diagnostic uncertainties, characterization of *PKHD1* mutations by direct sequencing is the only option for accurate genetic counseling and prenatal diagnosis. Prenatal diagnoses of ARPKD based on *PKHD1* mutation analysis has been successfully accomplished [48], and clinical gene-based testing as well as preimplantation genetic diagnosis will become more accessible as the number of diagnostic centers increase.

Cellular pathophysiology of polycystic kidney disease

Despite the identification of the genes responsible for ADPKD and ARPKD, the precise function of these genes and their protein products remains incompletely characterized. This is because of the novel attributes of the genes, including the complexity of their structure, the large size of *PKD1* and *PKHD1,* the multiple transcripts produced by these genes, and the multiple sites of protein distribution. Despite these difficulties, the development of antibodies to the PKD proteins and the study of nonorthologous animal models of RCD have provided important novel insights suggesting common cystogenic pathways and cellular pathophysiology in many cystic diseases [23,49–56].

Observations initially made in animal models of RCD—that protein products (cystoproteins) of RCD genes such as polaris (*Tg737*), cystin (*cpk*) and inversin (*Nphp2*) were localized to common cellular sites, including the primary cilia of renal epithelia—were quite intriguing [53]. The unexpected association of the primary cilium with several inherited cystic kidney diseases led to the "primary cilia" hypothesis [53]. Simply stated, the hypothesis is that structural or functional abnormalities in the primary apical cilia of tubular epithelia play a role in renal cyst development and may represent a unifying mechanism of cyst formation [57]. Additional cystoproteins responsible for non-PKD forms of human RCD such as NPHP (nephrocystin-1, 2, 4, and 5) and Bardet-Biedl syndrome (BBS 1–10) are also partially expressed in the basal bodies or the primary cilia [3]. The ADPKD proteins, polycystin-1(PC-1), polycystin-2 (PC-2), and the ARPKD protein, fibrocystin, are also expressed in cilia in addition to other locations within the cell. These findings indicate a striking association between proteins involved in RCD (cystoproteins) and cilia [58].

The pathogenic link between cystoprotein expression in cilia, basal bodies, and centrosomes, on the one hand, and the renal cystic phenotype, on the other hand, remain unknown. Recent studies, however, have demonstrated that physical manipulation of the primary cilium, including bending or removal, elicits changes in Ca^{2+} flux [52,59–62]. It is of interest to note that the only binding partner for fibrocystin identified to date is calcium modulating cyclophilin ligand (CAML), a protein involved in Ca^{2+} signaling [63].

Cystic epithelia share common phenotypic abnormalities in spite of the different genetic mutations that underlie the diseases. Cyst development and progressive enlargement requires epithelial cell proliferation, transepithelial fluid secretion, and extracellular matrix remodeling [64]. In vitro analysis of epithelia from both human and animal models of RCD has demonstrated that CT and biliary cystic epithelia have enhanced survival when compared with controls. Aberrant integration of complex signaling events results in increased cellular proliferation, secretory abnormalities, and epithelial dedifferentiation leading to cyst formation and growth. A number of signal-transduction cascades implicated in cyst formation and progressive enlargement have been implicated in both ADPKD and ARPKD. Recent data suggest that multimeric, cystoprotein-containing complexes (localized to adherins junctions, and focal adhesions as well as apical membrane areas, including the ciliary basal bodies) may have a fundamental role in abnormal signaling in both ADPKD and ARPKD [22,65–67].

The molecular and cellular data regarding localization of cystoproteins to multimeric complexes suggest that many different abnormalities of such complex structure and function can lead to a predictable phenotypic pattern. Although little is known about ciliary structure and function, these data provide a unifying mechanism for cyst development. Such data provide the rationale to examine common components of the multiple pathways abnormally regulated in PKD in an effort to identify specific therapeutic targets for both ARPKD and ADPKD.

A brief description of the proliferative and secretory abnormalities identified in PKD demonstrates how emerging molecular and cellular knowledge of the pathophysiology can translate into unique future therapeutic approaches.

Cyclase-adenosine 3′, 5′-cyclic monophosphate-mediated proliferation

Mounting evidence suggests that the adenylyl cyclase-adenosine 3′, 5′-cyclic monophosphate (cAMP) pathway promotes both fluid secretion and cell proliferation in both ADPKD and ARPKD renal epithelia. Mutated PKD proteins are thought to disrupt intracellular Ca^{2+} homeostasis or Ca^{2+} signaling, leading to cellular dedifferentiation and hyperproliferation through an abnormal cAMP-mediated proliferative pathway.

In ADPKD, polycystin-1 and polycystin-2 complexes appear to be involved in calcium-dependent signaling, and recent evidence suggests that fibrocystin may function as part of this polycystin complex [68]. As noted above, the recent finding that fibrocystin may interact with CAML suggests that fibrocystin may also be involved in the regulation of Ca^{2+} homeostasis [63].

In normal human and mouse renal epithelial cells, cAMP has been shown to inhibit the Ras/Raf-1/MEK/ERK pathway at the level of Raf-1, resulting in decreased proliferation. In contrast, cAMP has been shown to stimulate B-Raf and activate the MEK/ERK pathway in ARPKD and ADPKD renal epithelia, leading to increased cell proliferation [69–73]. In renal epithelia, the switch in cAMP from an anti-mitogen to a mitogenic stimulus has been shown to directly correlate with decreased intracellular calcium levels (Ca^{2+}) and increased activity of Src [72].

These data suggest that the PKD proteins (PC1, PC2, and fibrocystin) play a role in maintaining Ca^{2+} homeostasis. Mutations in any of the PKD proteins may lead to reduction in intracellular Ca^{2+} and activate the cAMP mitogenic pathway through activation of the MEK/ERK pathway.

Epidermal growth factor receptor axis-mediated proliferation

Evidence from a number of laboratories demonstrates a significant role for the epidermal growth factor receptor (EGFR) axis in promoting epithelial hyperplasia in cystic epithelia, with resultant renal cyst formation and progressive enlargement in both murine and human ADPKD and ARPKD [74–85]. Renal cystic epithelia demonstrate both quantitative (overexpression) and qualitative (mislocalization) expression of one or more members of the ErbB family of receptors. In addition, evidence from rodent models (including the orthologous PCK rat) suggests that similar abnormalities of the EGFR axis may mediate biliary epithelial hyperplasia and biliary ductal ectasia (BDE) [77,84,86,87]. Epidermal growth factor (EGF) has an important role in the expansion of renal cysts. Cystic epithelial cells from patients who have both ARPKD and ADPKD are unusually susceptible to the proliferative stimulus of EGF. Moreover, cyst fluid of patients contains mitogenic concentrations of EGFR-ligands, and such cyst fluid ligands are present in concentration that can induce cellular proliferation [74,88–93]. In all animal models studied to date, as well as human ADPKD and ARPKD, abnormalities in expression and localization of members of the EGFR axis have been reported. Cyst-causing genes on different chromosomes, whether or not they are orthologous with human PKD genes, result in cystic epithelia with EGFR axis abnormalities.

These data indicate that abnormalities in the EGFR axis are a common cellular phenotype downstream from a number of different primary gene mutations. Despite interesting speculations, the precise mechanisms of the striking relationship remain unknown [7,79,83,84,94,95].

Traditionally, the EGFR axis is considered to act primarily through activation of the MAPK (RAS/RAF/MEK/ERK) pathway. It has become increasingly clear that the EGFR axis signaling is much more complex. Recent data suggest that there is considerable cross-talk between the MAPK pathway and the *cAMP* mediated pathway [96].

Secretion

ADPKD cysts have a fundamental structural difference from ARPKD cysts, as stated above and shown in Fig. 1. ADPKD cysts rapidly pinch off from urinary flow and continue to expand by transepithelial secretion. As stated above, ARPKD cysts remain open, maintaining both afferent and efferent tubular connections; however, secretion is still a necessary element of cyst formation in ARPKD, and the difference in cyst structure suggests a different secretory mechanism.

In ADPKD, the weight of the evidence indicates that Cl⁻ is secreted via a cAMP-mediated cotransport mechanism in the basolateral membrane, and CFTR in the apical membrane, leading to cyst expansion by transtubular secretion [69,97]. In contrast, however, cystic fibrosis transmembrane conductance regulator (CFTR) does not appear to be involved in secretory abnormalities in ARPKD [98]. Recent studies have implicated EGF-mediated alterations in amiloride sensitive absorption [99] and MAPK pathway [100] in ARPKD secretion.

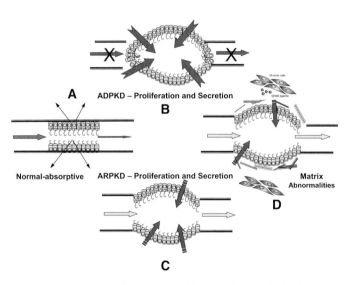

Fig. 1. Schematic representation of renal cysts. This figure depicts the fundamental structural differences between ADPKD and ARPKD. The development of PKD is characterized by a switch from a well-differentiated, nonproliferative, reabsorptive epithelia (*A*). In ADPKD (*B*), cysts rapidly pinch off from urinary flow and continue to expand by transepithelial secretion. In contrast, ARPKD cysts (*C*) remain open, maintaining both afferent and efferent tubular connections. Tubule (*D*) depicts the undefined nature of the contributions of interstitial cells and extracellular matrix components to cyst growth.

Cellular pathophysiology-translational implications

A critical test of the veracity of proposed pathophysiology is the effectiveness of targeted therapy on modulating disease. To date, there are no specific therapies in clinical use that limit renal cyst development and progressive enlargement or biliary ductal ectasia in ARPKD [101]; however, the studies noted above suggest that therapeutic targeting of the cAMP and EGFR axis abnormalities documented in cystic epithelia may translate into effective therapies for the proliferation and secretory abnormalities of ARPKD (and by analogy ADPKD).

To date, decreasing cAMP through vasopressin V2 receptor antagonism in renal CT has demonstrated efficacy in animal models of PKD orthologous to human diseases [102–104]; however, because of the restricted expression of the vasopressin 2 receptor (VPV2R) to renal principal cells, such approaches are limited to the renal lesions of NBPHP and such multisystem diseases as ADPKD, and ARPKD.

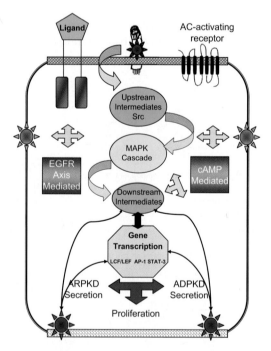

Fig. 2. Schematic representation of potential areas of therapeutic intervention. This figure depicts the areas where cystoproteins have been identified in multimeric protein complexes. The red stars represent the cilia and basal body localization of cystoproteins as well as signaling molecules. These cystoproteins also exist in adherins junctions (*blue stars*) and focal adhesions (*red stars*). The relationship of the signaling from these multiple complexes remains unknown. The figure, however, demonstrates the rationale of targeting common upstream or downstream intermediates of the multiple signaling cascades implicated in PKD. Many of these pathways have MAPK components as common elements of the signaling cascades.

Therapeutic targeting of the EGFR-axis has promise in ADPKD, and in particularly the dual renal and biliary cell abnormalities in ARPKD. To date, genetic complementation to decrease EGFR [81], inhibition of EGFR, c-ErbB2 and c-ErbB4 through small-molecule covalent inhibitors [84,86,105] and inhibition of EGFR ligand availability, alone and in combination with EGFR tyrosine kinase activity inhibitors [84,105], has demonstrated efficacy in ameliorating both renal CT abnormalities and biliary ductal ectasia in a variety of rodent ARPKD models. Similarly, therapeutic targeting of substrates downstream from EGFR such as MAPK/MEK5/ERK5/MEK1/2 has been effective in ameliorating biliary dysgenesis of PCK rat, in vitro [87].

Traditionally, the EGFR axis is considered to act primarily through activation of the MAPK (RAS/RAF/MEK/ERK) pathway. It has become increasingly clear that the EGFR axis is much more complex, and recent data suggest that there is considerable cross-talk between the MAPK pathway and the C-AMP mediated pathway [96].

A particularly promising approach appears to be specific targeting of intermediates common to both the cAMP and EGFR-axis mediated pathways. As shown in Fig. 2, c-Src (pp66Src) is one such component that interacts with identified cystic pathophysiological pathways, and exists at multiple locations in proximity to multermeric polycystic protein complexes. Preliminary studies targeting c-Src with a specific inhibitor (WY-606), [106,107] have been particularly effective in ameliorating both renal and biliary epithelial abnormalities in ARPKD models [64,108].

The delineation of the molecular and cellular pathophysiology of ARPKD has led to a new era of therapeutic innovation through targeting specific abnormalities of cystic epithelia. Such innovations bring great hope to patients who have RCD, and particularly to children devastated by the dual organ pathophysiology of ARPKD.

Appendix 1

Web-based resources for renal cystic disease

Polycystic Kidney Disease (PKD) Foundation. Available at: http://www.pkdcure.org. Accessed September 18, 2006.

GeneTests. Available at: http://www.genetests.org. Accessed September 18, 2006.

NIH/National Kidney and Urologic Diseases Information Clearinghouse. Available at: http://kidney.niddk.nih.gov. Accessed September 18, 2006.

March of Dimes. Available at: http://www.marchofdimes.com. Accessed September 18, 2006.

American Kidney Fund. Available at: http://www.kidneyfund.org. Accessed September 18, 2006.

National Kidney Foundation. Available at: http://www.kidney.org. Accessed September 18, 2006.

American Urological Association. Available at: http://www.afud.org. Accessed September 18, 2006.

National Center for Biotechnology Information. Available at: http://www.ncbi.nlm.nih.gov/. Accessed September 18, 2006.

Online Mendelian Inheritance in Man (OMIM). Available at: http://www.ncbi.nlm.nih.gov/entrez/query.fcgi?db=OMIM. Accessed September 18, 2006.

National Organization for Rare Disorders (NORD). Available at: http://www.rarediseases.org. Accessed September 18, 2006.

The Bartter Site. Available at: http://www.barttersite.com. Accessed September 18, 2006.

Laurence-Moon-Bardet-Biedl Society. Available at: http://www.lmbbs.org.uk. Accessed September 18, 2006.

Tuberous Sclerosis Alliance. Available at: http://www.tsalliance.org. Accessed September 18, 2006.

References

[1] Osathanondh V, Potter EL. Pathogenesis of polycystic kidneys. Survey of results of micro-dissection. Arch Pathol 1964;77:510–2.

[2] Osathanondh V, Potter EL. Pathogenesis of polycystic kidneys. Historical survey. Arch Pathol 1964;77:459–65.

[3] Hildebrandt F, Otto E. Cilia and centrosomes: a unifying pathogenic concept for cystic kidney disease? Nat Rev Genet 2005;6(12):928–40.

[4] Igarashi P, Shao X, McNally BT, et al. Roles of HNF-1beta in kidney development and congenital cystic diseases. Kidney Int 2005;68(5):1944–7.

[5] Ishikura K, Kamimaki I, Hamasaki Y, et al. Autosomal dominant polycystic kidney disease. Am J Kidney Dis 2006;47(6):A37, e73–5.

[6] Kerkar N, Norton K, Suchy FJ. The hepatic fibrocystic diseases. Clin Liver Dis 2006;10(1):55–71.

[7] Dell K, McDonald R, Watkins SL, et al. Polycystic kidney disease. In: Avner ED, Harmon WE, Niaudet P, editors. Pediatric nephrology. 4th editon. Philadelphia: Lippincott Williams & Wilkins; 2004. p. 675–99.

[8] Bernstein J. Glomerulocystic kidney disease—nosological considerations. Pediatr Nephrol 1993;7(4):464–70.

[9] Kaplan BS, Gordon I, Pincott J, et al. Familial hypoplastic glomerulocystic kidney disease: a definite entity with dominant inheritance. Am J Med Genet 1989;34(4):569–73.

[10] van Slegtenhorst M, de Hoogt R, Hermans C, et al. Identification of the tuberous sclerosis gene TSC1 on chromosome 9q34. Science 1997;277(5327):805–8.

[11] Wienecke R, Konig A, DeClue JE. Identification of tuberin, the tuberous sclerosis-2 product. Tuberin possesses specific Rap1GAP activity. J Biol Chem 1995;270(27):16409–14.

[12] Roach ES, Sparagana SP. Diagnosis of tuberous sclerosis complex. J Child Neurol 2004;19(9):643–9.

[13] Hyman MH, Whittemore VH. National Institutes of Health consensus conference: tuberous sclerosis complex. Arch Neurol 2000;57(5):662–5.

[14] Ong AC, Harris PC. Molecular pathogenesis of ADPKD: the polycystin complex gets complex. Kidney Int 2005;67(4):1234–47.

[15] Guay-Woodford LM, Muecher G, Hopkins SD, et al. The severe perinatal form of autosomal recessive polycystic kidney disease maps to chromosome 6p21.1-p12: Implications for genetic counseling. Am J Hum Genet 1995;56:1101–7.

[16] Onuchic LF, Furu L, Nagasawa Y, et al. PKHD1, the polycystic kidney and hepatic disease 1 gene, encodes a novel large protein containing multiple immunoglobulin-like plexin-transcription-factor domains and parallel beta-helix 1 repeats. Am J Hum Genet 2002; 70(5):1305–17.

[17] Ward CJ, Hogan MC, Rossetti S, et al. The gene mutated in autosomal recessive polycystic kidney disease encodes a large, receptor-like protein. Nat Genet 2002;30(3): 259–69.

[18] Harris PC, Rossetti S. Molecular genetics of autosomal recessive polycystic kidney disease. Mol Genet Metab 2004;81(2):75–85.

[19] Tahvanainen E, Tahvanainen P, Kaariainen H, et al. Polycystic liver and kidney diseases. Ann Med 2005;37(8):546–55.

[20] Sutters M. The pathogenesis of autosomal dominant polycystic kidney disease. Nephron Exp Nephrol 2006;103(4):e149–55.

[21] Consortium T. Polycystic kidney disease: the complete structure of the PKD1 gene and its protein. Cell 1995;81:289–98.

[22] Wilson PD. Polycystic kidney disease. N Engl J Med 2004;350(2):151–64.

[23] Witzgall R. New developments in the field of cystic kidney diseases. Curr Mol Med 2005; 5(5):455–65.

[24] Losekoot M, Haarloo C, Ruivenkamp C, et al. Analysis of missense variants in the PKHD1-gene in patients with autosomal recessive polycystic kidney disease (ARPKD). Hum Genet 2005;118(2):185–206.

[25] Sharp AM, Messiaen LM, Page G, et al. Comprehensive genomic analysis of PKHD1 mutations in ARPKD cohorts. J Med Genet 2005;42(4):336–49.

[26] Zerres K, Mücher G, Becker J, et al. Prenatal diagnosis of autosomal recessive polycystic kidney disease (ARPKD): molecular genetics, clinical experience, and fetal morphology. Am J Med Genet 1998;76:137–44.

[27] Blyth H, Ockenden BG. Polycystic disease of kidneys and liver presenting in childhood. J Med Genet 1971;8:257–84.

[28] Bernstein J, Slovis TL. Polycystic diseases of the kidney. In: Edelmann C, editor. Pediatric kidney diseases, vol. 2. Boston: Little, Brown; 1992. p. 1139–57.

[29] Osathanondh V, Potter EL. Pathogenesis of polycystic kidneys. Type 1 due to hyperplasia of interstitial portions of collecting tubules. Arch Pathol 1964;77:466–73.

[30] Jorgensen MJ. The ductal plate malformation. Acta Pathol Microbiol Scand Suppl 1977; 257:1–87.

[31] Desmet VJ. Congenital diseases of intrahepatic bile ducts: variations on the theme "ductal plate malformation." Hepatology 1992;16(4):1069–83.

[32] Dell K, Avner E. Autosomal recessive polycystic kidney disease. GeneReviews. Available at: http://www.genetests.org. Accessed March 26, 2006.

[33] Roy S, Dillon MJ, Trompeter RS, et al. Autosomal recessive polycystic kidney disease: long-term outcome of neonatal survivors. Pediatr Nephrol 1997;11(3):302–6.

[34] Guay-Woodford LM, Desmond RA. Autosomal recessive polycystic kidney disease: the clinical experience in North America. Pediatrics 2003;111:1072–80.

[35] Adeva M, El-Youssef M, Rosetti S, et al. Clinical and molecular characterizations defines a broadened spectrum of autosomal recessive polycystic kidney disease (ARPKD). Medicine 2006;85(1):1–21.

[36] Kaariainen H, Koskimies O, Norio R. Dominant and recessive polycystic kidney disease in children: evaluation of clinical features and laboratory data. Pediatr Nephrol 1988;2(3): 296–302.

[37] Kaplan BS, Fay J, Shah V, et al. Autosomal recessive polycystic kidney disease. Pediatr Nephrol 1989;3:43–9.

[38] Cole BR, Conley SB, Stapleton FB. Polycystic kidney disease in the first year of life. J Pediatr 1987;111(5):693–9.

[39] Guay-Woodford LM. Autosomal recessive polycystic kidney disease: clinical and genetic profiles. In: Watson ML, Torres VE, editors. Polycystic kidney disease. New York: Oxford University Press; 1996. p. 237–66.

[40] Davis ID, Ho M, Hupertz V, et al. Survival of childhood polycystic kidney disease following renal transplantation: the impact of advanced hepatobiliary disease. Pediatr Transplant 2003;7(5):364–9.

[41] Jafar TH, Stark PC, Schmid CH, et al. The effect of angiotensin-converting-enzyme inhibitors on progression of advanced polycystic kidney disease. Kidney Int 2005;67(1): 265–71.

[42] Zerres K, Rudnik-Schoneborn S, Steinkamm C, et al. Autosomal recessive polycystic kidney disease. Nephrol Dial Transplant 1996;11(Suppl 6):29–33.

[43] Bergmann C, Kupper F, Dornia C, et al. Algorithm for efficient PKHD1 mutation screening in autosomal recessive polycystic kidney disease (ARPKD). Hum Mutat 2005;25(3): 225–31.

[44] Bergmann C, Senderek J, Windelen E, et al. Clinical consequences of PKHD1 mutations in 164 patients with autosomal-recessive polycystic kidney disease (ARPKD). Kidney Int 2005;67(3):829–48.

[45] Rossetti S, Torra R, Coto E, et al. A complete mutation screen of PKHD1 in autosomal-recessive polycystic kidney disease (ARPKD) pedigrees. Kidney Int 2003;64(2): 391–403.

[46] Bergmann C, Senderek J, Sedlacek B, et al. Spectrum of mutations in the gene for autosomal recessive polycystic kidney disease (ARPKD/PKHD1). J Am Soc Nephrol 2003;14(1): 76–89.

[47] Furu L, Onuchic LF, Gharavi A, et al. Milder presentation of recessive polycystic kidney disease requires presence of amino acid substitution mutations. J Am Soc Nephrol 2003; 14(8):2004–14.

[48] Zerres K, Senderek J, Rudnik-Schoneborn S, et al. New options for prenatal diagnosis in autosomal recessive polycystic kidney disease by mutation analysis of the PKHD1 gene. Clin Genet 2004;66(1):53–7.

[49] Pazour GJ, Dickert BL, Vucica Y, et al. Chlamydomonas IFT88 and its mouse homologue, polycystic kidney disease gene tg737, are required for assembly of cilia and flagella. J Cell Biol 2000;151(3):709–18.

[50] Pazour GJ, San Agustin JT, Follit JA, et al. Polycystin-2 localizes to kidney cilia and the ciliary level is elevated in orpk mice with polycystic kidney disease. Curr Biol 2002; 12(11):R378–80.

[51] Yoder BK, Hou X, Guay-Woodford LM. The polycystic kidney disease proteins, polycystin-1, polycystin-2, polaris, and cystin, are co-localized in renal cilia. J Am Soc Nephrol 2002;13(10):2508–16.

[52] Praetorius HA, Frokiaer J, Nielsen S, et al. Bending the primary cilium opens Ca^{2+}-sensitive intermediate-conductance K^+ channels in MDCK cells. J Membr Biol 2003; 191(3):193–200.

[53] Guay-Woodford LM. Murine models of polycystic kidney disease: molecular and therapeutic insights. Am J Physiol Renal Physiol 2003;285(6):F1034–49.

[54] Nauli SM, Zhou J. Polycystins and mechanosensation in renal and nodal cilia. Bioessays 2004;26(8):844–56.

[55] Phillips CL, Miller KJ, Filson AJ, et al. Renal cysts of inv/inv mice resemble early infantile nephronophthisis. J Am Soc Nephrol 2004;15(7):1744–55.

[56] Sun Z, Amsterdam A, Pazour GJ, et al. A genetic screen in zebrafish identifies cilia genes as a principal cause of cystic kidney. Development 2004;131(16):4085–93.

[57] Pazour GJ, Rosenbaum JL. Intraflagellar transport and cilia-dependent diseases. Trends Cell Biol 2002;12(12):551–5.

[58] Igarashi P, Somlo S. Genetics and pathogenesis of polycystic kidney disease. J Am Soc Nephrol 2002;13(9):2384–98.

[59] Praetorius HA, Praetorius J, Nielsen S, et al. Beta1-integrins in the primary cilium of MDCK cells potentiate fibronectin-induced Ca2 + signaling. Am J Physiol Renal Physiol 2004;287(5):F969–78.

[60] Praetorius HA, Spring KR. Bending the MDCK cell primary cilium increases intracellular calcium. J Membr Biol 2001;184(1):71–9.

[61] Praetorius HA, Spring KR. The renal cell primary cilium functions as a flow sensor. Curr Opin Nephrol Hypertens 2003;12(5):517–20.

[62] Praetorius HA, Spring KR. Removal of the MDCK cell primary cilium abolishes flow sensing. J Membr Biol 2003;191(1):69–76.

[63] Nagano J, Kitamura K, Hujer KM, et al. Fibrocystin interacts with CAML, a protein involved in Ca(2+) signaling. Biochem Biophys Res Commun 2005;338(2):880–9.

[64] Sweeney WE Jr, Avner ED. Molecular and cellular pathophysiology of autosomal recessive polycystic kidney disease (ARPKD). Cell Tissue Res 2006; in press.

[65] Parnell SC, Magenheimer BS, Maser RL, et al. The polycystic kidney disease protein, polycystic-1, binds and activates heteromeric G-proteins. J Am Soc Nephrol 1998;9:380A.

[66] Li HP, Geng L, Burrow CR, et al. Identification of phosphorylation sites in the PKD1-encoded protein C-terminal domain. Biochem Biophys Res Commun 1999; 259(2):356–63.

[67] Bhunia AK, Piontek K, Boletta A, et al. PKD1 induces p21(waf1) and regulation of the cell cycle via direct activation of the JAK-STAT signaling pathway in a process requiring PKD2. Cell 2002;109(2):157–68.

[68] Anyatonwu GI, Ehrlich BE. Calcium signaling and polycystin-2. Biochem Biophys Res Commun 2004;322(4):1364–73.

[69] Sullivan LP, Grantham JJ. Mechanisms of fluid secretion by polycystic epithelia. Kidney Int 1996;49:1586–91.

[70] Yamaguchi T, Pelling JC, Ramaswamy NT, et al. cAMP stimulates the in vitro proliferation of renal cyst epithelial cells by activating the extracellular signal-regulated kinase pathway [see comments]. Kidney Int 2000;57(4):1460–71.

[71] Yamaguchi T, Nagao S, Wallace DP, et al. Cyclic AMP activates B-Raf and ERK in cyst epithelial cells from autosomal-dominant polycystic kidneys. Kidney Int 2003;63(6): 1983–94.

[72] Yamaguchi T, Wallace DP, Magenheimer BS, et al. Calcium restriction allows cAMP activation of the B-Raf/ERK pathway, switching cells to a cAMP-dependent growth-stimulated phenotype. J Biol Chem 2004;279(39):40419–30.

[73] Yamaguchi T, Hempson SJ, Reif GA, et al. Calcium restores a normal proliferation phenotype in human polycystic kidney disease epithelial cells. J Am Soc Nephrol 2006;17(1): 178–87.

[74] Neufield TK, Douglass D, Grant M, et al. In vitro formation and expansion of cysts derived from human renal cortex epithelial cells. Kidney Int 1992;41:1222–36.

[75] Lowden DA, Lindemann GW, Merlino G, et al. Renal cysts in transgenic mice expressing transforming growth factor-alpha [see comments]. J Lab Clin Med 1994;124(3): 386–94.

[76] Orellana SA, Sweeney WE, Neff CD, et al. Epidermal growth factor receptor expression is abnormal in murine polycystic kidney. Kidney Int 1995;47(2):490–9.

[77] Nauta J, Sweeney WE, Rutledge JC, et al. Biliary epithelial cells from mice with congenital polycystic kidney disease are hyperresponsive to epidermal growth factor. Pediatr Res 1995; 37(6):755–63.

[78] Pugh JL, Sweeney WE Jr, Avner ED. Tyrosine kinase activity of the EGF receptor in murine metanephric organ culture. Kidney Int 1995;47(3):774–81.

[79] Du J, Wilson PD. Abnormal polarization of EGF receptors and autocrine stimulation of cyst epithelial growth in human ADPKD. Am J Physiol 1995;269:C487–95.

[80] Gattone VH 2nd, Kuenstler KA, Lindemann GW, et al. Renal expression of a transforming growth factor-alpha transgene accelerates the progression of inherited, slowly progressive polycystic kidney disease in the mouse. J Lab Clin Med 1996;127(2):214–22.

[81] Richards WG, Sweeney WE, Yoder BK, et al. Epidermal growth factor receptor activity mediates renal cyst formation in polycystic kidney disease. J Clin Invest 1998;101(5):935–9.

[82] Sweeney WE Jr, Avner ED. Functional activity of epidermal growth factor receptors in autosomal recessive polycystic kidney disease. Am J Physiol 1998;275:F387–94.

[83] Lu W, Fan X, Babakanlou H, et al. Late onset of renal and hepatic cysts in Pkd1-targeted heterozygotes. Nat Gen 1999;21:160–1.

[84] Sweeney WE Jr, Hamahira K, Sweeney J, et al. Combination treatment of PKD utilizing dual inhibition of EGF-receptor activity and ligand bioavailability. Kidney Int 2003; 64(4):1310–9.

[85] Torres VE. Therapies to slow polycystic kidney disease. Nephron Exp Nephrol 2004;98(1): e1–7.

[86] Sweeney WE, Chen Y, Nakanishi K, et al. Treatment of polycystic kidney disease with a novel tyrosine kinase inhibitor. Kidney Int 2000;57:33–40.

[87] Sato Y, Harada K, Kizawa K, et al. Activation of the MEK5/ERK5 cascade is responsible for biliary dysgenesis in a rat model of Caroli's disease. Am J Pathol 2005;166(1):49–60.

[88] Ye M, Grant M, Sharma M, et al. Cyst fluid from human autosomal dominant polycystic kidneys promotes cyst formation and expansion by renal epithelial cells in vitro. J Am Soc Nephrol 1992;3(4):984–94.

[89] Klingel R, Dippold W, Storkel S, et al. Expression of differentiation antigens and growth-related genes in normal kidney, autosomal dominant polycystic kidney disease, and renal cell carcinoma. Am J Kidney Dis 1992;19(1):22–30.

[90] Lakshmanan J, Fisher DA. An inborn error in epidermal growth factor prohormone metabolism in a mouse model of autosomal recessive polycystic kidney disease. Biochem Biophys Res Commun 1993;196:892–901.

[91] Sullivan LP, Wallace DP, Grantham JJ. Chloride and fluid secretion in polycystic kidney disease. J Am Soc Nephrol 1998;9:903–16.

[92] Sweeney WE, Avner ED. BPK cyst fluid contains EGF and TGF-α like peptides which are motogenic and phosphorylate apical EGFR. J Am Soc Nephrol 1996;7:1606.

[93] Rohatgi R, Zavilowitz B, Vergara M, et al. Cyst fluid composition in human autosomal recessive polycystic kidney disease. Pediatr Nephrol 2005;20(4):552–3.

[94] Grantham JJ. Time to treat polycystic kidney diseases like the neoplastic disorders that they are [editorial comment]. Kidney Int 2000;57(1):339–40.

[95] Wilson PD. Polycystic kidney disease: new understanding in the pathogenesis. Int J Biochem Cell Biol 2004;36(10):1868–73.

[96] Grantham JJ. Renal cell proliferation and the two faces of cyclic adenosine monophosphate. J Lab Clin Med 1997;130:459–60.

[97] Belibi FA, Reif G, Wallace DP, et al. Cyclic AMP promotes growth and secretion in human polycystic kidney epithelial cells. Kidney Int 2004;66(3):964–73.

[98] Nakanishi K, Sweeney WE Jr, Macrae Dell K, et al. Role of CFTR in autosomal recessive polycystic kidney disease. J Am Soc Nephrol 2001;12(4):719–25.

[99] Veizis IE, Cotton CU. Abnormal EGF-dependent regulation of sodium absorption in ARPKD collecting duct cells. Am J Physiol Renal Physiol 2005;288(3):F474–82.

[100] Falin R, Veizis IE, Cotton CU. A role for ERK1/2 in EGF- and ATP-dependent regulation of amiloride-sensitive sodium absorption. Am J Physiol Cell Physiol 2005;288(5): C1003–11.

[101] Davis ID, MacRae Dell K, Sweeney WE, et al. Can progression of autosomal dominant or autosomal recessive polycystic kidney disease be prevented? Semin Nephrol 2001;21(5): 430–40.

[102] Gattone VH 2nd, Wang X, Harris PC, et al. Inhibition of renal cystic disease development and progression by a vasopressin V2 receptor antagonist. Nat Med 2003;9(10):1323–6.

[103] Torres VE, Wang X, Qian Q, et al. Effective treatment of an orthologous model of autosomal dominant polycystic kidney disease. Nat Med 2004;10(4):363–4.

[104] Torres VE. Vasopressin antagonists in polycystic kidney disease. Kidney Int 2005;68(5): 2405–18.

[105] Dell KM, Nemo R, Sweeney WE, et al. A novel inhibitor of tumor necrosis factor-alpha converting enzyme ameliorates polycystic kidney disease. Kidney Int 2001;60(4):1240–8.

[106] Boschelli DH, Wu B, Barrios Sosa AC, et al. Inhibition of Src kinase activity by 7-[(2,4-dichloro-5-methoxyphenyl)amino]-2-heteroaryl-thieno[3,2-b]pyridine-6-carbonitriles. Bioorg Med Chem Lett 2005;15:23.

[107] Boschelli DH, Wu B, Barrios Sosa AC, et al. Synthesis and Src kinase inhibitory activity of 2-phenyl- and 2-thienyl-7-phenylaminothieno[3,2-b]pyridine-6-carbonitriles. J Med Chem 2005;48(11):3891–902.

[108] Gunay-Aygun M, Avner ED, Bacallao RL, et al. Autosomal recessive polycystic kidney disease and congenital hepatic fibrosis: summary statement of the First National Institutes of Health/Office of Rare Diseases Conference. J Pediatr 2006;149:159–64.

ELSEVIER
SAUNDERS

Pediatr Clin N Am
53 (2006) 911–927

PEDIATRIC CLINICS
OF NORTH AMERICA

Defects in Surfactant Synthesis: Clinical Implications

F. Sessions Cole, MD[a],*, Lawrence M. Nogee, MD[b], Aaron Hamvas, MD[a]

[a]Division of Newborn Medicine in the Edward Mallinckrodt Department of Pediatrics, Washington University School of Medicine and St. Louis Children's Hospital, One Children's Place, St. Louis, MO 63110, USA
[b]Division of Neonatology in the Department of Pediatrics, Johns Hopkins University School of Medicine, 600 North Wolfe Street, Baltimore, MD 21287, USA

Neonatal respiratory distress syndrome is the most frequent respiratory cause of death and morbidity in the first year of life in the United States [1–3]. Pulmonary morbidity in survivors of neonatal respiratory distress syndrome is linked with significant cost: survivors of respiratory distress syndrome who have chronic respiratory disease consume 20 times more annualized health care dollars ($19,104 versus $955) and 5.9% of all dollars spent on children from 0 to 18 years of age [4,5]. More recent estimates from California and New York suggest that 80,000 cases of neonatal respiratory distress occur in the United States annually with 8500 resulting deaths at a hospital cost of $4.4 billion [6]. Although no estimate of the population-based frequencies of genetic defects in surfactant synthesis in older infants and children is available, increasing recognition of surfactant gene mutations in these populations suggests the importance of these defects beyond the neonatal period [7,8]. The authors outline an approach to evaluation of infants who have possible genetic defects in surfactant synthesis.

Supported in part by awards from the National Heart, Lung, and Blood Institute (HL-65174, FSC, AH, LMN; HL 65385, AH; HL-54703 and HL-56387, LMN) and the Eudowood Board (LMN).

* Corresponding author.
E-mail address: cole@kids.wustl.edu (F.S. Cole).

Genetic regulation of the pulmonary surfactant metabolic pathway

Since the original description of deficiency of the pulmonary surfactant in premature newborn infants by Avery and Mead in 1959, disruption of metabolism of the pulmonary surfactant most commonly has been attributed to developmental mechanisms [9–13]. The pulmonary surfactant is a mixture of phospholipids and protein synthesized, packaged, and secreted exclusively by type 2 pneumocytes that line the distal airways. This mixture forms a film at the air–liquid interface in the alveolus that lowers surface tension at end expiration of the respiratory cycle and thereby prevents atelectasis and ventilation–perfusion mismatch. In premature infants, type 2 pneumocytes do not appear before 32 to 34 weeks of gestation, and these infants lack the ability to produce mature or functional surfactant [9–13]. The report by Avery and Mead established that developmentally regulated surfactant deficiency attributable to reduction in the dominant surfactant phospholipid, phosphatidylcholine, causes neonatal respiratory distress syndrome in premature infants [14–17]. Studies of different ethnic groups, gender, targeted gene ablation in murine lineages, and recent clinical reports of monogenic causes of neonatal respiratory distress syndrome have suggested strongly that genetic mechanisms contribute significantly to risk for respiratory distress syndrome in newborn infants [18–46]. In addition, despite improvement in neonatal survival attributable to surfactant replacement therapy, long-term respiratory morbidity has persisted [4,47–52]. This persistence strongly suggests that genetic factors play an important pathogenic role [53,54]. By ameliorating developmentally regulated pulmonary surfactant dysfunction immediately after birth, surfactant replacement therapy has unmasked the contribution of genetic causes of disruption of pulmonary surfactant metabolism to morbidity and mortality in infancy [55,56]. In contrast to developmental disruption of pulmonary surfactant metabolism, which may improve as infants mature, genetic disruption results in both acute and chronic (and potentially irreversible) respiratory failure that is unresponsive to currently available therapies (eg, surfactant replacement therapy).

Genetic disruption of the pulmonary surfactant metabolic pathway

Although multiple genes regulate the pulmonary surfactant metabolic pathway, mutations in three genes are known to disrupt this pathway in human newborn infants and older children: autosomal recessive surfactant protein B gene (SFTPB) mutations reduce expression of a small (8 kd) hydrophobic protein critical for surfactant function; dominant mutations in the surfactant protein C gene (SFTPC) encode misfolded or mistargeted surfactant protein C that induces a global cellular response (the unfolded protein response) or interrupts the surfactant biosynthetic itinerary in type 2 cell pneumocytes; and autosomal recessive, ATP-binding cassette transporter

A3 (*ABCA3*) mutations likely disrupt transport of phospholipids into lamellar bodies in the type 2 pneumocyte [18,19,57–60].

Surfactant protein B deficiency

Surfactant protein B deficiency was the first recognized monogenic cause of disruption of pulmonary surfactant metabolism and has been the most extensively studied [46,57,61,62]. Rare homozygous loss-of-function mutations in *SFTPB* are unambiguously associated with lethal neonatal respiratory distress because of disruption of synthesis of surfactant protein B, a small hydrophobic protein required for function of the pulmonary surfactant [18,46,54,62–65]. The consistency of the clinical phenotype of surfactant protein B deficiency in infants from different ethnic backgrounds and the population-based frequency of the most common loss-of-function mutation in *SFTPB* (1/1000 individuals for the 121ins2 mutation) in two large cohort studies suggest that that these genotypes (homozygous or compound heterozygous loss-of-function mutations) are completely penetrant [43,57,61,64–66]. Despite the low population-based frequency of the 121ins2 mutation, surfactant protein B deficiency has been reported in 14% of term or near-term infants who have severe respiratory distress from a large international referral cohort [19]. Although not systematically studied, no cases of sporadic mutations have been reported. Analysis of the pulmonary surfactant isolated from surfactant protein B–deficient infants and mice has demonstrated undetectable surfactant protein B, deficient surfactant function, a tight metabolic linkage between surfactant protein B expression and surfactant protein C processing, and a decrease in the amount of phosphatidylglycerol, but no change in phosphatidylcholine, the phospholipid most critical for surfactant function [18,21,43,57,62,67–69]. Infants who have mutations on one or both alleles of *SFTPB* with reduced (<25%) *SFTPB* expression have exhibited both transient and lethal neonatal respiratory distress syndrome [70–72]. In human newborn infants not genetically deficient in surfactant protein B and in murine lineages genetically engineered to express surfactant protein B conditionally, reduction of surfactant protein B concentration below a quantitative threshold (<25% of normal surfactant protein B concentration in tracheal aspirates) results in surfactant deficiency not attributable to phospholipid deficiency [73–75]. Heterozygote knockout mice with 50% normal expression have also been shown to have decreased lung compliance, more air trapping, and to be more sensitive to oxygen toxicity, although no abnormalities detectable by pulmonary function testing have been observed in humans heterozygous for loss-of-function mutations [22,76–78]. These data suggest that *SFTPB*-dependent genetic disruption of pulmonary surfactant metabolism causes neonatal respiratory distress syndrome and chronic lung disease when expression of surfactant protein B decreases below 25% of normal expression [70,71,73–75,79].

Surfactant protein C disorders

In contrast to surfactant protein B deficiency, surfactant protein C disorders are attributable to dominant mutations in *SFTPC*, may be sporadic or inherited, and are associated with much more variable phenotypes, including interstitial lung disease and a wide spectrum of pulmonary disease phenotypes in newborn infants, older children, and adults [18,45,57,80–88]. The phenotypic heterogeneity observed in both humans and mice is likely attributable to undefined genetic and environmental factors, to reduction in surface activity encoded by genetic variants, and to the role of surfactant protein C in lung morphogenesis [18,57,86,89–94]. Unlike *SFTPB* mutations that reduce expression below a biosynthetic threshold, *SFTPC* mutations disrupt pulmonary surfactant metabolism by encoding toxic, gain-of-function misfolded or mistargeted forms of surfactant protein C that induce a global cellular response in type 2 pneumocytes (the unfolded protein response) or interrupt the surfactant biosynthetic itinerary [82,86,87,89–91,94–98]. Misfolding leads to retention in the endoplasmic reticulum in early endosomes or in aggresomes, which results in interruption of normal intracellular transport, lack of secretion, and aggregation of misfolded surfactant protein C that induces concurrent cellular injury by way of endoplasmic reticulum stress [18,45,57,81,82,87,98–101]. The mechanism through which the endoplasmic reticulum-associated degradation pathway's ubiquitin-mediated degradation of misfolded surfactant protein C results in the diverse pulmonary disease phenotypes of surfactant protein C deficiency likely involves the unfolded protein response [101,102]. This cellular response that has been preserved from yeast to mammals activates effector protein genes that encode chaperones to mediate disposal of misfolded proteins and to slow cellular protein translation. These responses may permit the cell to tolerate and survive conditions that cause excess misfolded protein accumulation [101]. Alternatively, the unfolded protein response may be pro-apoptotic and lead to cell death [103]. The mechanisms that regulate tolerant versus pro-apoptotic responses to misfolded proteins are not well understood. Besides misfolding, *SFTPC* mutations may encode mistargeting of surfactant protein C precursor protein [86,87,96,104]. It is likely that these mutations disrupt type 2 pneumocyte surfactant synthesis by mechanisms distinct from the unfolded protein response [86,87]. In contrast to the discrete effects of loss-of-function *SFTPB* mutations, *SFTPC* mutations disrupt pulmonary surfactant metabolism by way of global, toxic, or gain-of-function effects on type 2 pneumocyte biosynthetic function [86].

ABCA3 deficiency

Loss-of-function mutations in *ABCA3* disrupt pulmonary surfactant metabolism by altering composition of surfactant phospholipid in both newborn infants and older children [7,8,19,59,105]. ABCA3 is a 180- to 200-kd protein that is a member of a superfamily of proteins that transport macromolecules across membranes [7,106]. *ABCA3* encodes an ATP-binding cassette transporter that has been localized to the limiting membrane of lamellar bodies of type 2 pneumocytes [7,19]. It is likely that ABCA3 is involved in transport of phospholipids into the lamellar body in type 2 pneumocytes that may be required for assembly of the pulmonary surfactant [58]. Recent studies of lung tissue from 10 of 14 infants who had unexplained respiratory distress syndrome also suggest a role for ABCA3 in processing of surfactant proteins B and C [105]. Twelve distinct loss-of-function mutations in this gene have been reported recently in 16 of 21 patients who had severe, otherwise uncharacterized neonatal respiratory distress who were part of a larger cohort (n = 337 infants) with severe respiratory distress accumulated by national and international referral [19]. Dense lamellar body appearance, abnormalities in surfactant phospholipid composition, and severe surfactant dysfunction have been reported in an additional 8 infants with these mutations [59]. Older infants and children have been reported recently with *ABCA3* mutations, an observation that suggests greater genotype–phenotype diversity than observed in affected newborn infants [7,8,60]. The disruption of lamellar body organization is associated with disruption of processing rather than deficiencies of surfactant proteins B and C in a limited number of infants evaluated to date [59,105]. These data suggest that mutations in *ABCA3* disrupt the pulmonary surfactant metabolic pathway through effects on phospholipid transport.

Evaluation for genetic defects in surfactant synthesis

Newborn infants

Clinical characteristics and evaluation

Term or near-term ($\geq$ 36 weeks' gestation) infants who develop unexplained, severe, persistent respiratory distress (ie, without evidence of infection, pulmonary or cardiac defects, airway abnormalities, or chest wall or diaphragmatic problems) and who do not exhibit improvement within the first 7 to 10 days after birth should be evaluated within the first 2 weeks of life for genetic defects in surfactant synthesis in consultation with a center that is expert in the evaluation and care of these children as outlined in Fig. 1. This evaluation should be done promptly so that lung transplantation can be considered in the event that one of these disorders is present. Evaluation should include family history (including adult-onset symptoms) of unexplained pulmonary disease. Physical examination is notable for lack of extrapulmonary organ defects, evidence of impaired pulmonary compliance, and need for mechanical ventilation because of hypoxia and hypercarbia. Radiographic appearance of the chest may be consistent with surfactant deficiency (diffuse ground glass appearance with air bronchograms) or interstitial lung disease. The tenuous pulmonary status of these infants requires that the least invasive and most rapidly available diagnostic

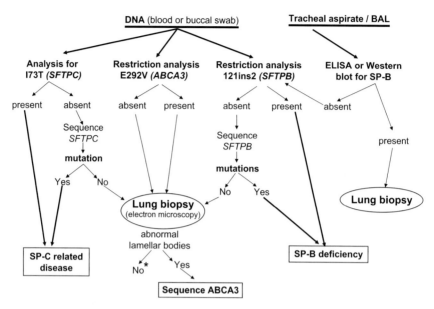

Fig. 1. Diagnostic approach to infants who have suspected genetic defects in surfactant synthesis. Genetic analyses in certified clinical laboratories provide a noninvasive initial approach to diagnosis. Research-based biochemical analysis of tracheal aspirate and consultation with a center experienced in evaluation of these infants should be strongly considered. If a genetic defect cannot be detected in a timely fashion, lung biopsy should be considered early in the evaluation. Note that lung biopsy should be processed to permit hematoxylin-eosin examination, complete microbiologic evaluation, immunohistochemical evaluation, in situ hybridization, and electron microscopic assessment. (*) indicates that the patient does not have any of the currently known inherited disorders of surfactant metabolism and conventional care should continue while the search for other explanations is ongoing.

steps be performed. Because of the complete penetrance of homozygous, loss-of-function *SFTPB* mutations, the authors suggest that evaluation begin with genetic analysis for common mutations in the surfactant-associated genes using genomic DNA extracted from EDTA anticoagulated blood or from buccal swabs (Fig. 1). These tests are available from certified clinical laboratories and therefore can be used in ongoing clinical management. Consultation with selected centers experienced in evaluation of these infants also may lead to concurrent use of research-based biochemical analysis for determination of the presence or absence of surfactant protein B in tracheal aspirate by ELISA or Western blot analysis. Surfactant protein B from natural surfactant replacement preparations can be detected by these analyses, and thus the authors recommend obtaining tracheal aspirate samples at least 48 hours after surfactant administration. These research-based biochemical analyses are not done in certified clinical laboratories and therefore cannot be used for clinical decision making. Selected centers, however, may incorporate these results into their approach to the chronology of genetic testing. Because the expression of surfactant protein C (SP-C) in the presence of *SFTPC* mutations is so variable, the presence or absence of pro- or mature SP-C in tracheal aspirate samples is neither sensitive nor specific for SP-C–related disease. Currently, there are no biochemical markers that can provide a noninvasive screen for ABCA3 deficiency. Tracheal aspirate samples sent to research laboratories may help to focus genetic diagnostic testing on surfactant protein B (SP-B) deficiency but do not permit the definitive diagnosis of genetic surfactant defects.

If surfactant protein B is undetectable, the authors test for the presence of the most common loss-of-function mutation in *SFTPB* (121ins2 muta- tion) by *SfuI* restriction enzyme analysis of amplified *SFTPB* exon 4 from the affected infant's genomic DNA, a test that can be performed within 48 hours (Fig. 2). If the infant is homozygous for the 121ins2 muta- tion, after confirmation by direct sequencing, the diagnosis, treatment op- tions, and prognosis of surfactant protein B deficiency are established and the infant's family may be counseled [61]. If the infant is heterozygous for the 121ins2 mutation or the 121ins2 mutation is not present, and lacks surfactant protein B in the tracheal aspirate, the infant's *SFTPB* should be sequenced completely at a certified clinical laboratory (eg, the DNA Diag- nostics Laboratory at Johns Hopkins Medical Institutions, http:// www.hopkinsmedicine.org/dnadiagnostic/services.htm) to search for rare loss-of-function mutations on the second allele. If such mutations are de- tected, diagnosis, treatment options, and prognosis can be discussed with the infant's family [61]. If *SFTPB* loss-of-function mutations cannot be con- firmed, consultation with a center experienced in evaluation of these infants should be considered; rare cases of a developmental or partial regulatory

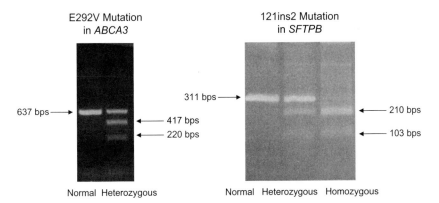

Fig. 2. Genetic defect diagnosis by restriction enzyme digestion. The E292V mutation in *ABCA3* and the 121ins2 mutation in *SFTPB* can each be rapidly diagnosed by amplification of genomic DNA from exon 7 of *ABCA3* (637 bp) or from exon 4 of *SFTPB* (311 bp) and digestion with restriction endonuclease *Bsrg1* (*ABCA3*) or *Sfu1* (*SFTPB*). Each mutation intro- duces a restriction enzyme site that results in cleavage of the amplified fragment when the mutation is present.

SFTPB defects that improve have been reported [71]. Consideration of lung biopsy should be initiated. In addition, the authors suggest concurrent examination of *SFTPC* and *ABCA3* initially by technically rapid testing for common mutations (allele-specific polymerase chain reaction or a TaqMan assay for the I173T mutations in exon 3 of *SFTPC* [107] and *BsrgI* restriction enzyme digestion of exon 7 of *ABCA3* to look for the E292V mutation) (Fig. 2). If these mutations are detected, confirmation by direct sequencing is required. If the clinical history suggests, the complete sequencing of *SFTPC* is indicated and feasible in a timely fashion because of the small size of the gene (~ 3.5 kb).

If the initial screening does not reveal a mutation in these genes, then the authors suggest expeditiously proceeding with lung biopsy, again so that appropriate counseling can be provided to the family. Before lung biopsy, the surgical, neonatal, and pathology teams should confer to prepare for obtaining and processing the lung biopsy. The authors also suggest consultation with a center experienced in evaluation of these infants. Clinical considerations (chest radiograph, chest tube placement, possible need for future lung transplantation) should help identify the location from which to obtain the biopsy. In addition, skilled pathologists who have experience in neonatal pulmonary lung diseases should be involved in planning for the lung biopsy. Although the histopathologic appearance of genetic surfactant defects is variable (Fig. 3), experienced pathologists can recognize a broad genetic defect phenotype that includes type 2 pneumocyte hyperplasia, alveolar proteinosis, and interstitial inflammation [45,46,82,108]. Processing of the specimen should permit not only routine examination but also relevant cultures and molecular microbial testing, preservation of tissue for electron microscopic examination, in situ hybridization, immunohistochemical staining, and RNA extraction (freezing of a portion of the sample in liquid nitrogen). Examination of the lung ultrastructure with electron microscopy is essential for analyzing lamellar body morphology that may suggest ABCA3 deficiency [19,59] (Fig. 4). If lamellar body morphology suggests surfactant metabolic disruption (disorganized or dense lamellar bodies) (Fig. 4), amplification and sequencing of *ABCA3* are indicated, but the genomic size of ABCA3 (30 translated exons and more than 80 kb) requires significantly more time for analysis (weeks to months). Although advances in sequencing technology will likely permit more rapid identification of pathologic sequence variants in ABCA3, sequencing time required by current technology limits the ability to rely on identification of such pathologic variants in the care of infants who have severe progressive respiratory failure. In addition, because most of the mutations in these genes are missense mutations, distinguishing true disease-causing mutations from rare, yet benign, sequence variants may be difficult. Even if the evaluation for the currently known inherited disorders is uninformative, the lung biopsy tissue should be preserved for future molecular and proteomic analyses as new mechanisms of lung disease are identified.

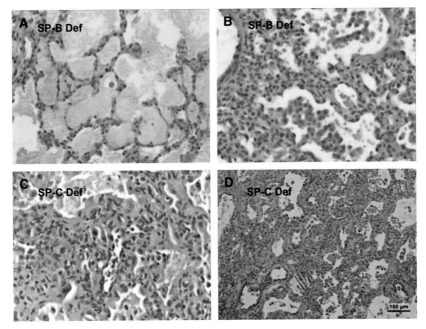

Fig. 3. Variable histopathologic appearance of genetic defects in surfactant synthesis. (*A*) Alveolar proteinosis in an infant homozygous for the 121ins2 mutation in *SFTPB* (×200). (*B*) Desquamative interstitial pneumonitis-like appearance with numerous intra-alveolar macrophages and mild pneumocyte hyperplasia is present in a second infant homozygous for the 121ins2 mutation in *SFTPB* (×400). (*C*) Alveoli with macrophages and a small amount of finely granular eosinophilic material, extension of smooth muscle into alveolar septa, and pneumocyte hyperplasia are present in an infant who has C189G mutation in *SFTPC* (×400). (*D*) Prominent pneumocyte hyperplasia and alveolar remodeling with smooth muscle extension into septa and fibrosis, a mild chronic inflammatory infiltrate, and alveoli with multinucleated macrophages, cholesterol clefts, and dense eosinophilic material in a child who has an I73T mutation in *SFTPC*. Bar, 100 μm.

Treatment options and prognosis

No specific treatments for genetic defects in *SFTPB*, *SFTPC*, and *ABCA3* are available currently. Genetic disruption of *SFTPB* expression will not improve with conventional therapy. Attempts at surfactant replacement therapy in an infant who had surfactant protein B deficiency were unsuccessful [109]. The treatment options for these infants include evaluation for lung transplantation and compassionate care [61]. In our experience, approximately 50% of families choose to proceed with evaluation for lung transplantation and 50% opt for compassionate care. The infant's medical condition and extrapulmonary organ function must be sustainable for the anticipated average wait for lung donation of approximately 2 to 3 months. Outcomes of transplanted infants are comparable to those of infants transplanted for other reasons in the first year of life [110].

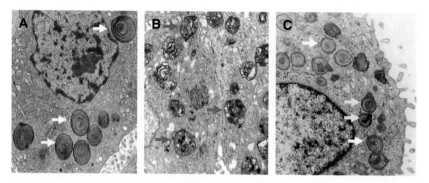

Fig. 4. Lamellar body appearance in genetic surfactant defects. (*A*) Normal-appearing lamellar bodies (*white arrows*) from the lung of an infant who has pulmonary vascular disease and no genetic surfactant defect. (*B*) Disorganized, granular lamellar bodies (*red arrows*) in an infant homozygous for the 121ins2 mutation in *SFTPB*. (*C*) Normal-appearing (*white arrows*) and dense lamellar bodies that lack normal lamellated structure (*yellow arrows*) in an infant who has ABCA3 deficiency.

The clinical phenotypes of infants who have genetic disruption of *SFTPC* or *ABCA3* are more diverse than those who have homozygous loss-of-function *SFTPB* mutations [45,60]. If a mechanistically significant *SFTPC* mutation or homozygous loss-of-function *ABCA3* mutation is confirmed, the severity and rate of deterioration of the infant's clinical status should contribute significantly to the decision to offer evaluation for lung transplantation. For infants who have interstitial lung disease associated with *SFTPC* mutations, hydroxychloroquine or glucocorticoids have been used empirically with variable success but have not been studied systematically [111]. The unpredictable natural history of SP-C–associated lung disease and ABCA3 deficiency dictates that lung transplantation be reserved for patients who have progressive and refractory respiratory failure who would otherwise qualify for transplantation irrespective of their diagnosis. To date, although several children who had progressive lung disease attributable to *SFTPC* or *ABCA3* mutations have undergone transplantation [82] (Aaron Hamvas, MD, unpublished data, 2006), outcomes of infants transplanted for *SFTPC* or *ABCA3* mutations have not been studied systematically. Once transplanted, the 5-year survival for the infants who have mutations in *SFTPB*, *SFTPC*, or *ABCA3* is approximately 50% to 60%, which is similar to the survival for all children undergoing lung transplantation regardless of diagnosis or age at transplant [112–114] (Aaron Hamvas, MD, unpublished data, 2006). In the authors' experience, the causes of morbidity and mortality and the pulmonary and developmental outcomes for these infants are similar to those of children who have undergone lung transplantation for other reasons, an observation that suggests that lung transplantation reconstitutes genetic SP-B, SP-C, or ABCA3 defects in pulmonary surfactant metabolism, and that the pulmonary manifestations of these disorders do not result from systemic disease unmasked by survival attributable to transplantation-based improvement in pulmonary function [110].

Postmortem diagnosis

Postmortem diagnosis may be complicated by lack of availability of autopsy tissue useful for electron microscopy, lack of access to genomic DNA from the affected child, and by the differences in frequency of sporadic mutations in *SFTPB*, *SFTPC*, and *ABCA3*. Because no sporadic mutations in *SFTPB* and *ABCA3* have been reported to date, access to parental DNA permits screening for *ABCA3* and *SFTPB* mutations first by restriction enzyme digestion as described above (Fig. 2). Because of the frequency of sporadic mutations in *SFTPC* (60%), parental DNA may not be useful if a disorder of surfactant protein C is suspected. If suggested by the clinical history and the histopathologic examination of lung biopsy or autopsy lung tissue, complete sequencing of *SFTPB* and *SFTPC* may be indicated. If no mutations are detected and histopathologic examination suggests a disorder of surfactant metabolism the authors advise complete sequencing of *ABCA3*.

Older infants and children

Older children who have interstitial lung disease without a clearly defined mechanism should be evaluated for defects in surfactant synthesis also, because SP-C–associated disease and ABCA3 deficiency may present at older ages with chronic respiratory insufficiency [8,60,115]. Initial studies should include restriction enzyme digestion for the E292V mutation in *ABCA3* and allele-specific polymerase chain reaction or TaqMan assay for the I173T mutation in *SFTPC* followed by direct sequencing of *SFTPC* if the I73T mutation is not detected. If these mutations are not detected, lung biopsy should be considered with preparation as described above. If histopathology or lamellar body phenotype is consistent with a genetic defect in surfactant synthesis, complete sequencing of *SFTPC* and *ABCA3* is indicated.

Summary

The pulmonary surfactant has a complex metabolic cycle that includes synthesis with post-translational processing, secretion, clearance, reuptake, and recycling. The authors and others have shown that mutations in *SFTPB*, *SFTPC*, and *ABCA3* disrupt different steps in this cycle, alter surfactant function, and cause respiratory distress with diverse clinical presentations in newborn infants, older children, and adults. Currently available genetic diagnostic methods permit rapid evaluation of common pathologic mutations. Lung biopsy may be necessary if initial genetic diagnosis is inconclusive. As other genes involved in the surfactant metabolic cycle are characterized, genetic evaluation for defects in surfactant synthesis will expand. New, high throughput genomic technologies will permit rapid screening of multiple genomic sites in large numbers of genes and will suggest novel therapeutic targets to improve outcomes for affected infants and children.

Acknowledgments

The authors thank F. White, MD, for photomicrographs from infants and children with genetic defects in surfactant synthesis.

References

[1] Guyer B, Freedman MA, Strobino DM, et al. Annual summary of vital statistics: trends in the health of Americans during the 20th century. Pediatrics 2000;106(6):1307–17.

[2] Hoyert D, Freedman MA, Strobino DM, et al. Annual summary of vital statistics: 2000. Pediatrics 2001;108(6):1241–55.

[3] Arias E, MacDorman MF, Strobino DM, et al. Annual summary of vital statistics: 2002. Pediatrics 2003;112(6 Pt 1):1215–30.

[4] Jobe AH, Bancalari E. Bronchopulmonary dysplasia. Am J Respir Crit Care Med 2001; 163(7):1723–9.

[5] Ireys H, Anderson GF, Shaffer TJ, et al. Expenditures for care of children with chronic illnesses enrolled in the Washington State Medicaid program, fiscal year 1993. Pediatrics 1997;100(2 Pt 1):197–204.

[6] Angus D, Linde-Zwirble WT, Clermont G, et al. Epidemiology of neonatal respiratory failure in the United States: projections from California and New York. Am J Respir Crit Care Med 2001;164(7):1154–60.

[7] van der Deen M, de Vries EG, Timens W, et al. ATP-binding cassette (ABC) transporters in normal and pathological lung. Respir Res 2005;6(1):59.

[8] Hartl D, Griese M. Interstitial lung disease in children–genetic background and associated phenotypes. Respir Res 2005;6(1):32.

[9] Avery M, Mead J. Surface properties in relation to atelectasis and hyaline membrane disease. AMA J Dis Child 1959;97(5, Pt 1):517–23.

[10] Clements JA. Lung surfactant: a personal perspective. Annu Rev Physiol 1997;59:1–21.

[11] Clements JA, Avery ME. Lung surfactant and neonatal respiratory distress syndrome. Am J Respir Crit Care Med 1998;157(4 Pt 2):S59–66.

[12] Whitsett JA, Stahlman MT. Impact of advances in physiology, biochemistry, and molecular biology on pulmonary disease in neonates. Am J Respir Crit Care Med 1998;157(4 Pt 2): S67–71.

[13] Haller T, Ortmayr J, Friedrich F, et al. Dynamics of surfactant release in alveolar type II cells. Proc Natl Acad Sci USA 1998;95(4):1579–84.

[14] Clements JA. Functions of the alveolar lining. Am Rev Respir Dis 1977;115(6 Pt 2):67–71.

[15] King RJ, Clements JA. Surface active materials from dog lung. II. Composition and physiological correlations. Am J Physiol 1972;223(3):715–26.

[16] Ingenito EP, Mora R, Mark L. Pivotal role of anionic phospholipids in determining dynamic behavior of lung surfactant. Am J Respir Crit Care Med 2000;161(3 Pt 1):831–8.

[17] Veldhuizen R, Nag K, Orgeig S, et al. The role of lipids in pulmonary surfactant. Biochim Biophys Acta 1998;1408(2–3):90–108.

[18] Whitsett JA, Weaver TE. Hydrophobic surfactant proteins in lung function and disease. N Engl J Med 2002;347(26):2141–8.

[19] Shulenin S, Nogee LM, Annilo T, et al. ABCA3 gene mutations in newborns with fatal surfactant deficiency. N Engl J Med 2004;350(13):1296–303.

[20] Clark DA, Pincus LG, Oliphant M, et al. HLA-A2 and chronic lung disease in neonates. JAMA 1982;248(15):1868–9.

[21] Clark JC, Wert SE, Bachurski CJ, et al. Targeted disruption of the surfactant protein B gene disrupts surfactant homeostasis, causing respiratory failure in newborn mice. Proc Natl Acad Sci USA 1995;92(17):7794–8.

[22] Clark JC, Weaver TE, Iwamoto HS, et al. Decreased lung compliance and air trapping in heterozygous SP-B-deficient mice. Am J Respir Cell Mol Biol 1997;16(1):46–52.

[23] Evans M, Palta M, Sadek M, et al. Associations between family history of asthma, bronchopulmonary dysplasia, and childhood asthma in very low birth weight children. Am J Epidemiol 1998;148(5):460–6.

[24] Floros J, Veletza SV, Kotikalapudi P, et al. Dinucleotide repeats in the human surfactant protein-B gene and respiratory-distress syndrome. Biochem J 1995;305(Pt 2):583–90.

[25] Floros J, DiAngelo S, Koptides M, et al. Human SP-A locus: allele frequencies and linkage disequilibrium between the two surfactant protein A genes. Am J Respir Cell Mol Biol 1996; 15(4):489–98.

[26] Floros J, Kala P. Surfactant proteins: molecular genetics of neonatal pulmonary diseases. Annu Rev Physiol 1998;60:365–84.

[27] Fujikura T, Froehlich LA. The influence of race and other factors on pulmonary hyaline membranes. A report from the Collaborative Study of Cerebral Palsy. Am J Obstet Gynecol 1966;95(4):572–8.

[28] Hulsey TC, Alexander GR, Robillard PY, et al. Hyaline membrane disease: the role of ethnicity and maternal risk characteristics. Am J Obstet Gynecol 1993;168(2):572–6.

[29] Jaskoll T, Hu CC, Melnick M. Mouse major histocompatibility complex and lung development: haplotype variation, H-2 immunolocalization, and progressive maturation. Am J Med Genet 1991;39(4):422–36.

[30] Kala P, Koptides M, Diangelo S, et al. Characterization of markers flanking the human SP-B locus. Dis Markers 1997;13(3):153–67.

[31] Kala P, Ten Have T, Nielsen H, et al. Association of pulmonary surfactant protein A (SP-A) gene and respiratory distress syndrome: interaction with SP-B. Pediatr Res 1998;43(2): 169–77.

[32] Karinch AM, deMello DE, Floros J. Effect of genotype on the levels of surfactant protein A mRNA and on the SP-A2 splice variants in adult humans. Biochem J 1997;321(Pt 1): 39–47.

[33] Korfhagen TR, Bruno MD, Ross GF, et al. Altered surfactant function and structure in SP-A gene targeted mice. Proc Natl Acad Sci USA 1996;93(18):9594–9.

[34] McCormick SM, Boggaram V, Mendelson CR. Characterization of mRNA transcripts and organization of human SP-A1 and SP-A2 genes. Am J Physiol 1994;266(4 Pt 1):L354–66.

[35] Miller HC, Futrakul P. Birth weight, gestational age, and sex as determining factors in the incidence of respiratory distress syndrome of prematurely born infants. J Pediatr 1968; 72(5):628–35.

[36] Mason RJ, Greene K, Voelker DR. Surfactant protein A and surfactant protein D in health and disease. Am J Physiol 1998;275(1 Pt 1):L1–13.

[37] Perelman RH, Palta M, Kirby R, et al. Discordance between male and female deaths due to the respiratory distress syndrome. Pediatrics 1986;78(2):238–44.

[38] Richardson DK, Torday JS. Racial differences in predictive value of the lecithin/sphingomyelin ratio. Am J Obstet Gynecol 1994;170(5 Pt 1):1273–8.

[39] Robillard PY, Hulsey TC, Alexander GR, et al. Hyaline membrane disease in black newborns: does fetal lung maturation occur earlier? Eur J Obstet Gynecol Reprod Biol 1994; 55(3):157–61.

[40] Tokieda K, Whitsett JA, Clark JC, et al. Pulmonary dysfunction in neonatal SP-B-deficient mice. Am J Physiol 1997;273(4 Pt 1):L875–82.

[41] Veletza SV, Rogan PK, Ten Have T, et al. Racial differences in allelic distribution at the human pulmonary surfactant protein B gene locus (SP-B). Exp Lung Res 1996;22(4):489–94.

[42] Ikegami M, Korfhagen TR, Whitsett JA, et al. Characteristics of surfactant from SP-A-deficient mice. Am J Physiol 1998;275(2 Pt 1):L247–54.

[43] Weaver TE, Conkright JJ. Function of surfactant proteins B and C. Annu Rev Physiol 2001;63:555–78.

[44] Hallman M. Lung surfactant, respiratory failure, and genes. N Engl J Med 2004;350(13): 1278–80.

[45] Nogee LM, Dunbar AE 3rd, Wert SE, et al. A mutation in the surfactant protein C gene associated with familial interstitial lung disease. N Engl J Med 2001;344(8):573–9.

[46] Nogee LM, de Mello DE, Dehner LP, et al. Brief report: deficiency of pulmonary surfactant protein B in congenital alveolar proteinosis. N Engl J Med 1993;328(6):406–10.

[47] Rodriguez RJ. Management of respiratory distress syndrome: an update. Respir Care 2003; 48(3):279–86 [discussion: 286–7].

[48] Merrill JD, Ballard RA. Pulmonary surfactant for neonatal respiratory disorders. Curr Opin Pediatr 2003;15(2):149–54.

[49] Avery ME, Tooley WH, Keller JB, et al. Is chronic lung disease in low birth weight infants preventable? A survey of eight centers. Pediatrics 1987;79(1):26–30.

[50] McColley S. Bronchopulmonary dysplasia. Impact of surfactant replacement therapy. Pediatr Clin N Amer 1998;45:573–86.

[51] Finer N. Surfactant use for neonatal lung injury: beyond respiratory distress syndrome. Paediatr Resp Rev 2004;5(Suppl A):S289–97.

[52] Smith VC, Zupancic JA, McCormick MC, et al. Trends in severe bronchopulmonary dysplasia rates between 1994 and 2002. J Pediatr 2005;146(4):469–73.

[53] Parker RA, Lindstrom DP, Cotton RB. Evidence from twin study implies possible genetic susceptibility to bronchopulmonary dysplasia. Semin Perinatol 1996;20(3):206–9.

[54] Cole F, Hamvas A, Nogee LM. Genetic disorders of neonatal respiratory function. Pediatr Res 2001;50(2):157–62.

[55] Hamvas A, Wise PH, Yang RK, et al. The influence of the wider use of surfactant therapy on neonatal mortality among blacks and whites. N Engl J Med 1996;334(25):1635–40.

[56] Frisbie W, Song SE, Powers DA, et al. The increasing racial disparity in infant mortality: respiratory distress syndrome and other causes. Demography 2004;41(4):773–800.

[57] Nogee LM. Alterations in SP-B and SP-C expression in neonatal lung disease. Annu Rev Physiol 2004;66:601–23.

[58] Cheong N, Madesh M, Gonzales LW, et al. Functional and trafficking defects in ATP binding cassette A3 mutants associated with respiratory distress syndrome. J Biol Chem 2006; 281(14):9791–800.

[59] Garmany TH, Moxley MA, White FV, et al. Surfactant composition and function in patients with ABCA3 mutations. Pediatr Res 2006;59:801–5.

[60] Bullard JE, Wert SE, Whitsett JA, et al. ABCA3 mutations associated with pediatric interstitial lung disease. Am J Respir Crit Care Med 2005;172(8):1026–31.

[61] Hamvas A. Surfactant protein B deficiency: insights into inherited disorders of lung cell metabolism. Curr Probl Pediatr 1997;27(9):325–45.

[62] Nogee LM, Garnier G, Dietz HC, et al. A mutation in the surfactant protein B gene responsible for fatal neonatal respiratory disease in multiple kindreds. J Clin Invest 1994;93(4): 1860–3.

[63] Hawgood S, Derrick M, Poulain F. Structure and properties of surfactant protein B. Biochim Biophys Acta 1998;1408(2–3):150–60.

[64] Nogee LM, Wert SE, Proffit SA, et al. Allelic heterogeneity in hereditary surfactant protein B (SP-B) deficiency. Am J Respir Crit Care Med 2000;161(3 Pt 1):973–81.

[65] Cole FS, Hamvas A, Rubinstein P, King E, Trusgnich M, Nogee LM, et al. Population-based estimates of surfactant protein B deficiency. Pediatrics 2000;105(3 Pt 1):538–41.

[66] Hamvas A, Trusgnich MA, Brice H, et al. Population-based screening for rare mutations: high-throughput DNA extraction and molecular amplification from Guthrie cards. Pediatr Res 2001;50(5):666–8.

[67] Li J, Hosia W, Hamvas A, et al. N-terminally extended surfactant protein (SP) C isolated from SP-B-deficient children has reduced surface activity and inhibited lipopolysaccharide binding. Biochemistry 2004;43(13):3891–8.

[68] Hamvas A, Nogee LM, Mallory GB Jr, et al. Lung transplantation for treatment of infants with surfactant protein B deficiency. J Pediatr 1997;130(2):231–9.

[69] Beers MF, Hamvas A, Moxley MA, et al. Pulmonary surfactant metabolism in infants lacking surfactant protein B. Am J Respir Cell Mol Biol 2000;22(3):380–91.

[70] Ballard PL, Nogee LM, Beers MF, et al. Partial deficiency of surfactant protein B in an infant with chronic lung disease. Pediatrics 1995;96(6):1046–52.

[71] Klein JM, Thompson MW, Snyder JM, et al. Transient surfactant protein B deficiency in a term infant with severe respiratory failure. J Pediatr 1998;132(2):244–8.

[72] Dunbar AE 3rd, Wert SE, Ikegami M, et al. Prolonged survival in hereditary surfactant protein B (SP-B) deficiency associated with a novel splicing mutation. Pediatr Res 2000; 48(3):275–82.

[73] Ballard PL, Merrill JD, Godinez RI, et al. Surfactant protein profile of pulmonary surfactant in premature infants. Am J Respir Crit Care Med 2003;168(9):1123–8.

[74] Merrill JD, Ballard RA, Cnaan A, et al. Dysfunction of pulmonary surfactant in chronically ventilated premature infants. Pediatr Res 2004;56(6):918–26.

[75] Melton KR, Nesslein LL, Ikegami M, et al. SP-B deficiency causes respiratory failure in adult mice. Am J Physiol Lung Cell Mol Physiol 2003;285(3):L543–9.

[76] Tokieda K, Ikegami M, Wert SE, et al. Surfactant protein B corrects oxygen-induced pulmonary dysfunction in heterozygous surfactant protein B-deficient mice. Pediatr Res 1999; 46(6):708–14.

[77] Tokieda K, Iwamoto HS, Bachurski C, et al. Surfactant protein-B-deficient mice are susceptible to hyperoxic lung injury. Am J Respir Cell Mol Biol 1999;21(4):463–72.

[78] Yusen RD, Cohen AH, Hamvas A. Normal lung function in subjects heterozygous for surfactant protein-B deficiency. Am J Respir Crit Care Med 1999;159(2):411–4.

[79] Cole FS. Surfactant protein B: unambiguously necessary for adult pulmonary function. Am J Physiol Lung Cell Mol Physiol 2003;285(3):L540–2.

[80] Amin R, Wert SE, Baughman RP, et al. Surfactant protein deficiency in familial interstitial lung disease. J Pediatr 2001;139(1):85–92.

[81] Thomas AQ, Lane K, Phillips J 3rd, et al. Heterozygosity for a surfactant protein C gene mutation associated with usual interstitial pneumonitis and cellular nonspecific interstitial pneumonitis in one kindred. Am J Respir Crit Care Med 2002;165(9):1322–8.

[82] Hamvas A, Nogee LM, White FV, et al. Progressive lung disease and surfactant dysfunction with a deletion in surfactant protein C gene. Am J Respir Cell Mol Biol 2004;30(6): 771–6.

[83] Chibbar R, Shih F, Baga M, et al. Nonspecific interstitial pneumonia and usual interstitial pneumonia with mutation in surfactant protein C in familial pulmonary fibrosis. Mod Pathol 2004;17(8):973–80.

[84] Tredano M, Griese M, Brasch F, et al. Mutation of SFTPC in infantile pulmonary alveolar proteinosis with or without fibrosing lung disease. Am J Med Genet A 2004; 126(1):18–26.

[85] Nogee LM, Dunbar AE, Askin F, et al. Mutations in the surfactant protein C gene associated with interstitial lung disease. Chest 2002;121(3 Suppl):20S–1S.

[86] Beers MF, Mulugeta S. Surfactant protein C biosynthesis and its emerging role in conformational lung disease. Annu Rev Physiol 2005;67:663–96.

[87] Stevens PA, Pettenazzo A, Brasch F, et al. Nonspecific interstitial pneumonia, alveolar proteinosis, and abnormal proprotein trafficking resulting from a spontaneous mutation in the surfactant protein C gene. Pediatr Res 2005;57(1):89–98.

[88] Lahti M, Marttila R, Hallman M. Surfactant protein C gene variation in the Finnish population - association with perinatal respiratory disease. Eur J Hum Genet 2004;12(4): 312–20.

[89] Nogee LM. Abnormal expression of surfactant protein C and lung disease. Am J Respir Cell Mol Biol 2002;26(6):641–4.

[90] Glasser SW, Burhans MS, Korfhagen TR, et al. Altered stability of pulmonary surfactant in SP-C-deficient mice. Proc Natl Acad Sci USA 2001;98(11):6366–71.

[91] Glasser SW, Detmer EA, Ikegami M, et al. Pneumonitis and emphysema in sp-C gene targeted mice. J Biol Chem 2003;278(16):14291–8.

[92] Perez-Gil J, Keough KM. Interfacial properties of surfactant proteins. Biochim Biophys Acta 1998;1408(2–3):203–17.

[93] Johansson J. Structure and properties of surfactant protein C. Biochim Biophys Acta 1998; 1408(2–3):161–72.

[94] Bridges JP, Wert SE, Nogee LM, et al. Expression of a human surfactant protein C mutation associated with interstitial lung disease disrupts lung development in transgenic mice. J Biol Chem 2003;278(52):52739–46.

[95] Mulugeta S, Beers MF. Processing of surfactant protein C requires a type II transmembrane topology directed by juxtamembrane positively charged residues. J Biol Chem 2003;278(48):47979–86.

[96] Wang W, Mulugeta S, Russo SJ, et al. Deletion of exon 4 from human surfactant protein C results in aggregosome formation and generation of a dominant negative. J Cell Sci 2003; 116:683–92.

[97] Kabore AF, Wang WJ, Russo SJ, et al. Biosynthesis of surfactant protein C: characterization of aggresome formation by EGFP chimeras containing propeptide mutants lacking conserved cysteine residues. J Cell Sci 2001;114(Pt 2):293–302.

[98] Mulugeta S, Nguyen V, Russo SJ, et al. A surfactant protein C precursor protein BRI-CHOS domain mutation causes endoplasmic reticulum stress, proteasome dysfunction, and caspase 3 activation. Am J Respir Cell Mol Biol 2005;32(6):521–30.

[99] Hampton RY. ER-associated degradation in protein quality control and cellular regulation. Curr Opin Cell Biol 2002;14(4):476–82.

[100] Oyadomari S, Araki E, Mori M. Endoplasmic reticulum stress-mediated apoptosis in pancreatic beta-cells. Apoptosis 2002;7(4):335–45.

[101] Patil C, Walter P. Intracellular signaling from the endoplasmic reticulum to the nucleus: the unfolded protein response in yeast and mammals. Curr Opin Cell Biol 2001;13(3):349–55.

[102] Zhang K, Kaufman RJ. Signaling the unfolded protein response from the endoplasmic reticulum. J Biol Chem 2004;279(25):25935–8.

[103] Niwa M, Walter P. Pausing to decide. Proc Natl Acad Sci USA 2000;97(23):12396–7.

[104] Johnson AL, Braidotti P, Pietra GG, et al. Post-translational processing of surfactant protein-C proprotein: targeting motifs in the NH(2)-terminal flanking domain are cleaved in late compartments. Am J Respir Cell Mol Biol 2001;24(3):253–63.

[105] Brasch F, Schimanski S, Muhlfeld C, et al. Alteration of the pulmonary surfactant system in full-term infants with hereditary ABCA3 deficiency. Am J Respir Crit Care Med 2006; 174(5):571–80.

[106] Dean M, Hamon Y, Chimini G. The human ATP-binding cassette (ABC) transporter superfamily. J Lipid Res 2001;42(7):1007–17.

[107] Holland PM, Abramson RD, Watson R, et al. Detection of specific polymerase chain reaction product by utilizing the 5′—-3′ exonuclease activity of Thermus aquaticus DNA polymerase. Proc Natl Acad Sci USA 1991;88(16):7276–80.

[108] Whitsett JA, Wert SE, Xu Y. Genetic disorders of surfactant homeostasis. Biol Neonate 2005;87(4):283–7.

[109] Hamvas A, Cole FS, deMello DE, et al. Surfactant protein B deficiency: antenatal diagnosis and prospective treatment with surfactant replacement. J Pediatr 1994;125(3):356–61.

[110] Palomar L, Nogee LM, Sweet SC, et al. Long-term outcomes after infant lung transplantation for surfactant protein B deficiency related to other causes of respiratory failure. J Pediatr, in press.

[111] Rosen DM, Waltz DA. Hydroxychloroquine and surfactant protein C deficiency. N Engl J Med 2005;352(2):207–8.

[112] Sweet SC. Pediatric lung transplantation: update 2003. Pediatr Clin North Am 2003;50(6): 1393–417 [ix].

[113] Harmon WE, McDonald RA, Reyes JD, et al. Pediatric transplantation, 1994–2003. Am J Transplant 2005;5(4 Pt 2):887–903.

[114] Meyers BF, de la Morena M, Sweet SC, et al. Primary graft dysfunction and other selected complications of lung transplantation: a single-center experience of 983 patients. J Thorac Cardiovasc Surg 2005;129(6):1421–9.

[115] Deterding R, Fan LL. Surfactant dysfunction mutations in children's interstitial lung disease and beyond. Am J Respir Crit Care Med 2005;172(8):940–1.

ELSEVIER
SAUNDERS

Pediatr Clin N Am
53 (2006) 929–959

PEDIATRIC CLINICS
OF NORTH AMERICA

The Cell Biology of Acute Childhood Respiratory Disease: Therapeutic Implications

Gerald M. Loughlin, MD, Anne Moscona, MD*

Department of Pediatrics, Weill Medical College of Cornell University, 515 East 71st Street, New York, NY, USA

Five diseases: acute respiratory infection (ARI), diarrhea, malaria, measles, and AIDS, are responsible for more than half of all deaths in children younger than age 5. ARI is now the leading cause of mortality in children younger than 5 years, accounting for nearly one fifth (20%) of childhood deaths worldwide, and killing between 2 and 3 million children each year. Because ARI often occurs with other diseases, including measles, malnutrition, and AIDS, childhood deaths attributed to other causes may actually be caused by ARI. The largest portion of ARI deaths occur in Africa and Southeast Asia, and, worldwide, mortality caused by ARI in children younger than 5 years is closely linked to poverty.

Croup, bronchiolitis, and pneumonia are the three major manifestations of ARI that affect young infants worldwide. Viruses belonging to the Paramyxoviridae family, particularly respiratory syncytial virus (RSV), the recently identified human metapneumovirus (HMPV) [1], and the human parainfluenza viruses (HPIVs), cause most cases of childhood croup, bronchiolitis, and pneumonia [2]. Influenza virus also causes a significant burden of disease in young children, although its significance in children was not fully recognized until recently [3]. Although influenza has received a large share of the research focus and funding allocated to the respiratory viruses, the pediatric pathogens RSV and parainfluenza have lagged far behind. For influenza, effective vaccines and antiviral drugs, although urgently needing

This work was supported in part by United States Public Health Service Grants AI31971 and AI056185 to Dr. Moscona from the National Institutes of Health.

* Corresponding author.

E-mail address: anm2047@med.cornell.edu (A. Moscona).

improvement, have been developed based on the scientific advances of the past several decades. Vaccine and antiviral development for RSV and parainfluenza has, in comparison, been strikingly neglected. The pediatric respiratory diseases have received some of the lowest levels of funding compared with other fields of health research [4]. Only limited resources have been devoted to RSV or parainfluenza virus vaccine or antiviral drug development, despite the huge impact of these diseases on illness and hospitalization of infants worldwide. It is therefore especially exciting to report important recent developments that result directly from scientific advances applied to prevention of acute respiratory disease.

This article is organized around several important individual pediatric pathogens that are responsible for croup, bronchiolitis, and pneumonia in children. Pathogens are discussed that have been studied for several decades, including respiratory syncytial virus and the parainfluenza viruses, and viral pathogens that are newly identified as of this writing are human metapneumovirus and human coronavirus NL63. In light of the escalating rate of emergence of new infectious agents, which is fortunately being met with equally rapid advancements in molecular methods of surveillance and pathogen discovery, new organisms will be added to the list in the near future. A section on therapies for bronchiolitis addresses several of the final common pathways that can result from infection with the diverse pathogens, highlighting the mechanisms that may be amenable to therapeutic approaches. The article concludes with a discussion of the overarching impact of new diagnostic strategies.

Respiratory syncytial virus infection

RSV is the leading cause of bronchiolitis and lower respiratory tract infection in young children, accounting for 50% to 90% of all hospitalizations from bronchiolitis. RSV is a member of the *Pneumovirus* genus within the Pneumovirinae subfamily of the Paramyxoviridae family of negative-stranded RNA viruses. RSV replicates initially in the nasopharyngeal epithelium and later spreads to the lower respiratory tract. Viral replication in the small airways causes inflammation, sloughing, and necrosis of the bronchiolar epithelium. The resultant edema and increased mucous secretion may, depending on the severity of disease, cause plugging of the small airways, atelectasis, airway narrowing, and obstruction. Primary infection with RSV in an immunologically naïve host tends to be the most severe, but whether this usually occurs because of immunopathologic mechanisms, immunologic immaturity, or the smaller vulnerable airways of infected infants, or a combination of factors is unclear. The contribution of the virus, the underlying genetic predisposition of the host, and the components of the inflammatory response form a complex picture in the genesis of severe RSV disease, in which the individual roles remain to be delineated.

Genetic susceptibility to severe respiratory syncytial virus

Several abnormal underlying conditions that predispose to severe forms of RSV disease have been enumerated, and include prematurity, preexisting lung disease, and various forms of immunodeficiency. However, one must understand why some apparently healthy infants and children proceed from initial infection to severe lower respiratory tract disease, whereas others experience a relatively mild, self-limited illness. Several groups have recently identified normal genetic variation among humans as a major factor in disease severity. Specific alleles of interleukin (IL)-4 [5] and the IL-4 receptor [6] were identified that are associated with more severe disease, and promoter variants of IL-10, IL-9, and tumor necrosis factor α (TNF-α) genes probably also influence disease severity [7]. Variations at the IL-10 gene locus are associated with a severe form of disease [8]. Ample evidence also exists for a relationship between a locus on the IL-8 gene and disease severity [9,10].

Recently identified variants of the chemokine receptor CCR5 also seem to predispose to severe RSV bronchiolitis [11], and a correlation was established between specific alleles of the genes for surfactant A and D and an increase in disease severity [12,13]. In light of this mounting evidence for specific genetic contributions to RSV disease severity and the possibility that similar or related genetic variation may underlie predisposition to asthma (and the link between respiratory virus infection and asthma [14]), understanding the mechanisms whereby these gene alterations influence pathogenesis will be critical. Early identification of vulnerable individuals could allow for targeted use of prophylactic strategies to protect those genetically at risk, as is currently practiced only for infants with abnormal underlying conditions. These preventative strategies could impact not only the morbidity and mortality of ARI but also the incidence of reactive airway disease.

Immunity to respiratory syncytial virus and inflammatory responses to respiratory syncytial virus infection

RSV primary infection does not confer permanent immunity; repeated re-infection with RSV within 1 year of the previous infection is common in young children, although subsequent infections are usually milder, suggesting some protection against severe disease after primary infection. In adults, secretory neutralizing antibodies (but not serum antibodies) correlate with protection against upper respiratory tract infection, whereas circulating serum antibodies, particularly against F and G glycoproteins, have been shown to protect from infection and decrease progression to the lower airways [15,16]. The limited degree of protection offered by maternal antibody is underscored by the fact that the peak incidence of serious RSV disease is seen in infants aged 2 to 5 months, when maternal antibody is still circulating within the infant.

RSV-induced lower respiratory tract disease (bronchiolitis and pneumonia) results from a balance between cellular damage mediated by the viral pathogen and injury caused by the immune response of the host [17–19]. Although the immunology and immunopathogenesis of RSV infection are not fully understood, humoral and cellular components of the immune system clearly contribute not only to protection from disease but also to pathogenesis of disease.

Mouse models of RSV disease have been used to dissect the contribution of different T-cell subsets and RSV proteins to the pathology of RSV infection and have shown different disease outcomes, depending on the RSV protein used to prime and the cellular response [20]. For example, in BALB/c mice the RSV surface protein G primes for an eosinophilic inflammatory response, mediated by Th2-type CD4+ T cells [21], reminiscent of the responses seen in the formalin-inactivated RSV vaccine model [22]. Although transfer of cytotoxic T lymphocytes (CTLs) to naïve mice resulted in accelerated viral clearance, immunopathology was also enhanced in mice with very active CTLs [23], indicating that CTLs associated with Th1-type responses also contribute to the immunopathology observed in RSV-infected mice. Recent studies have shown that the pattern recognition receptor CD14 (toll-like receptor 4) participates in the innate immune response to RSV [24–26], a response triggered by the F protein.

As in the animal models, cell-mediated immunity in children probably contributes to host defense against RSV but also causes much of the pathologic process, and inappropriate immune responses may drive pulmonary inflammation during naturally acquired infection [27]. Regulation of the response of T lymphocytes to RSV may be critical in determining the clinical outcome of RSV infection. Abnormal T-cell regulatory mechanisms may be related to a hyperactive IgE response, which contributes to an enhanced lung infiltrate [28,29]. Several proinflammatory cytokines detected in respiratory secretions from RSV-infected individuals, including IL-8, RANTES, and macrophage inflammatory protein 1 alpha (MIP-1α), mediate neutrophil and eosinophil chemotaxis, and these cell types can promote host defense and tissue damage. The contribution of Th1 cells to RSV disease in humans is supported by the findings that interferon gamma (IFNγ) is a prevalent cytokine produced by RSV-specific T-cells, and that the presence of IFNγ [30] and the levels of MIP-1α [31], rather than levels of Th2 cytokines, have been shown to correlate most closely with RSV disease severity.

The role of immunopathology in RSV was highlighted after children who had received formalin-inactivated RSV vaccine in 1967 developed enhanced RSV disease on exposure to virus [32]. The intense inflammatory infiltrate in the lungs of vaccinated children suggested an immunopathologic cause of enhanced disease. Animal models have been used successfully to study the immune correlates of pathology and the basis for enhanced disease [29]. The overexuberant inflammatory response, with lymphocytic and eosinophilic infiltration, has been ascribed to an imbalance in the ratio of Th1 to Th2 cells that could have resulted from poor preservation of F during formalin inactivation [33]. The resulting predominance of G in the formalin-inactivated vaccine was believed to cause a pathologic Th2 polarization of the immune response and pulmonary eosinophilia in children who were subsequently naturally infected with RSV.

CD4+ T cells play a major role in the immunopathogenesis of vaccine-enhanced RSV disease [34]. A marked increase in Th2-type cytokine expression (IL-5, IL-13, IL-10) and a reduction in IL-12 expression occurred in mice that were immunized with the formalin-inactivated vaccine, indicating a swing toward Th2 in the genesis of enhanced inflammation [35]. The presence of IL-5 correlated with an eosinophilic infiltration in the mouse lung. In contrast, priming with live RSV resulted in a Th1 pattern of cytokine production and prevented subsequent enhanced disease [36]. A recent study in mice suggests that immune complexes that fix complement also play a key role in the pathogenesis of enhanced disease; the augmented disease in mice is mediated by these immune complexes and abrogated in complement component C3 and B cell–deficient mice [37]. The bronchoconstriction component of the enhanced disease seems to be mediated by complement, whereas the enhanced pneumonia component of disease depends on Th2 effects.

These findings, which enhance understanding of protective immunity and destructive inflammation, suggest important elements to consider in RSV vaccine development [38]. Successful vaccines must induce neutralizing antibody and CD8+ virus-specific CTLs, and should elicit the CD4 cell response that corresponds to the response to natural infection. Although live attenuated vaccines can clearly achieve these goals directly, they are not appropriate for several populations. Therefore, novel strategies are also being applied to the development of nonreplicating vaccines.

Prevention of respiratory syncytial virus disease: active immunization

RSV vaccine development has been hampered in the past decades by the complex factors described earlier, the concerns that resulted from the history of the early formalin-inactivated vaccine trials, and the limited support for study of pediatric respiratory viruses and vaccine development [38,39]. Live-candidate attenuated RSV vaccines were never observed to cause enhanced RSV disease, and intranasal vaccination with live virus vaccines elicit better mucosal immunity than parenterally administered inactivated virus vaccines. Therefore, developing live attenuated vaccines for RSV-naïve populations, including infants, is a priority. However, live attenuated vaccines pose the challenge of finding a balance between overattenuation, with subsequent induction of inefficient immunologic responses, and underattenuation, which may result in disease especially in younger infants. It is therefore heartening to report that recent advances in molecular virology have allowed a live attenuated vaccine candidate to be developed that is well tolerated in infants and protects against challenge [40].

The recovery of infectious virus from cDNA clones of RSV [41,42], based on advances in molecular virology during the last decade, has completely changed the outlook for developing live attenuated RSV vaccines. New vaccine candidates can now be developed by introducing combinations of attenuating mutations into recombinant RSV through direct manipulation of the DNA intermediate. This new strategy is also advantageous for other pediatric respiratory viruses, which are discussed later. Specific mutations are introduced based on a rationale for their attenuating effects. This strategy, based on understanding the genetic basis of attenuation and applying it to the design of vaccines, is referred to as *reverse genetics* and will begin to replace the methods of serial passage of viruses or chemical mutagenesis, strategies that have been classically used to generate attenuating mutations [43].

Live cold-passaged (cp), temperature-sensitive (ts) RSV vaccines (cpts vaccines) containing many attenuating mutations were attractive candidates for live attenuated RSV vaccines. One cpts, the 248/404 vaccine candidate, was safe and immunogenic in RSV-seronegative infants as young as 6 months but was not sufficiently attenuated in 4- to 12-week-old infants. Therefore, additional attenuating mutations were added using the novel technology, and one new vaccine candidate (rA2cp248/404/1030SH) contains five new independent attenuating genetic elements.

In 2005, Karron and colleagues [40] evaluated recombinant RSV vaccines in clinical trials for the first time. The candidate vaccine rA2cp248/404/1030SH was well tolerated and responsible mainly for mild illness (the lower respiratory tract illness observed was associated with other viral infections). Administration of a second dose of this vaccine showed restriction of viral replication, proving that this vaccine could induce protective immunity. Consistent with the mechanisms of natural immunity, the antibody responses to this live attenuated virus were not the primary mediators of protection induced by the vaccine. Thus, rA2cp248/404/1030SH seems to be the first RSV vaccine candidate that is appropriately attenuated for young infants, including infants 1 to 2 months of age. Although half of the youngest infants did not show antibody responses, the limited replication of the second dose suggests that the infants were protected, which is critical because these infants are the most vulnerable and have presented the most challenges to vaccine development. This successful trial provides a map for future trials of recombinant vaccines against RSV and other pediatric respiratory pathogens.

Subunit vaccines, while not viable for infants and therefore of limited use in the normal population, may provide a suitable approach to vaccination in immunosuppressed populations at high risk of severe RSV infection including high risk children, the elderly, and possibly for maternal immunization [38]. One viral surface glycoprotein, the fusion protein (F), has been used as the antigen for developing subunit vaccines (purified F protein [PFP]-1, PFP-2, and PFP-3). These F subunit vaccines have been shown to be moderately immunogenic and well tolerated in healthy seropositive children older than 12 months, children older than 12 months who have cystic fibrosis, and children older than 12 months who have chronic lung disease of prematurity. A meta-analysis of PFP-1 and PFP-2 studies suggested that these vaccines reduced the incidence of RSV infections but not lower respiratory tract infection [44]. The PFP-2 vaccine may show more promise in pregnant women; in a recent trial, it produced fourfold increases in neutralizing antibody titers in mothers and infants at birth and at 2 months of age [45]. Another subunit vaccine candidate is BBG2Na, a peptide from the G (receptor-binding) glycoprotein of RSV that is conjugated to the albumin-binding domain of streptococcal protein G [46,47]. This vaccine is well tolerated, induces neutralizing antibody responses in healthy young adults, and is immunogenic in elderly individuals. Finally, subunit vaccines containing copurified F, G, and M proteins formulated with an alum adjuvant are being investigated [38,48]. However, the likely targets for these vaccines will be elderly adults and those at high risk for severe RSV infection.

Prevention of respiratory syncytial virus disease: passive immunization

Until effective vaccines for RSV are widely available, passive immuno-prophylaxis with RSV antibody preparations is important to protect children at high risk for severe RSV disease. A humanized monoclonal antibody (palivizumab) directed against the RSV fusion protein affords moderate protection to premature infants at high risk for severe RSV disease [49]. Palivizumab is administered monthly through intramuscular injection during the RSV season. Duration of therapy and indications for prophylaxis depend on gestational age, presence or absence of chronic lung disease, and environmental risk factors that increase RSV risk [50].

Another RSV-specific monoclonal antibody derived from palivizumab, MEDI-524 was developed. Compared with palivizumab, this antibody has an 80-fold greater finding affinity for the RSV F protein [51], is 23 times more potent at neutralizing RSV in vitro [51], and more effectively reduces RSV titers in the cotton rat model [51,52]. This preparation is currently in phase 3 trials in children at high risk for RSV and may be preferable to palivizumab in the future. Similar approaches using other monoclonal antibodies are in different stages of clinical development.

Antiviral strategies for respiratory syncytial virus

The role of antivirals in treating RSV infection remains uncertain. Although some studies have failed to show a correlation between viral load and disease severity, others suggest that reduced viral levels correlate with improved clinical outcomes. These findings are not surprising considering the significant role that proinflammatory responses play in the pathogenesis of this virus. Ribavirin is currently the only antiviral agent available for treating children who have RSV lower respiratory tract disease. Although ribavirin is a nucleoside analog that has good activity against RSV in vitro, clinical studies examining its effect in children conflict. Therefore, its use in children remains highly controversial and should only be considered for certain target populations.

Several new antiviral strategies against RSV are currently being investigated, including the promising approach of F protein fusion inhibitors. The RSV F (fusion) glycoprotein, like the F of all paramyxoviruses, mediates fusion between the viral and host cell membranes during infection [53,54]. The F protein forms a trimer during synthesis and is cleaved during transit to the cell surface to produce the final membrane-distal and membrane-anchored subunits. The carboxyl terminal of the membrane-anchored subunit of paramyxovirus F proteins is anchored to the viral membrane, whereas the newly exposed amino terminal contains the fusion peptide that inserts into target membranes during fusion, which occurs at neutral pH [55]. Initially, the paramyxovirus fusion peptide lies deep within the hydrophobic core of the F protein, and for the virion to fuse with the target membrane and effect viral entry, the F protein must undergo an activation step exposing the fusion peptide [56]. For the paramyxovirus HPIV-3, the authors found that the F protein is activated when the adjacent receptor-binding protein, hemagglutinin-neuraminidase (HN), binds to a sialic acid–containing receptor, permitting fusion to occur. On receptor binding, the receptor-binding protein triggers F to fuse [57,58] but must interact with its respective receptor for fusion to occur [53,57,59–61].

This mechanism has now been shown to be true for paramyxoviruses in general [56]; for RSV, G (the receptor binding glycoprotein) must be present and trigger F to fuse. Fig. 1 contains a schematic of the structural transitions that occur once F is activated, and that mediate membrane merger. The ectodomain of the membrane-anchored subunit of F protein contains two hydrophobic domains: the fusion peptide that inserts into the cellular target membrane during fusion and the transmembrane-spanning domain. The fusion peptide is adjacent to the N-terminal heptad repeat (HRN) and the transmembrane domain is adjacent to the C-terminal heptad repeat (HRC). The transient intermediate of F that is anchored to viral and cell membranes is believed to refold and assemble into a fusogenic six-helix bundle (6HB) structure as the HRN and HRC associate into a tight complex with N- and C-peptides aligned in an antiparallel arrangement. The refolding relocates the fusion peptide and transmembrane anchor to the same side, pulling the viral and cell membranes into close proximity and driving fusion [62].

The refolding step of F provides an attractive target for antivirals. The ability of heptad repeat peptides to interfere with the analogous fusion process for HIV has led to a clinically effective peptide inhibitor of HIV infection (T-20, enfuvirtide) [63–65]. Peptides derived from the HRC-peptide regions of several paramyxoviruses, including Sendai, measles, Newcastle disease virus, RSV, and PIV5, can interfere with fusion intermediates of paramyxovirus F proteins [63,66–71] and can inhibit viral infectivity in vitro [66–68,71–75]. It has been proposed that this inhibition occurs because the

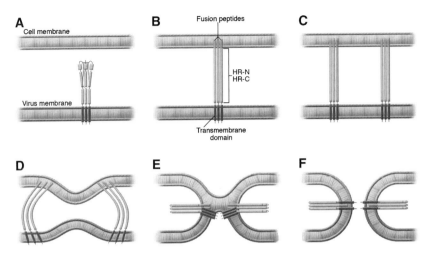

Fig. 1. Model of paramyxovirus fusion protein–mediated membrane fusion. The trimeric F protein (*A*) contains two hydrophobic domains: the fusion peptide and the transmembrane-spanning domain. Each is adjacent to one of two heptad repeat (HR) regions, HR-N and HR-C. The F protein binds to a receptor on the host cell membrane, and a conformational change leads to insertion of the hydrophobic fusion peptide into the host cell membrane (*B*). Multiple trimers of F mediate the fusion process (*C*). Protein refolding occurs as host and viral cell membranes bend toward each other (*D*) and the lipids on the outer part of the membranes begin to interact (*E*). As protein refolding finishes (*F*), the fusion peptide and the transmembrane domain are antiparallel in the same membrane. (*From* Moscona A. Entry of parainfluenza virus into cells as a target for interrupting childhood respiratory disease. J Clin Invest 2005;115:1688–98; with permission.)

peptides bind to their complementary heptad repeat region, thereby preventing HRN and HRC from refolding into the 6HB stable structure required for fusion [56,62,69].

In a related approach, it was recently observed that the *C*-terminal of the HRN trimer contains a hydrophobic pocket that provides a potential binding site for small molecules that might interfere with the stability of the hairpin structure [76], and could provide advantages over the use of peptides in clinical use. A low molecular weight molecule that is highly effective in inhibiting RSV fusion was recently shown to bind this hydrophobic pocket of HRN, suggesting that a small molecule that disrupts the hairpin can derail the RSV fusion process [77]. Inhibition of the F-triggering process by peptides or other small molecules that interact with the heptad repeat regions is a promising area for development of antiviral therapies and awaits further study.

Several other novel experimental approaches to inhibit RSV replication include the use of antisense oligonucleotides and RNA interference technology. These approaches, although promising, are still in early stages of development [78].

Parainfluenza viruses

The HPIV types 1, 2, and 3 (HPIV-1, -2, and -3) are the major cause of croup. Although RSV ranks as the most common agent of bronchiolitis and pneumonia, with HMPV also possibly contributing significantly [1], parainfluenza viruses also follow closely behind [2]. HPIV-3 alone is responsible for approximately 11% of pediatric respiratory hospitalizations in the United States [79,80] and is the predominant cause of croup in young infants. HPIV-1 and -3 belong to the *Respirovirus* genus within the Paramyxovirinae subfamily of the Paramyxoviridae family of negative-stranded RNA viruses, whereas HPIV-2 belongs to the *Rubulavirus* genus.

Although vaccination programs and antiviral use have helped suppress other causes of respiratory disease in children, such as influenza and measles, children are still unaided in their battle against the major cause of croup. While for RSV effective strategies of prophylaxis are available to protect the groups at most risk [81], no weapons are currently available against the parainfluenza viruses.

Immunity to parainfluenza viruses and inflammatory responses to infection

Parainfluenza viruses replicate in the epithelium of the upper respiratory tract and spread to the lower respiratory tract within 3 days. Croup results from inflammatory obstruction of the airway. Epithelial cells of the small airways may become infected, with resultant necrosis and inflammatory infiltrates. The interplay between virus-induced cell damage, beneficial immune responses, and inflammatory responses that contribute to HPIV-3 disease has not been as well studied as for RSV. However, as with RSV, disease severity is often probably increased, and the pathology of clinical disease actually caused, by the inflammatory response rather than the cytopathic effects of the virus. This fundamental concept is highlighted by the fact that virus titers in the infected hosts are generally waning when disease symptoms become apparent [2] and that virus titer does not correlate with the severity of lower respiratory disease. The pathologic changes in children who died from parainfluenza infection suggest exaggerated inflammation [82,83] rather than simply tissue destruction by virus.

HPIV primary infection does not confer permanent immunity. However, although reinfection occurs, immunity is usually sufficient to restrict virus replication from the lower respiratory tract and prevent severe disease. Mucosal IgA levels correlate with protection from replication of parainfluenza viruses in humans [84,85]. Cell-mediated immunity also contributes importantly to preventing disease. For example, HPIV-3 infection in infants who are T-cell–deficient can cause a fatal giant-cell pneumonia [84,85], and HPIV pneumonia has a 30% mortality in bone marrow transplant recipients [86].

A cotton rat (*Sigmodon hispidus*) model of disease has been useful in analyzing factors affecting the pathogenesis of HPIV-3 in vivo. Experimental infection of the cotton rat with HPIV-3 leads to infection of bronchiolar epithelial cells, bronchiolitis, and interstitial pneumonia, mimicking human disease and making it a relevant model for HPIV-3 lower respiratory infection [87]. The authors studied cotton rats infected with either wild-type HPIV-3 or variant viruses containing HN molecules with individual mutations that conferred high receptor-binding avidity or low neuraminidase (receptor-cleaving) activity [88]. The infected animals experienced normal clearance of the variant viruses as opposed to the wild-type viruses; however, each of the HN protein alterations led to striking differences in the ability of HPIV-3 to cause extensive disease in the cotton rat lung. The variants caused alveolitis and an interstitial infiltrate, whereas the wild-type virus only caused peribronchiolitis, and the enhanced disease caused by the HN variants was manifested by greatly increased inflammatory cell infiltrate in the alveoli and interstitial spaces in the lung. This finding suggested that the differences between variants were caused by modulation of the inflammatory response through the different HN protein activity of the variants, and are dissociated from viral replication or infectivity. The authors hypothesize that mutations in the HN protein that alter either its affinity for receptor or its receptor-cleaving activity may modify the nature of the inflammatory response of the host. By using HN variants to dissect the etiology of enhanced disease it may be possible to identify which component(s) of the immune system's response to HPIV3 contributes to disease. Experiments are underway to determine whether HPIV-3 HN protein alterations that enhance disease specifically alter chemokine expression. The results will provide information that could be used to develop therapies to modulate an overactive inflammatory response after HPIV infection.

Prevention of parainfluenza disease: vaccine development

The development of a vaccine for the parainfluenza viruses has been hampered by the need to induce an immune response in young infants whose immature immune systems and maternal antibodies interfere with the development of an adequate immune response. An inactivated HPIV-1, -2, -3 vaccine used in infants in the late 1960s was immunogenic but did not offer protection from infection [89,90]. Experimental vaccines are being evaluated, and a vaccine for HPIV-3 and perhaps also HPIV-1 is anticipated [91–95]. This progress has benefited greatly from the recent advances in molecular virology.

Two different strategies are being developed for HPIV-3 vaccines. One is a live-attenuated bovine parainfluenza type 3 (BPIV-3) vaccine, and the other is a vaccine based on a cold-adapted attenuated strain. The BPIV-3 vaccine is attenuated in humans by nature of host range. The bovine virus itself, when used to infect humans, was well tolerated but did not induce similar levels of antibody titers seen in infection with the human virus. Therefore, the reverse genetics approach was used to generate a set of HPIV-3 variants that carry individual genes from the bovine virus (*chimeric viruses*). These strains elicited an improved antibody response and, in monkeys, protected against HPIV-3 infection. Two of the chimeric viruses, one containing the HN gene from the bovine virus in a human virus background and the other containing the F and HN glycoprotein genes from the human virus in the bovine virus background are now viewed as the strongest vaccine candidates for human trials [96–98]. The latter candidate combines the host range restriction of BPIV-3 with the major antigenic determinants of HPIV-3, permitting efficient replication in vitro (which is beneficial for vaccine development) along with host range phenotype and excellent antigenicity. The bovine/human chimeric approach is also being used to create a strategy for vaccinating simultaneously against HPIV-3 and RSV, and possibly also HMPV. The chimeric virus that contains the HPIV-3 F and HN glycoprotein genes in the BPIV-3 background was engineered to also express protective antigens to RSV and HMPV, and this strategy will lead to bivalent vaccines against HPIV-3/RSV or HPIV-3/HMPV using a single virus. The BPIV-3/HPIV-3 chimera that also expresses RSV F is in clinical trials.

The HPIVs are also theoretically well suited as vaccine vectors for other pediatric pathogen vaccines, especially those that use the respiratory portal for entry, because the intranasal route of administration is highly advantageous. HPIV-3–based vaccines would immunize within the first 6 months of life because the virus infects in early infancy, whereas vaccines using HPIV-1 or HPIV-2 backbones could be used in the second half of the first year of life. Taking the strategy of reverse genetics using HPIV as a backbone vaccine one step further, HPIVs could thereby be used as vaccine vectors for other viruses that infect through the respiratory portal, including severe acute respiratory syndrome (SARS) and Ebola. A BPIV-3/HPIV-3 virus expressing the spike glycoprotein of SARS–coronavirus elicited a neutralizing antibody response and protection against challenge with SARS in African green monkeys [99]. HPIV-3 expressing the glycoprotein of Ebola was highly effective in a guinea pig model [100] and is being evaluated in primates. These types of vaccines could be developed to protect children against emerging infections.

The second attenuated virus being developed for HPIV-3 vaccines, cp45, is based on a live cpts vaccine containing many attenuating mutations. This vaccine is both well-tolerated and immunogenic in children and infants, even those as young as 1 to 2 months [91,93,101,102] and is being further evaluated in clinical trials [93]. Given the promise of this candidate, an attenuated RSV vaccine (the 248/404 cpts vaccine) was tested in combination with the HPIV-3 cp45 vaccine. Although some interference occurred between the two virus vaccines, the results justify further evaluation of combination vaccines [101].

Antiviral strategies for parainfluenza

Several features of the viral lifecycle make parainfluenza viruses vulnerable to attack (Fig. 2). The parainfluenza viruses enter their target cell by binding to a receptor molecule and then fusing their viral envelope with the cell membrane to gain access to the cytoplasm. Because binding and fusion are critical steps for infection to proceed, interfering with these critical processes at the entry stage of the viral lifecycle would prevent disease. The HPIV-3 F protein was found to be fully activated only when the adjacent receptor-binding protein HN binds to sialic acid–containing receptor, permitting fusion to occur. On receptor binding, HN actively triggers F to fuse [57,58,61]. This mechanism is true for most paramyxoviruses [56]. The receptor-binding protein of these viruses, including HPIV-1 and HPIV-2, RSV, measles virus, Hendra virus, and Nipah virus, must interact with its respective receptor for fusion to occur [53,57,59–61].

The authors identified and functionally characterized specific receptor-interacting sites on the HPIV-3 HN molecule [60,103,104], and once the three-dimensional crystal structure of the HN protein was solved [105], they mapped these functional sites onto the HN structure [106]. With this information, binding inhibitors can now be designed specifically to fit into the binding pocket on the globular head of HN (Fig. 2B) [107,108]. In addition to interfering with receptor binding by the HN protein, this blockade will interfere with the F-triggering function of the HN protein, which can only occur when the HN protein is in contact with its receptor.

The F-triggering function provides a target for several antiviral strategies. First, based on a recent analysis of the F-triggering process, peptides corresponding to the HR domains of F (see Fig. 1) can be designed to prevent the F protein from reaching its fusion-active state (Fig. 2C). The authors are performing computational modeling, based on the three-dimensional structure of the related parainfluenza virus 5 (PIV5, previously called Simian Virus 5 or SV5) F [109], to predict which peptides will be most active, and will then test these predictions experimentally. This strategy has been effective at improving the design of antiviral peptides for paramyxoviruses [71]. Preliminary studies in the authors' laboratory also suggest that the normal triggering process may be subverted, causing the F protein to become activated before it reaches the target host cell and incapacitating F before it can mediate viral entry. The authors have shown that specific mutations in the stalk region of HN affect HN's ability to trigger F protein [57], and that specific features of the globular head region of HN modulate this triggering function [61]. However, how the signal for activation is transmitted from HN to F protein is unknown. For example, if HN's receptor binding induces a conformational change in HN, how does this change lead to activation of F? A more detailed understanding of this pathway should lead to additional targets for interruption of viral entry.

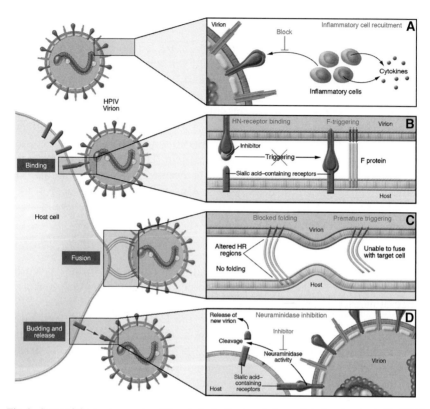

Fig. 2. Steps of the paramyxovirus lifecycle that offer targets for antiviral molecules (with HPIV as the model virus). (*A*) Agents that block HN's recruitment of inflammatory cells to the lung and resultant cytokine expression may reduce the inflammatory response to infection and lessen disease severity. (*B*) Molecules that fit into the binding pocket on HN's head region may inhibit HN-receptor binding and thereby inhibit the F-triggering mediated by HN's stalk. The diagram on the left shows HN with an inhibitor bound, precluding the next step shown on the right, in which HN's receptor-binding has led to F-activation. (*C*) F peptides may prevent the refolding of F that is necessary for fusion during virus entry into the host cell. In addition, the F protein may be triggered too early and thus be put out of action before it reaches the target host cell membrane. (*D*) HN's neuraminidase activity cleaves sialic acid moieties of the cellular receptors, allowing release of new virions from the host cell. Specific inhibition of neuraminidase may prevent virion entry into additional uninfected cells. (*From* Moscona A. Entry of parainfluenza virus into cells as a target for interrupting childhood respiratory disease. J Clin Invest 2005;115:1688–98; with permission.)

Because HPIV-3 pathogenesis is probably largely caused by the inflammatory response to infection, the findings that specific alterations in HN protein correlate with enhanced pathology and that HN may play a role in eliciting inflammatory responses suggest that approaches to modulating the inflammatory response may ameliorate disease (Fig. 2A).

Finally, the HN molecule, in addition to binding to receptors, contains neuraminidase (receptor-cleaving) activity, and cleaves the sialic acid moieties of cellular receptors, allowing new virions to be released from the host cell surface and infection to spread. Although neuraminidase inhibition is unlikely to be as effective an antiviral strategy for parainfluenza viruses as it has been for influenza virus [58,104,110,111], specific inhibition of this activity could prevent virion entry into additional uninfected cells (Fig. 2D). These several potential therapeutic targets are being actively pursued with the hope that they will open new avenues for parainfluenza infection interference; certainly, strategies to protect and treat children with parainfluenza virus infection are urgently needed.

Human metapneumovirus

HMPV is a newly identified respiratory virus that is associated with lower respiratory tract disease in infants and children. This virus was first reported in the Netherlands in 2001 [112] by investigators who identified sequences of the virus after performing randomly primed reverse transcription–polymerase chain reaction (RT-PCR) analysis of respiratory secretions from children who had lower respiratory tract disease. HMPV belongs to the *Metapneumovirus* genus within the Pneumovirinae subfamily of the Paramyxoviridae family of negative-stranded RNA viruses. HMPV may account for much of the lower respiratory disease in young children that was of previously unknown origin [1,113], and a significant portion of upper respiratory infection [114]. It may also cause wheezing episodes in late winter to spring [115] and, less frequently, croup or pneumonia.

Immunity to metapneumovirus and development of vaccine strategies

Although significant information about HMPV has accrued in the 5 years since the virus was recognized as a cause of respiratory disease, much remains to be learned about the incidence of HPMV in specific populations, its basic virology, the strain variation, and the mechanisms of pathogenesis and immunity. Little is known about the correlates of immunity to HMPV infection or about the host–pathogen balance in lung disease, but features are probably shared with RSV and parainfluenza. Infection induces serum-neutralizing antibodies in experimentally infected animals, and protection against reinfection has been induced through primary infection in several animal models [116–118].

A cotton rat model was recently developed for HMPV, with similar features to the cotton rat model for HPIV-3 [118]. Cotton rats were inoculated intranasally with HMPV. The infected cotton rat lungs exhibited the histopathologic changes of peribronchial inflammatory infiltrates, and immunohistochemical staining detected virus at the luminal surfaces of respiratory epithelial cells throughout the respiratory tract. The cotton rats mounted neutralizing antibody responses against HPMV, and on subsequent rechallenge with HMPV, the animals exhibited partial protection in terms of viral replication and lung disease. Therefore, the cotton rat will probably be a useful small animal model of HMPV infection that, as for RSV and HPIV-3, reflects the disease and the correlates of immunity or immunopathology in children [81,87,119,120]. This model will now facilitate the in vivo studies of pathogenesis that lead to development of vaccine and antiviral candidates.

For HPMV, vaccine strategies immediately benefited from the advances in reverse genetics and vaccine technology that were developed for RSV and HPIV-3 and allow recombinant engineered viruses to be generated from DNA clones of viral genes. As a result, live attenuated virus vaccine development for HPMV is already in progress. Recombinant HMPV strains were generated, representing rescue of strains from Canada (strain CAN97-83) and the Netherlands (strains NL/1/00 and NL/1/99) entirely from cDNA [121]. Several chimeric viruses were generated that are considered suitable vaccine candidates. For example, HPMV viruses in which several individual genes (the small hydrophobic protein gene *SH*, the receptor-binding protein gene *G*, or the *M2* gene) or open reading frames were deleted were assessed for their ability to replicate and their efficacy as intranasal vaccines in African green monkeys [122]. Each gene-deletion recombinant virus, although highly attenuated, was also very immunogenic and protected the monkeys against challenge with HMPV. Two of these viruses (*G*-deleted and *M2*-deleted) are promising vaccine candidates [122]. In a different recombinant approach, chimeras were generated by replacing the nucleoprotein or phosphoprotein (P) open reading frame of HMPV with the corresponding gene from the avian metapneumovirus subgroup C [123]. When tested in African green monkeys immunized intranasally and intratracheally, both chimeras were comparable to wild-type HMPV in their immunogenicity and protective efficacy, and the P chimera, although it exhibited excellent growth in vitro (making it feasible for vaccine development) was also highly attenuated. Thus, the P chimera could be a superb vaccine candidate that combines good growth in vitro with attenuation in vivo and excellent protection in a primate model [123]. Candidate vaccines will probably emerge from clinical trials fairly soon, underscoring the importance of recent advances in molecular virology of respiratory viruses in accelerating clinical vaccine development.

Human coronavirus NL63: a new coronavirus cause of croup

Several newly identified members of the coronavirus family cause lower respiratory disease. One is SARS–coronavirus, the etiologic agent of SARS, first detected after cases of a severe atypical pneumonia of unknown origin were reported in late 2002. The disease rapidly spread to more than 25 countries and sickened thousands of individuals by April 2003, and the global medical and scientific communities engaged in a striking cooperative effort that led to rapid progress in identifying the SARS–coronavirus and diagnosing this severe disease [124–127]. Outbreaks have been effectively contained, and research is underway to develop protective measures against this infrequent but fatal disease.

The second novel coronavirus, human coronavirus NL63 (HCoV-NL63), is less virulent but seems to be far more common and a frequent cause of lower respiratory tract disease in young children. Two different groups identified the virus in 2004 [128,129]. The following year, HCoV-NL63–specific quantitative real-time PCR was used to define the clinical spectrum of disease by analyzing more than 900 samples from a prospective study on lower respiratory tract infection in children younger than 3 years [130]. HCoV-NL63 was found to be the third most frequently detected pathogen after RSV and HPIV-3. The infection was strongly associated with croup (rather than bronchiolitis), suggesting a causal relationship, and therefore was probably somewhat less pathogenic than RSV [130]. Thus, another significant cause of respiratory disease in children was added to the list.

Receptor identification for human coronavirus NL63

Cell tropism and receptor use of HCoV-NL63 have been recently analyzed [131]. Receptor identification was performed using the new technology of pseudotyping viruses, in which the surface proteins of one virus can be incorporated into the membrane of another viral particle (eg, HPIV-3 glycoproteins in a retrovirus particle). Thus, binding and entry assays can be performed using the well-characterized and molecularly malleable retrovirus particle. The pseudotype allows engineering of any desired variant of the viral envelope protein being studied, and provides reporter assays for assessment of the envelope protein's ability to mediate binding, fusion, and entry. To identify the HCoV-NL63 receptor, the HCoV-NL63 spike (S) protein was incorporated into the membrane of retroviral particles to analyze cell tropism and receptor engagement of HCoV-NL63 [131]. The NL63 S protein was found to bind angiotensin-converting enzyme 2 (ACE2), the receptor for SARS–coronavirus, and to use ACE2 as a receptor for infection of target cells. Potent neutralizing activity directed against HCoV-NL63's S protein was detected in most sera from individuals aged 8 years or older, suggesting that HCoV-NL63 infection of humans is commonly acquired during childhood. The facts that SARS–coronavirus and HCoV-NL63 use the same receptor but differ greatly in pathogenicity, and HCoV-NL63 infection in children seems to be such a frequent event, raise the concern that pathogenic variants could evolve and highlight the need for coronavirus vaccine development.

Antiviral strategies for HCoV-NL63

Investigation into antiviral strategies began in 2006, 2 years after the new viral agent was identified [132]. Several existing antiviral drugs and new synthetic compounds were tested preliminarily as inhibitors of HCoV-NL63, and several potential strategies were identified for further study, including HR peptides that could interfere with the fusion protein's function and several small interfering RNAs [132]. Identifying common themes in strategies for inhibiting a diverse array of pediatric respiratory viruses (eg, using HR peptides to interfere with fusion during entry) will likely allow advances in the study of one virus to benefit antiviral strategies for other viruses. The scientific progress in understanding viral replication, entry, and fusion for other respiratory viruses will likely benefit the search for antiviral strategies for this newest member of the group of viruses that cause respiratory disease in children.

Treating the final common pathways: new therapies for bronchiolitis

In 1963, two leading pediatricians summarized the "state of the art" of bronchiolitis treatment: "To sum up, oxygen is vitally important and there is little convincing evidence that any other therapy is consistently or even occasionally useful" [133]. Unfortunately, more than 40 years later, this statement is largely still true and few real advances have been made in the pharmacologic treatment of bronchiolitis. The occurrence of wheezing in both RSV-induced bronchiolitis and asthma, coupled with the observation that many infants hospitalized with bronchiolitis caused by RSV or other respiratory viruses are at increased risk for recurrent wheezing episodes in early childhood [134–137], has largely directed the most drug development to focus on acute bronchiolitis to various asthma therapies. In fact, genetic factors governing airway size and control of airway function and variability in the inflammatory response to the viral infection, together with environmental exposures, appear to contribute not only to the pattern of disease seen in acute bronchiolitis but also to the predisposition to recurrent wheezing/asthma [138,139].

Although understanding the mechanisms linking viral bronchiolitis and asthma is critical in light of the implications for therapy, this association remains elusive. As a result, treating bronchiolitis with the same strategies for treating an acute asthma episode has not yielded consistent benefit over the past few decades. Corticosteroids (systemic or inhaled), β agonists, mixed α and β agonists, anticholinergics, and theophylline have been tried and have been generally largely ineffective [140–142]. In light of the pathology of airway obstruction associated with bronchiolitis (desquamation of the respiratory epithelium and airway wall edema), this lack of effectiveness is not surprising. Acute reversible airways obstruction, although common in children who have asthma, is not a constant finding in some patients who have viral bronchiolitis [143], and may relate to the type of immune response generated by the infection. Advances in knowledge of the immunologic and inflammatory factors that contribute to disease may suggest new approaches to treatment and facilitate understanding of the relationship between viral bronchiolitis and recurrent wheezing [19].

Inhibition of leukotrienes

Cysteinyl leukotriene (LTC4, LTD4, and LTE4) concentrations were recently found to be elevated in upper and lower respiratory tract secretions from infants who had RSV bronchiolitis [144,145]. These leukotrienes play a key role in the airway obstruction associated with asthma by mediating mucosal edema, mucus hyper-secretion, recruitment of eosinophils, and smooth muscle contraction. Bisgaard and colleagues [146] showed that a 4-week course of the cysteinyl leukotriene blocker montelukast in infants who had acute RSV bronchiolitis reduced daytime cough and increased the number of symptom-free days. Although this study population included children up to 36 months of age experiencing first-time wheezing, a detailed analysis of these data suggests that the effect was most pronounced in the younger subjects, an observation that correlates well with the evidence for higher levels of leukotriene levels in infants younger than 6 months [145,146]. The study design focused on long-term rather than acute effects, and insufficient data support the use of montelukast for treating milder forms of the disease, or for relieving airways obstruction in the acute setting. As those authors and an accompanying editorial note, further investigation in an appropriate study population with documented RSV infection are needed to gauge the benefit of this therapy [147].

DNase treatment

The observation that secretions composed primarily of desquamated epithelial cells obstruct the small airways in children who have bronchiolitis suggested the use of recombinant human deoxyribonuclease I, a treatment that has been effective in patients who have cystic fibrosis. In one study of hospitalized infants who had acute RSV bronchiolitis, the chest radiographs at discharge showed that recombinant human DNase treatment was associated with significant improvement [148]. However, therapy did not affect other clinical features, such as respiratory rate, wheezing, and retractions. A similar, smaller intervention study in more severely ill patients also showed this therapy to be effective in correcting massive atelectasis and avoiding the need for mechanical ventilation in patients who had impending respiratory failure [149]. As with leukotrienes, more studies are needed to define the usefulness of this therapy. This intervention is one of few that focus on addressing the problem of airway obstruction.

Surfactant replacement

Decreased levels of surfactant protein (SP)-A, -B, and -D have been reported in infants who have RSV bronchiolitis [150]. In mice, surfactant deficiency confers an increased susceptibility to inflammation during RSV infection [151,152]. If this increased susceptibility is also found in humans, identifying infants deficient in SP-A or -D who would be at risk for more severe RSV disease would be beneficial to target for prevention and therapy. Therefore, surfactant replacement is logical not only because of its effect on improving lung function but also because of the potential benefits of decreasing inflammation. In a small study of ventilated patients who had RSV bronchiolitis, the patients experiencing respiratory failure who were treated with two doses of bovine surfactant showed improved static compliance (indicative of decreased hyperinflation) and decreased airways resistance compared with the untreated patients [153]. No acute improvement in gas exchange occurred, but the group treated with surfactant showed improved oxygenation and ventilation indices over the first 60 hours of mechanical ventilation. Unfortunately, surfactant currently must be delivered through endotracheal intubation, and therefore this therapy is reserved for children in respiratory failure. Larger studies are needed to assess the effects of surfactant on the duration of mechanical ventilation and on viral clearance [154].

Rapid diagnostic strategies for respiratory viruses

The development of accurate and rapid diagnostic assays for respiratory viruses is key for two seemingly separate but rapidly converging arenas. Diagnosis will become increasingly important to clinical management of individual children, and is urgently needed for global public health, including pathogen surveillance. In recent years significant progress has been made in applying advances in molecular biology to respiratory virus diagnosis, and some of the new strategies are already clinically useful [155–157]. For the practitioner, guidelines and clear data are needed regarding the situations in which specific kinds of assays may be appropriate. The transition of these technologies from the development stage to the clinically useful stage is still in flux. However, one may look forward to a situation in which public health institutions will be rapidly responsive to pathogens arising in the community and practitioners will be able to use detailed information to guide prevention or therapy.

MassTag polymerase chain reaction: a paradigm for new detection strategies for early recognition and containment of a wide range of respiratory pathogens

Recently, Briese and colleagues [158] described the development of a MassTag PCR for differential diagnosis of respiratory disease. MassTag PCR is a multiplex assay in which the pathogen gene targets are coded by a library of 64 distinct mass tags. The microbial RNA or DNA is amplified by multiplex RT-PCR using up to 64 primers. Each primer is labeled with a different molecular weight tag, which is attached to the primer with a photo-cleavable link. After amplification, the mass tags are released from the amplified material with UV irradiation, and the identity of the tag is determined with mass spectrometry. The identity of the organism is determined from the presence of its two specific tags, one from each primer. The technology was successfully applied to respiratory disease in its first test case [158]. The multiplex primer sets were designed to identify up to 22 respiratory pathogens in a single MassTag PCR reaction, and the method was found to be highly sensitive and specific for diagnosing these viral and bacterial agents in clinical samples. The tests were performed using blinded analysis of previously diagnosed clinical specimens (banked sputum, nasal swabs, and lung washes), and the MassTag PCR was highly effective at identifying all pathogens, including RSV; HPIV-1, -2, and -3; HMPV; influenza; and coronavirus-SARS (HCoV-NL63 was not included in the study). This technology probably will be used most immediately in the public health setting for identifying outbreaks and global surveillance. As the technology becomes streamlined and mass spectrometry becomes more easily accessible, this method has great potential for individual patient management.

Diagnosing respiratory syncytial virus and paramyxovirus human parainfluenza virus in the clinical setting

RSV and HPIV antigens can be rapidly identified in individual patients using commercially available rapid screening kits with sensitivities and specificities of 80% to 90%. These tests are performed directly on nasopharyngeal secretions using either fluorescent-conjugated antibody or ELISA with a monoclonal antibody [155]. Multiplex quantitative RT-PCR–enzyme hybridization assays can identify a panel of respiratory viruses and differentiate between RSV viral subtypes A and B and HPIV-1, -2 and -3 [159–161]. The Hexaplex assay (Prodesse, Inc., Milwaukee, Wisconsin) [159] is a multiplex RT-PCR assay for detecting HPIV-1, -2, and -3; RSV A and B; and influenza virus types A and B. Although the sensitivity, specificity, and positive and negative predictive values are excellent [159], confirmation with viral culture (either rapid or traditional) is still important, especially with a negative result in an ill child. PCR-based technology may provide a useful contribution to diagnosis and subtyping of RSV and HPIV-3 in the future [157].

These assay kits, and those for antigen detection, allow simple screening of children and will likely be used more commonly in the future as more therapies for pediatric respiratory viruses become available. However, it is hoped that the importance of accurate viral diagnosis gains wider acceptance among practitioners, especially during influenza season, when prompt specific treatment for influenza can effectively shorten the duration and lessen the severity of disease in children [110]. Identification of the etiologic agent, even if no specific therapy is available, is critical in containing respiratory virus outbreaks and avoiding transmission to vulnerable individuals.

Diagnosing newly identified pathogens: human metapneumovirus and coronavirus NL63

Although HMPV was included among the 22 respiratory pathogens successfully identified in the single MassTag PCR described earlier [158], clinical diagnosis of this recently identified pathogen is still less developed than for RSV and HPIV. However, molecular methods have been developed recently [162–164]. HMPV virus in respiratory secretions is best identified with RT-PCR. Several of the original clinical reports on this virus used RT-PCR assays that used PCR primers hybridizing to the polymerase (L) gene, and used the L gene PCR product sequence to identify the virus. Faster and specific real-time RT-PCR tests were developed over the past 2 years that can also detect viruses from the four known genetic lineages of HMPV [163–165].

Diagnostic strategies for HCoV-NL63 were developed for use in population studies to assess the incidence of infection with this virus and its association with respiratory disease [130,166]. Whether HCoV-NL63 diagnosis will have a place in practice, or whether identifying this agent will be most important in the public health setting, is unclear. A "pan-coronavirus" RT-PCR assay was recently developed and used to assess respiratory disease in hospitalized children [166]. The original consensus RT-PCR assay, which was designed to amplify all known coronaviruses, is unable to detect HCoV-NL63 because of mismatches with the primer sequences [167]. For the new assay, the consensus primers were modified based on an alignment with the HCoV-NL63 prototype sequence. In addition to HCoV-NL63 and SARS–coronavirus, the two other human coronaviruses known to infect the respiratory tract, OC43 (HCoV-OC43) and 229E (HCoV-229E), were included in the optimized pan-coronavirus RT-PCR assay. In addition to identifying the specific viral infections, sequence analysis of amplified gene segments showed that the HCoV-NL63 isolates could be classified into the two subtypes corresponding to the two prototype HCoV-NL63 sequences.

The pan-coronavirus assay was tested not only on the four known human coronaviruses, but also on three animal coronaviruses: feline infectious peritonitis virus, porcine hemagglutinating encephalomyelitis virus, and murine hepatitis virus. The results suggest that the assay efficiently amplifies a broad range of coronaviruses, both human and animal. This pan-coronavirus RT-PCR assay could be especially useful for its ability to identify previously unknown coronaviruses.

Acknowledgments

Support has been generously provided to Dr. Moscona's laboratory for portions of the work discussed here by United States Public Health Service Grants AI31971 and AI056185. Dr. Moscona would like to thank Carole Heilman, Sonnie Kim, Fran Rubin, and Cristina Cassetti and their colleagues at the National Institutes of Allergy and Infectious Diseases for their unwavering support of pediatric respiratory virus research.

References

[1] Williams JV, Harris PA, Tollefson SJ, et al. Human metapneumovirus and lower respiratory tract disease in otherwise healthy infants and children. N Engl J Med 2004;350(5): 443–50.

[2] Collins P, Chanock R, McIntosh K. Parainfluenza viruses. In: Fields B, Knipe DM, Howley P, editors. Fields virology. Philadelphia: Lippincott-Raven Publishers; 1996. p. 1205–41.

[3] Poehling KA, Edwards KM, Weinberg GA, et al. The underrecognized burden of influenza in young children. N Engl J Med 2006;355(1):31–40.

[4] Michaud CM, Murray CJ, Bloom BR. Burden of disease–implications for future research. JAMA 2001;285(5):535–9.

[5] Choi EH, Lee HJ, Yoo T, Chanock SJ. A common haplotype of interleukin-4 gene IL4 is associated with severe respiratory syncytial virus disease in Korean children. J Infect Dis 2002;186(9):1207–11.

[6] Hoebee B, Rietveld E, Bont L, et al. Association of severe respiratory syncytial virus bronchiolitis with interleukin-4 and interleukin-4 receptor alpha polymorphisms. J Infect Dis 2003;187(1):2–11.

[7] Hoebee B, Bont L, Rietveld E, van, et al. Influence of promoter variants of interleukin-10, interleukin-9, and tumor necrosis factor-alpha genes on respiratory syncytial virus bronchiolitis. J Infect Dis 2004;189(2):239–47.

[8] Wilson J, Rowlands K, Rockett K, et al. Genetic variation at the IL10 gene locus is associated with severity of respiratory syncytial virus bronchiolitis. J Infect Dis 2005;191(10): 1705–9.

[9] Hull J, Ackerman H, Isles K, et al. Unusual haplotypic structure of IL8, a susceptibility locus for a common respiratory virus. Am J Hum Genet 2001;69(2):413–9.

[10] Hull J, Rowlands K, Lockhart E, et al. Haplotype mapping of the bronchiolitis susceptibility locus near IL8. Hum Genet 2004;114(3):272–9.

[11] Hull J, Rowlands K, Lockhart E, et al. Variants of the chemokine receptor CCR5 are associated with severe bronchiolitis caused by respiratory syncytial virus. J Infect Dis 2003; 188(6):904–7.

[12] Lahti M, Lofgren J, Marttila R, et al. Surfactant protein D gene polymorphism associated with severe respiratory syncytial virus infection. Pediatr Res 2002;51(6):696–9.

[13] Lofgren J, Ramet M, Renko M, et al. Association between surfactant protein A gene locus and severe respiratory syncytial virus infection in infants. J Infect Dis 2002; 185(3):283–9.

[14] Ehlenfield DR, Cameron K, Welliver RC. Eosinophilia at the time of respiratory syncytial virus bronchiolitis predicts childhood reactive airway disease. Pediatrics 2000;105(1 Pt 1): 79–83.

[15] Anderson LJ, Heilman CA. Protective and disease-enhancing immune responses to respiratory syncytial virus. J Infect Dis 1995;171(1):1–7.

[16] Falsey AR, Walsh EE. Relationship of serum antibody to risk of respiratory syncytial virus infection in elderly adults. J Infect Dis 1998;177(2):463–6.

[17] Welliver RC. Immunology of respiratory syncytial virus infection: eosinophils, cytokines, chemokines and asthma. Pediatr Infect Dis J 2000;19(8):780–3 [discussion: 784–5; 811–3].

[18] van Schaik SM, Obot N, Enhorning G, et al. Role of interferon gamma in the pathogenesis of primary respiratory syncytial virus infection in BALB/c mice. J Med Virol 2000;62(2): 257–66.

[19] van Schaik SM, Welliver RC, Kimpen JL. Novel pathways in the pathogenesis of respiratory syncytial virus disease. Pediatr Pulmonol 2000;30(2):131–8.

[20] Srikiatkhachorn A, Braciale TJ. Virus-specific memory and effector T lymphocytes exhibit different cytokine responses to antigens during experimental murine respiratory syncytial virus infection. J Virol 1997;71(1):678–85.

[21] Alwan WH, Kozlowska WJ, Openshaw PJ. Distinct types of lung disease caused by functional subsets of antiviral T cells. J Exp Med 1994;179(1):81–9.

[22] Openshaw PJ, Clarke SL, Record FM. Pulmonary eosinophilic response to respiratory syncytial virus infection in mice sensitized to the major surface glycoprotein G. Int Immunol 1992;4(4):493–500.

[23] Cannon MJ, Openshaw PJ, Askonas BA. Cytotoxic T cells clear virus but augment lung pathology in mice infected with respiratory syncytial virus. J Exp Med 1988;168(3):1163–8.

[24] Haeberle HA, Takizawa R, Casola A, et al. Respiratory syncytial virus-induced activation of nuclear factor-kappaB in the lung involves alveolar macrophages and toll-like receptor 4-dependent pathways. J Infect Dis 2002;186(9):1199–206.

[25] Haynes LM, Moore DD, Kurt-Jones EA, et al. Involvement of toll-like receptor 4 in innate immunity to respiratory syncytial virus. J Virol 2001;75(22):10730–7.

[26] Kurt-Jones EA, Popova L, et al. Pattern recognition receptors TLR4 and CD14 mediate response to respiratory syncytial virus. Nat Immunol 2000;1(5):398–401.

[27] Scott R, Kaul A, Scott M, et al. Development of in vitro correlates of cell-mediated immunity to respiratory syncytial virus infection in humans. J Infect Dis 1978;137(6):810–7.

[28] Welliver RC, Kaul TN, Sun M, et al. Defective regulation of immune responses in respiratory syncytial virus infection. J Immunol 1984;133(4):1925–30.

[29] Openshaw PJ, Culley FJ, Olszewska W. Immunopathogenesis of vaccine-enhanced RSV disease. Vaccine 2001;20(Suppl 1):S27–31.

[30] Bont L, Heijnen CJ, Kavelaars A, et al. Local interferon-gamma levels during respiratory syncytial virus lower respiratory tract infection are associated with disease severity. J Infect Dis 2001;184(3):355–8.

[31] Garofalo RP, Patti J, Hintz KA, et al. Macrophage inflammatory protein-1alpha (not T helper type 2 cytokines) is associated with severe forms of respiratory syncytial virus bronchiolitis. J Infect Dis 2001;184(4):393–9.

[32] Kim HW, Canchola JG, Brandt CD, et al. Respiratory syncytial virus disease in infants despite prior administration of antigenic inactivated vaccine. Am J Epidemiol 1969;89(4):422–34.

[33] Graham BS. Pathogenesis of respiratory syncytial virus vaccine-augmented pathology. Am J Respir Crit Care Med 1995;152(4 Pt 2):S63–6.

[34] Connors M, Kulkarni AB, Firestone CY, et al. Pulmonary histopathology induced by respiratory syncytial virus (RSV) challenge of formalin-inactivated RSV-immunized BALB/c mice is abrogated by depletion of CD4+ T cells. J Virol 1992;66(12):7444–51.

[35] Waris ME, Tsou C, Erdman DD, et al. Respiratory syncytial virus infection in BALB/c mice previously immunized with formalin-inactivated virus induces enhanced pulmonary inflammatory response with a predominant Th2-like cytokine pattern. J Virol 1996;70(5):2852–60.

[36] Waris ME, Tsou C, Erdman DD, et al. Priming with live respiratory syncytial virus (RSV) prevents the enhanced pulmonary inflammatory response seen after RSV challenge in BALB/c mice immunized with formalin-inactivated RSV. J Virol 1997;71(9):6935–9.

[37] Polack FP, Teng MN, Collins PL, et al. A role for immune complexes in enhanced respiratory syncytial virus disease. J Exp Med 2002;196(6):859–65.

[38] Polack FP, Karron RA. The future of respiratory syncytial virus vaccine development. Pediatr Infect Dis J 2004;23(1 Suppl):S65–73.

[39] Englund J. In search of a vaccine for respiratory syncytial virus: the saga continues. J Infect Dis 2005;191(7):1036–9.

[40] Karron RA, Wright PF, Belshe RB, et al. Identification of a recombinant live attenuated respiratory syncytial virus vaccine candidate that is highly attenuated in infants. J Infect Dis 2005;191(7):1093–104.

[41] Collins P, Mink M, Stec D. Rescue of synthetic analogs of respiratory syncytial virus genomic RNA and effect of truncations and mutations on the expression of a foreign reporter gene. Proc Natl Acad Sci U S A 1991;88:9663–7.

[42] Collins PL, Hill MG, Camargo E, et al. Production of infectious human respiratory syncytial virus from cloned cDNA confirms an essential role for the transcription elongation factor from the 5′ proximal open reading frame of the M2 mRNA in gene expression and provides a capability for vaccine development. Proc Natl Acad Sci U S A 1995;92(25): 11563–7.

[43] Murphy BR, Collins PL. Live-attenuated virus vaccines for respiratory syncytial and parainfluenza viruses: applications of reverse genetics. J Clin Invest 2002;110(1):21–7.

[44] Simoes EA, Tan DH, Ohlsson A, et al. Respiratory syncytial virus vaccine: a systematic overview with emphasis on respiratory syncytial virus subunit vaccines. Vaccine 2001; 20(5–6):954–60.

[45] Munoz FM, Piedra PA, Glezen WP. Safety and immunogenicity of respiratory syncytial virus purified fusion protein-2 vaccine in pregnant women. Vaccine 2003;21(24): 3465–7.

[46] Plotnicky-Gilquin H, Robert A, Chevalet L, et al. CD4(+) T-cell-mediated antiviral protection of the upper respiratory tract in BALB/c mice following parenteral immunization with a recombinant respiratory syncytial virus G protein fragment. J Virol 2000; 74(8):3455–63.

[47] Power UF, Nguyen TN, Rietveld E, et al. Safety and immunogenicity of a novel recombinant subunit respiratory syncytial virus vaccine (BBG2Na) in healthy young adults. J Infect Dis 2001;184(11):1456–60.

[48] Ison MG, Johnston SL, Openshaw P, et al. Current research on respiratory viral infections: Fifth International Symposium. Antiviral Res 2004;62(3):75–110.

[49] Prevention of respiratory syncytial virus infections: indications for the use of palivizumab and update on the use of RSV-IGIV. American Academy of Pediatrics Committee on Infectious Diseases and Committee of Fetus and Newborn. Pediatrics 1998;102(5): 1211–6.

[50] Meissner HC, Long SS. Revised indications for the use of palivizumab and respiratory syncytial virus immune globulin intravenous for the prevention of respiratory syncytial virus infections. Pediatrics 2003;112(6 Pt 1):1447–52.

[51] Wu H, Pfarr DS, Tang Y, et al. Ultra-potent antibodies against respiratory syncytial virus: effects of binding kinetics and binding valence on viral neutralization. J Mol Biol 2005; 350(1):126–44.

[52] Mejias A, Chavez-Bueno S, Rios AM, et al. Asthma and respiratory syncytial virus. New opportunities for therapeutic intervention. An Pediatr (Barc) 2004;61(3):252–60 [in Spanish].

[53] Lamb R. Paramyxovirus fusion: a hypothesis for changes. Virology 1993;197:1–11.

[54] Plemper RK, Lakdawala AS, Gernert KM, et al. Structural features of paramyxovirus F protein required for fusion initiation. Biochemistry 2003;42(22):6645–55.

[55] Hernandez LD, Hoffman LR, Wolfsberg TG, et al. Virus-cell and cell-cell fusion. Annu Rev Cell Dev Biol 1996;12:627–61.

[56] Colman PM, Lawrence MC. The structural biology of type I viral membrane fusion. Nat Rev Mol Cell Biol 2003;4(4):309–19.

[57] Porotto M, Murrell M, Greengard O, et al. Triggering of human parainfluenza virus 3 fusion protein(F) by the hemagglutinin-neuraminidase (HN): an HN mutation diminishing the rate of F activation and fusion. J Virol 2003;77(6):3647–54.

[58] Moscona A. Entry of parainfluenza virus into cells as a target for interrupting childhood respiratory disease. J Clin Invest 2005;115(7):1688–98.

[59] Moscona A, Peluso RW. Fusion properties of cells persistently infected with human parainfluenza virus type 3: Participation of hemagglutinin-neuraminidase in membrane fusion. J Virol 1991;65:2773–7.

[60] Moscona A, Peluso RW. Relative affinity of the human parainfluenza virus 3 hemagglutinin-neuraminidase for sialic acid correlates with virus-induced fusion activity. J Virol 1993; 67:6463–8.

[61] Porotto M, Murrell M, Greengard O, et al. Influence of the human parainfluenza virus 3 attachment protein's neuraminidase activity on its capacity to activate the fusion protein. J Virol 2005;79(4):2383–92.

[62] Russell CJ, Jardetzky TS, Lamb RA. Membrane fusion machines of paramyxoviruses: capture of intermediates of fusion. EMBO J 2001;20(15):4024–34.

[63] Wild CT, Shugars DC, Greenwell TK, et al. Peptides corresponding to a predictive alpha-helical domain of human immunodeficiency virus type 1 gp41 are potent inhibitors of virus infection. Proc Natl Acad Sci U S A 1994;91(21):9770–4.

[64] Wild C, Oas T, McDanal C, et al. A synthetic peptide inhibitor of human immunodeficiency virus replication: correlation between solution structure and viral inhibition. Proc Natl Acad Sci U S A 1992;89(21):10537–41.

[65] Eckert DM, Kim PS. Design of potent inhibitors of HIV-1 entry from the gp41 N-peptide region. Proc Natl Acad Sci U S A 2001;98(20):11187–92.

[66] Rapaport D, Ovadia M, Shai Y. A synthetic peptide corresponding to a conserved heptad repeat domain is a potent inhibitor of Sendai virus-cell fusion: an emerging similarity with functional domains of other viruses. EMBO J 1995;14(22):5524–31.

[67] Lambert DM, Barney S, Lambert AL, et al. Peptides from conserved regions of paramyxovirus fusion (F) proteins are potent inhibitors of viral fusion. Proc Natl Acad Sci U S A 1996;93(5):2186–91.

[68] Yao Q, Compans RW. Peptides corresponding to the heptad repeat sequence of human parainfluenza virus fusion protein are potent inhibitors of virus infection. Virology 1996; 223(1):103–12.

[69] Baker KA, Dutch RE, Lamb RA, et al. Structural basis for paramyxovirus-mediated membrane fusion. Mol Cell 1999;3(3):309–19.

[70] Lu M, Blacklow SC, Kim PS. A trimeric structural domain of the HIV-1 transmembrane glycoprotein. Nat Struct Biol 1995;2(12):1075–82.

[71] Porotto M, Doctor L, Carta P, et al. Inhibition of Hendra virus membrane fusion. J Virol 2006; In press.

[72] Joshi SB, Dutch RE, Lamb RA. A core trimer of the paramyxovirus fusion protein: parallels to influenza virus hemagglutinin and HIV-1 gp41. Virology 1998;248(1):20–34.

[73] Wild TF, Buckland R. Inhibition of measles virus infection and fusion with peptides corresponding to the leucine zipper region of the fusion protein. J Gen Virol 1997;78(Pt 1): 107–11.

[74] Young JK, Hicks RP, Wright GE, et al. Analysis of a peptide inhibitor of paramyxovirus (NDV) fusion using biological assays, NMR, and molecular modeling. Virology 1997; 238(2):291–304.

[75] Young JK, Li D, Abramowitz MC, et al. Interaction of peptides with sequences from the newcastle disease virus fusion protein heptad repeat regions. J Virol 1999;73(7): 5945–56.

[76] Chan DC, Chutkowski CT, Kim PS. Evidence that a prominent cavity in the coiled coil of HIV type 1 gp41 is an attractive drug target. Proc Natl Acad Sci U S A 1998;95(26):15613–7.

[77] Cianci C, Langley DR, Dischino DD, et al. Targeting a binding pocket within the trimer-of-hairpins: small-molecule inhibition of viral fusion. Proc Natl Acad Sci U S A 2004;101(42): 15046–51.

[78] Maggon K, Barik S. New drugs and treatment for respiratory syncytial virus. Rev Med Virol 2004;14(3):149–68.

[79] Chanock RM. Control of pediatric viral diseases: past successes and future prospects. Pediatr Res 1990;27(6 Suppl):S39–43.

[80] Murphy BR. Current approaches to the development of vaccines effective against parainfluenza viruses. Bull World Health Organ 1988;66(3):391–7.

[81] Groothuis J, Simoes E, Levin M, et al. Prophylactic administration of respiratory syncytial virus immune globulin to high-risk infants and young children. N Engl J Med 1993;329: 1524–30.

[82] Aherne W, Bird T, Court S, et al. Pathological changes in virus infections of the lower respiratory tract in children. J Clin Pathol 1970;23:7–18.

[83] Downham M, Gardner P, McQuillin J, et al. Role of respiratory viruses in childhood mortality. Br Med J 1975;1:235–9.

[84] Smith C, Purcell R, Bellanti J, et al. Protective effect of antibody to parainfluenza type 1 virus. N Engl J Med 1966;275:1145–52.

[85] Tremonti L, Lin J, Jackson G. Neutralizing activity in nasal secretions and serum in resistance of volunteers to parainfluenza virus type 2. J Immunol 1968;101:572–7.

[86] Wendt C, Weisdorf D, Jordan M, et al. Parainfluenza virus respiratory infection after bone marrow transplantation. N Engl J Med 1992;326:921–6.

[87] Porter D, Prince G, Hemming V, et al. Pathogenesis of human parainfluenza virus 3 infection in two species of cotton rat: *Sigmodon hispidus* develops bronchiolitis, while *Sigmodon fulviventer* develops interstitial pneumonia. J Virol 1991;65:103–11.

[88] Prince GA, Ottolini MG, Moscona A. Contribution of the human parainfluenza virus type 3 HN-receptor interaction to pathogenesis in vivo. J Virol 2001;75(24):12446–51.

[89] Chin J, Magoffin R, Shearer L, et al. Field evaluation of a respiratory syncytial virus vaccine and a trivalent parainfluenza virus vaccine in a pediatric population. Am J Epidemiol 1969; 89:449–63.

[90] Fulginiti V, Eller J, Sieber O, et al. Respiratory virus immunization. I. A field trial of two inactivated respiratory virus vaccines; an aqueous trivalent parainfluenza virus vaccine and an alum-precipitated respiratory syncytial virus vaccine. Am J Epidemiol 1969; 89:435–48.

[91] Belshe RB, Newman FK, Tsai TF, et al. Phase 2 evaluation of parainfluenza type 3 cold passage mutant 45 live attenuated vaccine in healthy children 6–18 months old. J Infect Dis 2004;189(3):462–70.

[92] Karron RA, Belshe RB, Wright PF, et al. A live human parainfluenza type 3 virus vaccine is attenuated and immunogenic in young infants. Pediatr Infect Dis J 2003;22(5): 394–405.

[93] Madhi SA, Cutland C, Zhu Y, et al. Transmissibility, infectivity and immunogenicity of a live human parainfluenza type 3 virus vaccine (HPIV3cp45) among susceptible infants and toddlers. Vaccine 2006;24(13):2432–9.

[94] Greenberg DP, Walker RE, Lee MS, et al. A bovine parainfluenza virus type 3 vaccine is safe and immunogenic in early infancy. J Infect Dis 2005;191(7):1116–22.

[95] Newman JT, Riggs JM, Surman SR, et al. Generation of recombinant human parainfluenza virus type 1 vaccine candidates by importation of temperature-sensitive and attenuating mutations from heterologous paramyxoviruses. J Virol 2004;78(4):2017–28.

[96] Haller AA, Miller T, Mitiku M, et al. Expression of the surface glycoproteins of human parainfluenza virus type 3 by bovine parainfluenza virus type 3, a novel attenuated virus vaccine vector. J Virol 2000;74(24):11626–35.

[97] Pennathur S, Haller AA, MacPhail M, et al. Evaluation of attenuation, immunogenicity and efficacy of a bovine parainfluenza virus type 3 (PIV-3) vaccine and a recombinant chimeric bovine/human PIV-3 vaccine vector in rhesus monkeys. J Gen Virol 2003;84(Pt 12): 3253–61.

[98] Schmidt AC, McAuliffe JM, Huang A, et al. Bovine parainfluenza virus type 3 (BPIV3) fusion and hemagglutinin-neuraminidase glycoproteins make an important contribution to the restricted replication of BPIV3 in primates. J Virol 2000;74(19):8922–9.

[99] Bukreyev A, Lamirande EW, Buchholz UJ, et al. Mucosal immunisation of African green monkeys (Cercopithecus aethiops) with an attenuated parainfluenza virus expressing the SARS coronavirus spike protein for the prevention of SARS. Lancet 2004;363(9427): 2122–7.

[100] Bukreyev A, Yang L, Zaki SR, et al. A single intranasal inoculation with a paramyxovirus-vectored vaccine protects guinea pigs against a lethal-dose Ebola virus challenge. J Virol 2006;80(5):2267–79.

[101] Belshe RB, Newman FK, Anderson EL, et al. Evaluation of combined live, attenuated respiratory syncytial virus and parainfluenza 3 virus vaccines in infants and young children. J Infect Dis 2004;190(12):2096–103.

[102] Karron R, Wright P, Newman F, et al. A live human parainfluenza type 3 virus vaccine is attenuated and immunogenic in healthy infants and children. J Infect Dis 1995;172: 1445–50.

[103] Huberman K, Peluso R, Moscona A. The hemagglutinin-neuraminidase of human parainfluenza virus type 3: role of the neuraminidase in the viral life cycle. Virology 1995;214: 294–300.

[104] Murrell M, Porotto M, Weber T, et al. Mutations in human parainfluenza virus type 3 HN causing increased receptor binding activity and resistance to the transition state sialic acid analog 4-GU-DANA (zanamivir). J Virol 2003;77:309–17.

[105] Lawrence MC, Borg NA, Streltsov VA, et al. Structure of the haemagglutinin-neuraminidase from human parainfluenza virus type III. J Mol Biol 2004;335(5):1343–57.

[106] Porotto M, Murrell M, Greengard O, et al. Inhibition of parainfluenza type 3 and Newcastle disease virus hemagglutinin-neuraminidase receptor binding: effect of receptor avidity and steric hindrance at the inhibitor binding sites. J Virol 2004;78(24):13911–9.

[107] Porotto M, Fornabaio M, Greengard O, et al. Paramyxovirus receptor-binding molecules: engagement of one site on the hemagglutinin-neuraminidase protein modulates activity at the second site. J Virol 2006;80(3):1204–13.

[108] Alymova IV, Portner A, Takimoto T, et al. The novel parainfluenza virus hemagglutinin-neuraminidase inhibitor BCX 2798 prevents lethal synergism between a paramyxovirus and Streptococcus pneumoniae. Antimicrob Agents Chemother 2005;49(1): 398–405.

[109] Yin HS, Wen X, Paterson RG, et al. Structure of the parainfluenza virus 5 F protein in its metastable, perfusion conformation. Nature 2006;439(7072):38–44.

[110] Moscona A. Neuraminidase inhibitors for influenza. N Engl J Med 2005;353:1363–73.

[111] Porotto M, Greengard O, Poltoratskaia N, et al. Human parainfluenza virus type 3 HN-receptor interaction: the effect of 4-GU-DANA on a neuraminidase-deficient variant. J Virol 2001;76:7481–8.

[112] van den Hoogen BG, de Jong JC, Groen J, et al. A newly discovered human pneumovirus isolated from young children with respiratory tract disease. Nat Med 2001;7(6): 719–24.

[113] Boivin G, Abed Y, Pelletier G, et al. Virological features and clinical manifestations associated with human metapneumovirus: a new paramyxovirus responsible for acute respiratory-tract infections in all age groups. J Infect Dis 2002;186(9):1330–4.

[114] Williams JV, Wang CK, Yang CF, et al. The role of human metapneumovirus in upper respiratory tract infections in children: a 20-year experience. J Infect Dis 2006;193(3): 387–95.

[115] Jartti T, van den Hoogen B, Garofalo RP, et al. Metapneumovirus and acute wheezing in children. Lancet 2002;360(9343):1393–4.

[116] Skiadopoulos MH, Biacchesi S, Buchholz UJ, et al. The two major human metapneumovirus genetic lineages are highly related antigenically, and the fusion (F) protein is a major contributor to this antigenic relatedness. J Virol 2004;78(13):6927–37.

[117] MacPhail M, Schickli JH, Tang RS, et al. Identification of small-animal and primate models for evaluation of vaccine candidates for human metapneumovirus (hMPV) and implications for hMPV vaccine design. J Gen Virol 2004;85(Pt 6):1655–63.

[118] Williams JV, Tollefson SJ, Johnson JE, et al. The cotton rat (Sigmodon hispidus) is a permissive small animal model of human metapneumovirus infection, pathogenesis, and protective immunity. J Virol 2005;79(17):10944–51.

[119] Prince GA, Curtis SJ, Yim KC, et al. Vaccine-enhanced respiratory syncytial virus disease in cotton rats following immunization with Lot 100 or a newly prepared reference vaccine. J Gen Virol 2001;82(Pt 12):2881–8.

[120] Niewiesk S, Prince G. Diversifying animal models: the use of cotton rats (*Sigmodon hispidus*) in infectious diseases. Lab Anim 2002;36:357–72.

[121] Biacchesi S, Skiadopoulos MH, Tran KC, et al. Recovery of human metapneumovirus from cDNA: optimization of growth in vitro and expression of additional genes. Virology 2004;321(2):247–59.

[122] Biacchesi S, Pham QN, Skiadopoulos MH, et al. Infection of nonhuman primates with recombinant human metapneumovirus lacking the SH, G, or M2–2 protein categorizes each as a nonessential accessory protein and identifies vaccine candidates. J Virol 2005;79(19): 12608–13.

[123] Pham QN, Biacchesi S, Skiadopoulos MH, et al. Chimeric recombinant human metapneumoviruses with the nucleoprotein or phosphoprotein open reading frame replaced by that of avian metapneumovirus exhibit improved growth in vitro and attenuation in vivo. J Virol 2005;79(24):15114–22.

[124] Ksiazek TG, Erdman D, Goldsmith CS, et al. A novel coronavirus associated with severe acute respiratory syndrome. N Engl J Med 2003;348(20):1953–66.

[125] Rota PA, Oberste MS, Monroe SS, et al. Characterization of a novel coronavirus associated with severe acute respiratory syndrome. Science 2003;300(5624):1394–9.

[126] Drosten C, Gunther S, Preiser W, et al. Identification of a novel coronavirus in patients with severe acute respiratory syndrome. N Engl J Med 2003;348(20):1967–76.

[127] Fouchier RA, Kuiken T, Schutten M, et al. Aetiology: Koch's postulates fulfilled for SARS virus. Nature 2003;423(6937):240.

[128] Fouchier RA, Hartwig NG, Bestebroer TM, et al. A previously undescribed coronavirus associated with respiratory disease in humans. Proc Natl Acad Sci U S A 2004;101(16): 6212–6.

[129] van der Hoek L, Pyrc K, Jebbink MF, et al. Identification of a new human coronavirus. Nat Med 2004;10(4):368–73.

[130] van der Hoek L, Sure K, Ihorst G, et al. Croup is associated with the novel coronavirus NL63. PLoS Med 2005;2(8):e240.

[131] Hofmann H, Pyrc K, van der Hoek L, et al. Human coronavirus NL63 employs the severe acute respiratory syndrome coronavirus receptor for cellular entry. Proc Natl Acad Sci U S A 2005;102(22):7988–93.

[132] Pyrc K, Bosch BJ, Berkhout B, et al. Inhibition of human coronavirus NL63 infection at early stages of the replication cycle. Antimicrob Agents Chemother 2006;50(6): 2000–8.

[133] Reynolds EO, Cook CD. The Treatment Of Bronchiolitis. J Pediatr 1963;63:1205–7.

[134] Sigurs N, Bjarnason R, Sigurbergsson F, et al. Respiratory syncytial virus bronchiolitis in infancy is an important risk factor for asthma and allergy at age 7. Am J Respir Crit Care Med 2000;161(5):1501–7.

[135] Sigurs N, Gustafsson PM, Bjarnason R, et al. Severe respiratory syncytial virus bronchiolitis in infancy and asthma and allergy at age 13. Am J Respir Crit Care Med 2005;171(2): 137–41.

[136] Lemanske RF Jr. Viruses and asthma: inception, exacerbation, and possible prevention. J Pediatr 2003;142(2 Suppl):S3–7 [discussion S7–8].

[137] Gern JE, Lemanske RF Jr. Infectious triggers of pediatric asthma. Pediatr Clin North Am 2003;50(3):555–75.

[138] Moore ML, Peebles RS Jr. Respiratory syncytial virus disease mechanisms implicated by human, animal model, and in vitro data facilitate vaccine strategies and new therapeutics. Pharmacol Ther 2006, epub ahead of print.

[139] Martinez FD. Respiratory syncytial virus bronchiolitis and the pathogenesis of childhood asthma. Pediatr Infect Dis J 2003;22(2 Suppl):S76–82.

[140] Patel H, Platt R, Lozano JM, et al. Glucocorticoids for acute viral bronchiolitis in infants and young children. Cochrane Database Syst Rev 2004;3:CD004878.
[141] Hartling L, Wiebe N, Russell K, et al. Epinephrine for bronchiolitis. Cochrane Database Syst Rev 2004;1:CD003123.
[142] Gadomski A, Bhasale A. Bronchodilators for bronchiolitis. Cochrane Database Syst Rev 2006;3:CD001266.
[143] Soto ME, Sly PD, Uren E, et al. Bronchodilator response during acute viral bronchiolitis in infancy. Pediatr Pulmonol 1985;1(2):85–90.
[144] Kim CK, Koh JY, Han TH, et al. Increased levels of BAL cysteinyl leukotrienes in acute RSV bronchiolitis. Acta Paediatr 2006;95(4):479–85.
[145] Piedimonte G, Renzetti G, Auais A, et al. Leukotriene synthesis during respiratory syncytial virus bronchiolitis: influence of age and atopy. Pediatr Pulmonol 2005;40(4):285–91.
[146] Bisgaard H, Study Group on Montelukast and Respiratory Syncytial Virus. A randomized trial of montelukast in respiratory syncytial virus postbronchiolitis. Am J Respir Crit Care Med 2003;167(3):379–83.
[147] Szefler SJ, Simoes EA. Montelukast for respiratory syncytial virus bronchiolitis: significant effect or provocative findings? Am J Respir Crit Care Med 2003;167(3):290–1.
[148] Nasr SZ, Strouse PJ, Soskolne E, et al. Efficacy of recombinant human deoxyribonuclease I in the hospital management of respiratory syncytial virus bronchiolitis. Chest 2001;120(1):203–8.
[149] Merkus PJ, de Hoog M, van Gent R, et al. DNase treatment for atelectasis in infants with severe respiratory syncytial virus bronchiolitis. Eur Respir J 2001;18(4):734–7.
[150] Kerr MH, Paton JY. Surfactant protein levels in severe respiratory syncytial virus infection. Am J Respir Crit Care Med 1999;159(4 Pt 1):1115–8.
[151] LeVine AM, Gwozdz J, Stark J, et al. Surfactant protein-A enhances respiratory syncytial virus clearance in vivo. J Clin Invest 1999;103(7):1015–21.
[152] LeVine AM, Elliott J, Whitsett JA, et al. Surfactant protein-d enhances phagocytosis and pulmonary clearance of respiratory syncytial virus. Am J Respir Cell Mol Biol 2004;31(2):193–9.
[153] Tibby SM, Hatherill M, Wright SM, et al. Exogenous surfactant supplementation in infants with respiratory syncytial virus bronchiolitis. Am J Respir Crit Care Med 2000;162(4 Pt 1):1251–6.
[154] Ventre K, Haroon M, Davison C. Surfactant therapy for bronchiolitis in critically ill infants. Cochrane Database Syst Rev 2006;3:CD005150.
[155] Henrickson KJ. Advances in the laboratory diagnosis of viral respiratory disease. Pediatr Infect Dis J 2004;23(1 Suppl):S6–10.
[156] Henrickson KJ. Cost-effective use of rapid diagnostic techniques in the treatment and prevention of viral respiratory infections. Pediatr Ann 2005;34(1):24–31.
[157] Puppe W, Weigl JA, Aron G, et al. Evaluation of a multiplex reverse transcriptase PCR ELISA for the detection of nine respiratory tract pathogens. J Clin Virol 2004;30(2):165–74.
[158] Briese T, Palacios G, Kokoris M, et al. Diagnostic system for rapid and sensitive differential detection of pathogens. Emerg Infect Dis 2005;11(2):310–3.
[159] Kehl SC, Henrickson KJ, Hua W, et al. Evaluation of the Hexaplex assay for detection of respiratory viruses in children. J Clin Microbiol 2001;39(5):1696–701.
[160] Fan J, Henrickson KJ, Savatski LL. Rapid simultaneous diagnosis of infections with respiratory syncytial viruses A and B, influenza viruses A and B, and human parainfluenza virus types 1, 2, and 3 by multiplex quantitative reverse transcription-polymerase chain reaction-enzyme hybridization assay (Hexaplex). Clin Infect Dis 1998;26(6):1397–402.
[161] Fan J, Henrickson KJ. Rapid diagnosis of human parainfluenza virus type 1 infection by quantitative reverse transcription-PCR-enzyme hybridization assay. J Clin Microbiol 1996;34(8):1914–7.
[162] Kuypers J, Wright N, Corey L, et al. Detection and quantification of human metapneumovirus in pediatric specimens by real-time RT-PCR. J Clin Virol 2005;33(4):299–305.

[163] Maertzdorf J, Wang CK, Brown JB, et al. Real-time reverse transcriptase PCR assay for detection of human metapneumoviruses from all known genetic lineages. J Clin Microbiol 2004;42(3):981-6.

[164] Mackay IM, Jacob KC, Woolhouse D, et al. Molecular assays for detection of human metapneumovirus. J Clin Microbiol 2003;41(1):100-5.

[165] Cote S, Abed Y, Boivin G. Comparative evaluation of real-time PCR assays for detection of the human metapneumovirus. J Clin Microbiol 2003;41(8):3631-5.

[166] Moes E, Vijgen L, Keyaerts E, et al. A novel pancoronavirus RT-PCR assay: frequent detection of human coronavirus NL63 in children hospitalized with respiratory tract infections in Belgium. BMC Infect Dis 2005;5(1):6.

[167] Stephensen CB, Casebolt DB, Gangopadhyay NN. Phylogenetic analysis of a highly conserved region of the polymerase gene from 11 coronaviruses and development of a consensus polymerase chain reaction assay. Virus Res 1999;60(2):181-9.

ELSEVIER
SAUNDERS

Pediatr Clin N Am
53 (2006) 961–987

PEDIATRIC CLINICS
OF NORTH AMERICA

Pulmonary Hypertension in Children: The Twenty-First Century

Stuart Berger, MD*, Girija G. Konduri, MD

Medical College of Wisconsin, Children's Hospital of Wisconsin, 9000 West Wisconsin Avenue, Milwaukee, WI 53226, USA

Pulmonary hypertension is an elevation in pulmonary artery pressure that is associated with a spectrum of diseases and causes. Its clinical severity and presentation are widely varied. The field of study has changed immensely over the past several years. Significant knowledge has been gained in the pathophysiology, genetics, and vascular biology associated with pulmonary hypertension. These discoveries have contributed to medical interventions that have improved outcomes associated with pulmonary hypertension. This article reviews pulmonary hypertension in children, focusing on idiopathic pulmonary hypertension. Because most information is associated with children who have this form of the disease, formerly classified as primary pulmonary hypertension, medical therapy is discussed with a focus on this patient group. Additional therapeutic concepts relevant to other causes of pulmonary hypertension are highlighted.

Definition and background and general history and physical examination

Pulmonary hypertension of any origin may be associated with significant morbidity and mortality. Regardless of origin, it can be progressive and severe and can lead to right ventricular failure, arrhythmias, and death. Pulmonary hypertension is defined as a mean pulmonary artery pressure greater than 25 mm Hg at rest.

The symptoms associated with pulmonary hypertension may vary depending on severity and age at presentation. At a critical level of pulmonary artery pressure elevation, the symptoms associated with pulmonary hypertension are typically related to low cardiac output, although they may be nonspecific. Therefore, infants may present with symptoms of poor appetite

---

* Corresponding author.
E-mail address: sberger@mcw.edu (S. Berger).

0031-3955/06/$ - see front matter © 2006 Elsevier Inc. All rights reserved.
doi:10.1016/j.pcl.2006.08.001   *pediatric.theclinics.com*

and growth and older children may present with nausea, vomiting, activity intolerance, lethargy, or diaphoresis. Syncope or sudden cardiac death at any age may be a presenting symptom in patients who have severely elevated pulmonary artery pressure.

Physical examination can identify pulmonary hypertension. Findings may be consistent with low cardiac output, including tachypnea and tachycardia. The pulmonic component of the second heart sound is accentuated and a right ventricular heave may be caused by right ventricular hypertrophy or dysfunction. Tricuspid regurgitation may be present, depending on the degree of pulmonary artery pressure elevation. Clinical signs of right ventricular failure may also be present, including hepatomegaly, ascites, and peripheral edema.

Classification

Until recently, pulmonary hypertension was classified as primary or secondary, with most secondary forms in children related to congenital heart disease or lung disease. Other secondary forms of pulmonary hypertension are seen more frequently in adults and include collagen vascular diseases, sarcoid disease, pulmonary embolic disease, liver disease, and HIV disease.

A new classification scheme, presented in Box 1, resulted from the Venice 2003 World Health Organization (WHO) conference. Because primary pulmonary hypertension is referred to as *idiopathic pulmonary hypertension*, Group 1 forms of pulmonary hypertension include idiopathic forms, familial forms, and associated forms of pulmonary hypertension (eg, collagen vascular disease, left-to-right shunt disease, HIV disease, portal hypertension, HIV-related, drug- or toxin-induced). Note that persistent pulmonary hypertension of the newborn is listed in Group 1. Groups 2, 3, and 4 include pulmonary hypertension associated with left heart disease, pulmonary hypertension associated with lung disease or hypoxemia, and pulmonary hypertension associated with chronic embolic disease, respectively. The rationale for this new classification scheme may be related to common underlying pathophysiologic mechanisms, although this has not yet been proven. Based on this classification system, drug therapies may be tailored relative to specific class and origin of the pulmonary hypertension. However, this strategy is also speculative, although many studies are in progress. Most, but not all, current studies target patients who have pulmonary hypertension who fall within WHO classification Group 1.

Incidence/epidemiology

The true incidence of idiopathic pulmonary hypertension is unknown. Although initially believed to be a rare disease, it is being diagnosed with greater frequency, perhaps because of a greater awareness of the disease

---

Box 1. WHO classification of pulmonary hypertension

1. Pulmonary artery hypertension
1.1 Idiopathic pulmonary hypertension
1.2 Familial
1.3 Pulmonary hypertension associated with
   a. Collagen vascular disease
   b. Congenital heart disease with left-to-right shunt
   c. Portal hypertension
   d. HIV disease
   e. Drugs: anorexigens or other toxins
   f. Thyroid disorders
   g. Other entities: Gaucher disease, hereditary hemorrhagic telangiectasia, hemoglobinopathies
1.4 Persistent pulmonary hypertension of the newborn
1.5 Pulmonary veno-occlusive disease

2. Pulmonary hypertension with left heart disease
2.1 Left atrial or left ventricular disease
2.2 Left-sided valvular disease

3. Pulmonary hypertension associated with respiratory disorders or hypoxemia
3.1 Chronic obstructive lung disease
3.2 Interstitial lung disease
3.3 Sleep-disordered breathing
3.4 Alveolar hypoventilation
3.5 Chronic exposure to high altitude
3.6 Neonatal lung disease
3.7 Alveolar–capillary dysplasia
3.8 Other

4. Pulmonary hypertension caused by chronic thrombotic/embolic disease
4.1 Thrombotic obstruction of proximal pulmonary arteries
4.2 Obstruction of distal pulmonary arteries
   • Pulmonary embolism (thrombus, tumor, parasites)
   • In situ thrombosis

5. Miscellaneous (eg, sarcoid)

---

rather than an increase in its frequency. The gender ratio of adult women to men has been reported to be 1.7:1, respectively. In children, variability in gender incidence has been reported. Some experts have suggested an equal frequency in children before adolescence, with a 1.5:1 male-to-female frequency in adolescence. Other studies have suggested a 1.5:1 female-to-male ratio at all ages of diagnosis [1].

Familial idiopathic pulmonary hypertension composes 6% to 12% of all cases of idiopathic pulmonary hypertension [2]. Autosomal dominant transmission seems to be the mode of inheritance with incomplete penetrance. The disease tends to present in subsequent generations at younger ages (genetic anticipation) [3,4]. The gene for familial idiopathic primary pulmonary hypertension was recently identified on chromosome 2q33. Because this gene is believed to cause defects in bone morphogenetic protein receptor 2 (BMPR-2) and may lead to abnormalities in vascular smooth muscle, including uncontrolled proliferation [5–7], first-degree relatives of patients who have idiopathic pulmonary hypertension should undergo clinical and genetic screening. Genetic screening is available for detecting BMPR-2 mutations, although their absence does not rule out the disease [6].

Pathophysiology

General

Regulating pulmonary vascular tone is complex and represents a continuous balance between dilator and constrictor stimuli. The vascular tone in pulmonary hypertension is shifted to vasoconstriction, regardless of the initiating event. Major advances in vascular biology have improved understanding of the adaptations that occur in pulmonary hypertension. Pediatric pulmonary hypertension can be broadly divided into three categories: (1) persistent pulmonary hypertension of the newborn (PPHN), (2) pulmonary hypertension secondary to congenital heart disease, and (3) systemic illnesses and idiopathic/familial pulmonary arterial hypertension (IPAH/FPAH). PPHN often is associated with and contributes to hypoxic respiratory failure and is often reversible. The presentation and clinical course of pulmonary hypertension associated with congenital heart defects and systemic illnesses, such as sickle cell disease and systemic sclerosis, vary with the underlying disease.

This article focuses on the mechanisms involved in PPHN and IPAH/FPAH. Some alterations in vascular biology are common to all three categories and are discussed together. The transitional changes that occur at birth and the growth of pulmonary circulation during early childhood largely influence the response of the lung and pulmonary vasculature to injury and disease process. These aspects of pediatric pulmonary hypertension are distinct from the pulmonary arterial hypertension (PAH) seen in adults. The nitric oxide (NO)–cyclic GMP (cGMP) system and prostacyclin–cAMP system are particularly active in the pulmonary circulation of neonates and infants [8,9], and alterations in this pathway are important causes of pulmonary vascular disease. A review of these two systems is important to understanding the pathobiology of PAH.

Perinatal transition in pulmonary circulation

The fetal pulmonary vascular resistance (PVR) is high and the lungs receive only 5% to 10% of right ventricular output, with the remainder moving across the patent ductus arteriosus to the descending aorta [10,11]. The PVR decreases rapidly at birth accompanied by a 10-fold increase in the pulmonary blood flow [10,11]. Prostaglandins and NO released by pulmonary vascular endothelium are the key mediators in the vasodilation that occurs at birth [12–14]. The influence of these dilator stimuli is opposed by several vasoconstrictors, such as endothelin-1, thromboxanes, and products of the cytochrome P450 pathway [5].

Cyclooxygenase and NO synthase, the key enzymes in the transition of pulmonary circulation, undergo developmental maturation during late gestation and at birth [8,9]. The activity of these enzymes increases dramatically in response to birth-related stimuli, with ventilation and oxygenation having specific effects [16,17]. In addition, oxygen specifically stimulates the activity of these enzymes by increasing the synthesis and release of ATP from oxygenated red blood cells in the pulmonary circulation during the perinatal transition [18,19]. NO is released (Fig. 1) as a byproduct of the conversion of L-arginine to L-citrulline by endothelial nitric oxide synthase (eNOS).

The biologic effects of NO are mediated by soluble guanylate cyclase in the vascular smooth muscle, which promotes conversion of guanosine triphosphate (GTP) to cGMP. The enzyme, phosphodiesterase-5 (PDE-5), catalyzes breakdown of cGMP to limit the duration of vasodilation observed with NO (see Fig. 1). Guanylate cyclase and phosphodiesterase undergo developmental maturation with marked increases in activity at term gestation and early postnatal life [20,21]. Prostacyclin (PGI_2), synthesized in endothelial cells from arachidonic acid and endoperoxides, stimulates adenylate cyclase–mediated conversion of ATP to cyclic AMP (cAMP) (see Fig. 1). A cAMP-specific phosphodiesterase (PDE-3) catalyzes breakdown of cAMP and limits the duration of vasodilator response to prostacyclin [22].

As shown in Fig. 1, increases in cGMP and cAMP levels in vascular smooth muscle are associated with relaxation and vasodilation. The cAMP-specific PDE is inhibited by cGMP, suggesting that synergy between these complementary systems is possible in PAH therapy [15]. Within the smooth muscle cell, the cyclic nucleotides activate specific protein kinases to decrease the Ca++ influx into the cell and decrease the Ca++ sensitivity of the contractile apparatus. In contrast, activation of signaling through the Rho GTPases and Rho kinase increase the Ca++ sensitivity and stimulate the contractile apparatus [15]. Current therapeutic approaches to pulmonary vasodilation focus on increasing the intracellular levels of these cyclic nucleotides through enhancing the availability of NO or prostacyclin; inhibiting the corresponding phosphodiesterases to preserve the biologic activity of cGMP or cAMP; decreasing the effects of endothelin, thromboxane, and

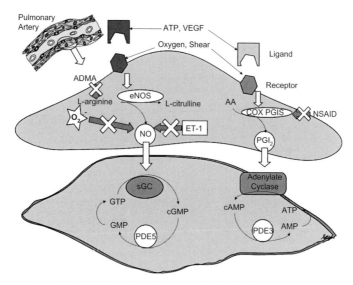

Fig. 1. Mechanism of endothelium-dependent vasodilation in the pulmonary artery. Endothelial nitric oxide synthase (eNOS) and cyclooxygenase (COX) are stimulated by physiologic agonists ATP and vascular endothelial growth factor (VEGF) and directly by oxygen and shear stress. Nitric oxide (NO) and prostacyclin (PGI_2) diffuse to vascular smooth muscle, where they activate soluble guanylate cyclase (sGC) and adenylate cyclase, respectively, to increase the levels of cGMP and cAMP. These cyclic nucleotides initiate smooth muscle relaxation. Specific phosphodiesterases (PDE) promote breakdown of the cyclic nucleotides. The arginine analog, asymmetric dimethyl arginine (ADMA), superoxide (O_2-), and endothelin (ET-1) decrease NO release and cause vasoconstriction. NSAID, nonsteroidal anti-inflammatory drug; PGIS, prostacyclin synthase.

other constrictors; and preventing quenching of NO by reactive oxygen species, such as superoxide.

Persistent pulmonary hypertension of newborn

PPHN occurs when the fetal pulmonary circulation fails to adapt to the normal postnatal circulation. PPHN is associated with persistence of high PVR and associated right-to-left shunts at the patent foramen ovale or patent ductus arteriosus. Most infants who have PPHN also have coexisting parenchymal lung diseases, such as meconium aspiration syndrome, pneumonia or sepsis, or respiratory distress syndrome, whereas 20% are classified as idiopathic. Case reports and epidemiologic studies suggest that the significant association of prenatal exposure to nonsteroidal anti-inflammatory drugs (NSAIDs) with resulting ductal constriction may cause PPHN [23–25]. Analysis of meconium for prenatal exposure showed a high prevalence of NSAID exposure in babies who had PPHN [26]. Ductal constriction in fetal lambs at near-term gestation (128–132 days of 145 days) has been shown to reproduce the hemodynamic and structural features of PPHN [27,28]. Investigation of altered vascular biology in this model showed a decrease in eNOS expression and NO release [29–31]. Studies in babies who had PPHN reported a decrease in eNOS gene expression [32] and levels of NO metabolites [33].

However, loss of NO availability only partly accounts for the impaired vasodilation in PPHN. Pulmonary arteries from fetal lambs with PPHN show an impaired response to NO [34]. Nearly 40% of babies with PPHN experience poor response to inhaled NO therapy [35]. Studies in the ductal ligation model have showed that an increase in oxidant stress impairs the vasodilator responses [34]. In addition, alterations in the turnover of the eNOS substrate, L-arginine, has been implicated in the impaired vasodilation in PPHN [33,36]. Increased levels of asymmetric dimethyl arginine (ADMA), a competitive endogenous inhibitor of NO release, have been shown in PPHN [33], and decreased endogenous synthesis of arginine from recycling of L-citrulline pathway has been shown in pulmonary hypertension [33]. Downstream signaling for the NO–cGMP pathway, including decreased guanylyl cyclase activity and increased PDE-5 activity that causes increased breakdown of cGMP, has been shown in the ductal ligation model of PPHN [37,38]. These data indicate that the adaptation in PPHN involves down-regulation of vasodilator mechanisms at multiple steps along the NO–cGMP pathway. A coordinated regulation of vasoconstrictor stimuli also occurs with increased endothelin release [31] and oxidative stress, contributing to vasoconstriction and vascular remodeling.

Oxidative stress in pulmonary arterial hypertension

Increasing evidence shows that reactive oxygen species (ROS) participate in pulmonary vasoconstriction and remodeling in PAH. Superoxide (O2−) is an oxygen free radical generated in pulmonary arteries in response to increased pressure load [34]. The pulmonary vessels contain multiple sources of superoxide, including xanthine oxidase, NADPH oxidase, and, in the endothelial cells, uncoupled eNOS [38]. Superoxide is converted to hydrogen peroxide by superoxide dismutases or to peroxynitrite by NO [38]. Both hydrogen peroxide and peroxynitrite are diffusible and contribute to smooth muscle hypertrophy and vascular remodeling [38,39]. Although the mechanism of the ROS induction is not fully known, the vasoconstrictors endothelin and angiotensin activate NADPH oxidase in the vascular smooth muscle [38,39]. Although eNOS is commonly known as the source of NO, it releases superoxide under some conditions [38]. Decreased availability of the substrate arginine, co-factor tetrahydrobiopterin (BH4), and its chaperone heat shock protein 90 (hsp90), can lead to uncoupled activity of eNOS and release of O_2- [40,41]. ADMA, an endogenous analog of arginine, competes with arginine for binding with eNOS and can cause uncoupling of eNOS (see Fig. 1). In pulmonary hypertension, ADMA levels increase because of its decrease clearance by the enzyme dimethylarginine dimethylaminohydrolase (DDAH), with a corresponding decreased availability of NO

[36]. Mice with deficient BH4 synthesis develop pulmonary hypertension and evidence of uncoupled eNOS activity and oxidant injury in pulmonary vessels [42]. PPHN is associated with decreased eNOS–hsp90 interactions and uncoupling of eNOS [41]. Superoxide dismutase improves the relaxation response of pulmonary vessels to NO in vitro and improves the oxygenation response and pulmonary vasodilation at birth in lambs with PPHN [43].

Idiopathic and familial pulmonary hypertension

The cause of idiopathic pulmonary hypertension in children is probably diverse and, in most patients, remains poorly understood. The proximate cause of vascular injury is difficult to identify because clinical recognition of disease often occurs after the process is fairly advanced. The initiating events are therefore obscured by the adaptations that occur in response to pulmonary hypertension. However, 6% to 12% of the patients who have PAH have a family history of the disease and are classified as having familial PAH, whereas the remainder can be classified as having idiopathic PAH [44]. Regardless of the initiating event, the elevated pulmonary artery pressure is caused by pulmonary vasoconstriction, obliteration of lumen in arteries and arterioles, and plexiform lesions [44]. A concentric thickening of pulmonary arteries occurs from intimal and medial hypertrophy and excessive proliferation of smooth muscle cells [44]. The plexiform lesions result from monoclonal proliferation of endothelial cells [45], migration and proliferation of smooth muscle cells, and accumulation of circulating macrophages and endothelial progenitor cells [44]. Several initiating events have been described in adults and children who have idiopathic and familial PAH, including exposure to anorexigens [46], viral and bacterial infections [47,48], and hypoxia [48].

Genetic basis of pulmonary hypertension

Most cases of familial PAH [48] and up to 22% of those involving children who have sporadic IPAH [49] are associated with mutations in the *BMPR-2* gene. Currently, more than 50 loss-of-function mutations are known to occur in the *BMPR-2* gene [44]. *BMPR-2* is a member of the transforming growth factor β (TGF-β) superfamily of proteins and receptors involved in regulating cell growth and differentiation. Bone morphogenic proteins (BMPs) are ligands released by many cells, including vascular endothelial cells and smooth muscle cells, that bind *BMPR-1* and -2, leading to activation of downstream signaling molecules called S_{mad}s. The BMP–S_{mad} signaling causes decreased proliferation and increased apoptosis of vascular smooth muscle cells. In contrast, BMP-S_{mad} signaling causes decreased apoptosis of endothelial cells to maintain the integrity of endothelial barrier to proteins and lipids, helping to preserve pulmonary arteries that are thin-walled with low resistance to flow. Loss of *BMPR-2* in the signaling cascade can potentially lead to endothelial injury, leakage of proteins into matrix, and hypertrophy of vascular smooth muscle (Fig. 2). The mutations are acquired by an autosomal dominant inheritance. However, the mutant alleles typically have a low penetrance and do not cause PAH unless accompanied by other gene mutations or environmental insult [48]. A loss of wild-type allele from a somatic mutation sometimes occurs in the vascular endothelium of plexiform lesions [50,51].

In addition to *BMPR-2* mutations, altered gene expression in several other signaling molecules involved in maintaining vascular tone have been identified in IPAH. These include serotonin receptors and transporters, activin-like kinase-1 (ALK-1) and endoglin, vascular voltage-gated K+ channels, and eNOS [52–54]. Exposure to anorexigens, infections, or hypoxia may be the second hit or environmental stress that initiates vascular injury [46–48]. This concept is supported by the fact that transgenic mice expressing dominant–negative *BMPR-2* gene in vascular smooth muscle,

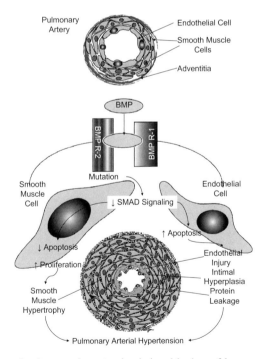

Fig. 2. Mechanism of pulmonary hypertension induced by loss of bone morphogenic protein receptor 2 (BMPR-2) signaling through gene mutations. Bone morphogenic proteins (BMPs) bind membrane receptors BMPR-1 and -2 and activate S_{mad} signaling. Normally this signaling inhibits vascular smooth muscle growth and promotes endothelial integrity. Loss of this signaling leads to uncontrolled proliferation of smooth muscle cells and endothelial injury, which leads to protein leak into matrix and further stimulation of smooth muscle growth. BMPR-2 mutant alleles have low penetrance and need another mutation in the signaling pathway or environmental factor to initiate the injury and pulmonary artery hypertension.

and heterozygous *BMPR-2+/−* knockout mice develop pulmonary hypertension only in response to hypoxia [55].

In response to hypoxia or exercise, unaffected family members of patients who have FPAH carrying *BMPR-2* mutations show signs of abnormal vascular function with larger increases in pulmonary artery pressure compared with relatives who have no mutations and unrelated controls [56]. In response to stress, endothelial progenitor cells from patients who have *BMPR-2* gene mutations show accelerated apoptosis compared with those of adults who have no mutations [57]. An interaction of genetic vulnerability with environmental factors is therefore required to initiate this disease. Once injury is initiated, the vessels undergo progressive thickening from intimal and medial hyperplasia.

Evaluation

General workup

Patients who have pulmonary hypertension should be evaluated to rule out associated entities, such as congenital heart disease, lung disease, and upper airway disease. The workup will also help determine the severity of pulmonary artery pressure elevation. Finally, cardiac catheterization and acute drug testing are important to determine the optimal pulmonary vasodilator therapy.

Box 2 summarizes the specific workup. Laboratory studies include complete blood count with differential, electrolytes, blood urea nitrogen, and serum creatinine; liver function studies; collagen vascular serologies; thyroid function studies; HIV studies; and brain natriuretic peptide levels. Radiographic imaging studies include posteroanterior and lateral chest radiographs and nuclear perfusion scan or spiral CT scan of the chest to rule out pulmonary embolic disease. A two-dimensional echocardiogram will rule out congenital heart disease, including both left-to-right shunt disease and left heart obstructive disease. An echocardiogram can also estimate the severity of the pulmonary artery pressure elevation and assess right ventricular function. Additional workup, such as upper airway studies, sleep studies, continuous oxygen saturation measurements, pulmonary function studies, and coagulation studies, are typically performed and can be guided by clinical suspicion.

Although some centers advocate performing quantitative pulmonary wedge angiography at cardiac catheterization using a distal balloon occlusion technique to provide additional information about the severity of the pulmonary vascular disease, this maneuver is not performed routinely at all centers. Other measurements have been applied to the angiograms generated by this technique to evaluate disease severity and progression. Specifically, Rabinovitch and colleagues [58] reported on the rate of taper, background filling of the peripheral vessels, and circulation time.

Box 2. Diagnostic workup for patients presenting with pulmonary hypertension

Chest radiograph
Electrocardiogram
Echocardiogram
Cardiac catheterization with acute vasodilator testing
Complete blood count
Urinalysis
Liver studies
  • Liver function studies
  • Hepatitis profile
  • Abdominal ultrasound
Collagen vascular studies
  • Antinuclear antibody
  • Rheumatoid factor
  • Erythrocyte sedimentation rate
  • Complement studies
Lung evaluation
  • Pulmonary function studies with appropriate studies to
    exclude obstructive lung disease
  • Sleep study and pulse oximetry
  • CT/chest MRI to rule out chronic pulmonary embolic disease
  • Ventilation–perfusion scan
  • Lung biopsy
HIV test
Thyroid function studies
Hypercoagulable evaluation
  • Disseminated intravascular coagulation screen
  • Factor V Leiden
  • Antithrombin III
  • Protein S
  • Protein C
  • Anticardiolipin IgG/IgM
Stress test/6-minute-walk study
Toxicology testing for stimulants such as cocaine
and methamphetamine
Brain natriuretic peptide level

Cardiac catheterization and acute vasodilator testing

A cardiac catheterization study must be performed in patients diagnosed with pulmonary hypertension. Acute drug testing is critical for assessing the pulmonary vascular reactivity and recommending an approach to pulmonary vasodilator therapy.

Catheterization is typically performed using a general anesthetic with endotracheal intubation in children, but can be also performed under deep sedation. General anesthesia often allows easier delivery of inhaled NO, which is a very potent selective pulmonary vasodilator, although some systems allow inhaled NO to be delivered without an endotracheal tube.

Saturations and pressures are obtained in the right heart chambers at catheterization and initially under baseline conditions. Thermodilution or the Fick principle measures pulmonary capillary wedge pressure and determines cardiac output. For accuracy, thermodilution requires the absence of intracardiac shunts, and the Fick principle requires the measurement of oxygen consumption rather than assuming a specific value. Blood gases are then obtained from the pulmonary artery circulation and the systemic circulation. Additional calculated variables are generated based on these measured variables, including transpulmonary pressure gradient, PVR, and PVR index.

Once the baseline parameters are obtained, parameters are repeated with the acute testing of medications to determine if pulmonary vascular reactivity is present. Various and multiple medications can be tested to determine the presence or absence of reactivity. Before the advent of many current medications, 100% oxygen was used. However, most laboratories use inhaled NO to test pulmonary vascular reactivity because it is a potent and selective pulmonary vasodilator. This drug can be tested at a concentration of 20 and 40 ppm. Its effect on the pulmonary vasculature occurs within minutes, and therefore repeat hemodynamic testing can occur within 5 minutes of delivery. Additional medications may also be tested in the catheterization laboratory, including intravenous prostacyclin, intravenous adenosine, oral sildenafil, oral nifedipine, or inhaled prostacyclin. Prostacyclin is given intravenously and started at 2 ng/kg/min. Its effect will also occur within minutes. The dose can be titrated by 2 ng until a beneficial effect is noted or systemic hypotension occurs. In children, the latter will typically occur in the 10 to 20 ng/kg/min range. Each medication does not need to be tested in the laboratory to determine whether pulmonary vascular reactivity is present; patients are unlikely to experience no response to inhaled NO but an acute response to another medication listed.

Finally, an *acute responder* is a patient who, with acute drug testing, experiences a 20% decrease in PVR with unchanged or increased cardiac output. Any patient who experiences a lesser response is considered a *nonresponder*.

Cardiac catheterization has risks, especially if the degree of pulmonary hypertension is severe. Therefore, adequate sedation is necessary to minimize stress and anxiety, and avoiding hypoxemia and hypovolemia is critical.

Management

General measures

The general care of children who have pulmonary hypertension is important, because the usual childhood illnesses that are relatively benign for most children can be devastating for those who have pulmonary hypertension. Therefore, respiratory illnesses can worsen ventilation–perfusion mismatching and result in hypoxemia or atelectasis, and will worsen the degree of pulmonary hypertension. Gastroenteritis can result in hypovolemia, which may also have an untoward effect on already borderline cardiac outputs in patients who have severe pulmonary hypertension. Similarly, fever can increase metabolic demands and should be controlled. To prevent illness, the usual regimen of immunizations is recommended, including annual influenza vaccination.

Anticoagulation

The efficacy of anticoagulation in children who have pulmonary hypertension has not been established; its use is based on studies in affected adult patients [59,60]. Before vasodilator agents were used, adults treated with warfarin to maintain an international normalized ratio (INR) in the 2.3 to 3.0 range had a survival advantage. This therapy was initially prompted by the observation of thrombosis in situ within the pulmonary vasculature either on lung biopsy or autopsy. Whether the latter was a primary or secondary finding is unclear. Neither antiplatelet therapy with aspirin or dipyridamole nor anticoagulation with heparin or enoxaparin seems to be as effective in preventing thrombosis in situ in areas of low flow within the pulmonary vascular bed. Therefore, the use of warfarin has been recommended in children who have pulmonary hypertension. Its use requires frequent blood sampling and dosage adjustments.

Vasodilator therapy

The use of pulmonary vasodilator agents is a rapidly evolving therapeutic field. Multiple agents are currently available, many untested in children, and newer agents are constantly introduced. This section reviews the currently available vasodilator agents and presents a logical approach to therapy based on the results of acute drug testing and the clinical presentation.

Historically, agents that relax the pulmonary vascular bed were postulated to have potential use because progression in vascular remodeling from medial hypertrophy to plexiform arteriopathy is noted in patients who have pulmonary hypertension [61]. Medial hypertrophy relates to vessel constriction, whereas plexiform arteriopathy is considered irreversible. Idiopathic pulmonary hypertension was believed to be initiated by increased reactivity of pulmonary vessels and vasoconstriction that later progressed to fixed obstruction. Because it is difficult to determine at which stage a patient may be in the disease process, acute drug testing is critical to guide chronic therapy. Barst and colleagues [62] showed that acute pulmonary vasodilation seems to be age-related, with the youngest patients best able to reverse the degree of pulmonary hypertension. However, multiple studies suggest that, even in the absence of response to acute drug testing, patients undergoing chronic vasodilator therapy experience enhanced survival compared with historical controls [62,63]. Experts have postulated that pulmonary vascular remodeling, even in the absence of a response to acute drug testing, can occur over time with chronic pulmonary vasodilator therapy.

Calcium channel blockers

Patients who experience acute response in the catheterization laboratory have been shown to respond to calcium channel blockers [62]. Therefore, common practice in this setting has been to initiate a trial of oral calcium channel blockers, usually nifedipine or diltiazem. However, initiating this therapy without showing an acute beneficial response in the catheterization laboratory is dangerous; a nonresponder can develop significant systemic vasodilation and hypotension rather than selective pulmonary vessel dilation.

Prostacyclin

Experts have postulated that an imbalance of thromboxane A_2 and prostacyclin synthesis is operative in some forms of pulmonary hypertension, including idiopathic pulmonary hypertension and the pulmonary hypertension associated with congenital heart disease [64]. Several studies have shown that long-term intravenous prostacyclin therapy is efficacious in children and adults, improving survival and quality of life [65,66] in acute responders and initial nonresponders. Experts have suggested that 5-year survival in children who have idiopathic pulmonary hypertension who are nonresponders may be higher than 80% (Fig. 3) [65].

However, continuous intravenous prostacyclin therapy has disadvantages and potential side-effects. Dose-dependent side-effects include nausea, anorexia, jaw pain, diarrhea, and nonspecific musculoskeletal aches and pains. In addition, the route of delivery (through central venous access) creates a risk for complications, including line sepsis and venous thrombosis. Because of tachyphylaxis, the dose of the drug requires intermittent increases. Finally, abrupt interruption of the medication can cause acute deterioration in some patients and is rarely associated with a severe rebound increase in pulmonary artery pressure and death.

Other prostacyclin analogs and routes of delivery

Seeking alternative routes for delivery of prostacyclin has obvious advantages.

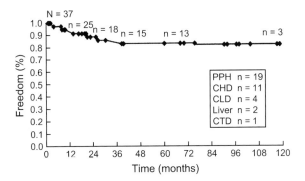

Fig. 3. Kaplan-Meier curve of long-term prostacyclin therapy in children who had pulmonary hypertension at The Children's Hospital Heart Institute/Pediatric Heart Lung Center in Denver, Colorado. PPH, primary pulmonary hypertension; CHD, congenital heart disease; CLD, chronic lung disease; CTD, connective tissue disease; Liver, liver disease. (*From* Rashid A, Ivy D. Severe paediatric pulmonary hypertension: new management strategies. Arch Dis Child 2005;90:92–8; with permission.)

Treprostinil. Treprostinil is a prostacyclin analog with similar hemodynamic effects to epoprostenol but a half-life of 45 minutes. Currently, it is primarily delivered subcutaneously, with some recent information suggesting that it might also be used intravenously. The subcutaneous delivery system is associated with pain and erythema at the delivery site. A recent multicenter, placebo-controlled, randomized study has shown beneficial effects on hemodynamics and exercise tolerance [67].

Iloprost. Initial trial results of the inhaled prostacyclin analog iloprost are promising, showing improved symptomatology and quality of life [68]. Because it is delivered through inhalation, iloprost has the advantage of relative selectivity on the pulmonary vasculature without a significant effect on systemic blood pressure. However, because it has a short half-life of 25 minutes, six to nine inhalations per day are required. Iloprost has been suggested to benefit children who have acute lung injury by redistributing pulmonary blood flow from nonventilated to ventilated lung regions, thereby improving gas exchange and decreasing pulmonary shunt [69,70].

Beroprost. Few data are available on the oral prostacyclin analog beroprost. It has been used in Europe, but is not currently available in the United States. It is a fast-acting medication with a half-life of 35 to 40 minutes. Its efficacy has not been tested [71].

The endothelin system

Endothelin is a potent vasoconstrictor peptide. The endothelins include a family of vasoactive peptides: ET-1, ET-2, and ET-3. ET-1 is a very potent vasoactive peptide. It is produced in the vascular endothelial cells and smooth muscle cells, and the two receptor subtypes, ET_A and ET_B, mediate its activity. ET_A receptors on smooth muscle cells are involved in the vaso-constrictor response, whereas ET_B receptors on endothelial cells are involved with release of NO or prostacyclin. These ET_B receptors also act as clearance receptors for ET-1 [83].

ET-1 expression is increased in the pulmonary arteries of patients who have pulmonary hypertension, suggesting that inhibiting this axis might be beneficial [83]. Bosentan is a dual ET receptor antagonist. Studies have shown that it is effective in lowering pulmonary artery pressure and PVR and improving exercise tolerance, while lengthening the time to clinical deterioration in adults who have pulmonary hypertension [72]. In addition, children who have pulmonary hypertension associated with congenital heart disease and those who have idiopathic pulmonary hypertension seem to benefit from bosentan therapy [73]. Specifically, pulmonary artery pressure and PVR improved in the latter group of patients.

Additional endothelin receptor blockers are being studied. Sitaxsentan is a selective ET_A receptor blocker that has the theoretical advantage of blocking the constrictor effect of the ET_A receptor with little or no effect on vasodilator and clearance modalities of the ET_B receptors. It has high oral availability and long duration of action. One study showed that 12 weeks of oral therapy resulted in beneficial effects on exercise capacity and hemodynamics in patients who had idiopathic pulmonary hypertension, pulmonary hypertension associated with connective tissue disorders, and pulmonary hypertension associated with congenital heart disease [74,83]. Additional studies are investigating other endothelin receptor blockers and their use for additional indications, such as pulmonary hypertension after repair of congenital cardiac defects [75,76].

Combination therapy for pulmonary hypertension is a reasonable course, especially when targeting multiple mechanisms of vasoconstriction. Therefore, concomitant use of epoprostenol and bosentan can be considered, and addition of bosentan to long-term epoprostenol therapy may allow a decrease in dose of epoprostenol with consequent diminution in its side effects [77].

The phosphodiesterase-5 inhibitors

Sildenafil, a PDE-5 inhibitor, is new in its use as a pulmonary vasodilator agent. Sildenafil causes an increase in cGMP levels, which have a role in causing pulmonary vasodilation. Sildenafil is as effective as inhaled NO and may be an oral analog of the latter [64,78]. Sildenafil has also been shown to facilitate weaning of inhaled NO postoperatively or in the setting of pulmonary hypertension and chronic lung disease [79–82].

Many anecdotal case reports document the benefit of sildenafil therapy in children in various clinical settings, including idiopathic pulmonary hypertension and pulmonary hypertension associated with chronic lung disease. Figs. 4A and B depict data from our experience with a 4-month-old infant who had severe chronic lung disease and severe pulmonary hypertension

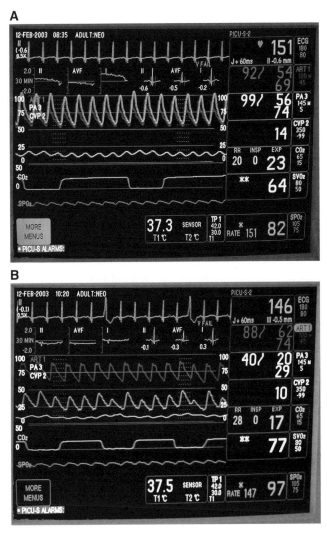

Fig. 4. (*A*) Baseline hemodynamic measurements in a 4-month-old who had severe lung disease and pulmonary hypertension associated with bronchopulmonary dysplasia. Monitoring includes continuous measurement of arterial blood pressure, pulmonary artery pressure (PA), central venous pressure (CVP), systemic venous saturation (SVO$_2$, measured continuously through oximetric catheter in the pulmonary artery), and systemic arterial oxygen saturation (SPO$_2$). (*B*) Hemodynamic measurements in a 4-month-old infant 30 minutes after a single dose of oral sildenafil, 0.5 mg/kg. Note the significant decrease in pulmonary artery pressure with concomitant increase in systemic venous oxygen saturation and systemic arterial oxygen saturation.

associated with bronchopulmonary dysplasia. This patient was continuously monitored with measurements of arterial blood pressure, pulmonary artery pressure, end-tidal carbon dioxide, pulmonary artery saturation (SVO$_2$) through an oximetric flow-directed pulmonary artery catheter, and pulse oximetry. A single dose of oral sildenafil resulted in a significant decrease in pulmonary artery pressure and a concomitant increase in pulmonary artery oxygen saturation and systemic arterial oxygen saturation. Although several case reports and small series document the beneficial effects of oral sildenafil therapy, a multicenter, placebo-controlled, double-blind study in children is currently underway.

Summary and approach to vasodilator therapy

We suggest a vasodilator treatment strategy such as Rashid and Ivy [83] describe, based on acute vasodilator testing in the catheterization laboratory (Fig. 5). For patients who experience acute response to inhaled NO or epoprostenol, beginning a trial of calcium channel blockers is reasonable and appropriate. Therapy with epoprostenol, treprostinil, or iloprost should be considered for nonresponders who experience symptoms of right heart failure with or without syncope; the choice depends on practitioner preference and experience and varies based on each patient's clinical situation and preference. In the absence of right heart failure, nonresponders may be started on bosentan or sildenafil, although some practitioners would also consider this group of patients for therapy with epoprostenol, treprostinil, or iloprost, depending on the degree of pulmonary artery pressure elevation. Finally, patients who undergo failed therapy with a calcium channel blocker can be switched to any other agent. Although the choice of agent is guided by symptoms, it may also be related to practitioner experience and comfort.

Digoxin

No data show the efficacy of digoxin in patients who have idiopathic pulmonary hypertension [84]. In the absence of evidence, most practitioners use digoxin in patients who have pulmonary hypertension and right ventricular

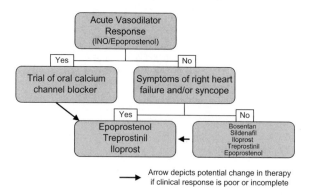

Fig. 5. Algorithm for treatment of pediatric pulmonary artery hypertension. (*Adapted from* Rashid A, Ivy D. Severe paediatric pulmonary hypertension: new management strategies. Arch Dis Child 2005;90:92–8.)

dysfunction. Although whether digoxin has a role in patients who have pulmonary hypertension and normal right heart function is even less clear, many practitioners also routinely prescribe digoxin in this setting.

Diuretics

As with digoxin, diuretic therapy is used in patients who have right heart failure. Although diuretics can be beneficial in this setting, hypovolemia must be prevented because it can diminish cardiac output that may be borderline at baseline.

Atrial septostomy

Exercise-induced syncope is presumably caused by systemic vasodilation and an inability to augment cardiac output. Recurrent syncope in patients who have pulmonary hypertension is concerning and is associated with a very poor long-term prognosis [85,86]. Atrial septostomy can be life-saving in the symptomatic patient who has severe pulmonary hypertension. Some data suggest that the presence of a patent foramen ovale in patients who have severe pulmonary hypertension may confer a survival benefit [87,88]. Specifically, the patent foramen ovale in this circumstance is believed to allow right-to-left shunting to maintain cardiac output, albeit at the expense of arterial oxygen desaturation. Successful palliation of symptoms after creation of an atrial-level communication is well documented. Several reports have documented significant clinical and hemodynamic improvement with resolution of right heart failure and symptoms of syncope. Kerstein and colleagues [89,90] noted improved oxygen delivery, cardiac output, 1- and 2-year survival rates, and quality of life. Our laboratory performs this maneuver using a transseptal puncture technique followed by static dilation of the atrial septum. The size of the balloon dilation catheter may vary. In a young adult, a 15-mm balloon dilation catheter will typically result in adequate atrial-level communication to decompress the right heart. In this circumstance, an arterial saturation range from high 80% to low 90% is desirable.

Lung transplantation

Lung transplantation may be offered to patients whose condition does not respond to long-term vasodilator therapy and who continue to experience symptoms or right heart failure. Advancements continue to be made in this arena, including the possibility of living-related lung transplantation, with recent reports suggesting improved long-term survival and decreased postoperative morbidity with this approach [91,92].

Newer approaches to treatment of pulmonary hypertension

Several promising therapies take advantage of improved understanding of vascular biology in PAH. Recognition of oxidative stress as a major cause of vascular dysfunction has lead to the investigation of superoxide dismutase (SOD) and its mimetics in experimental pulmonary hypertension. Steinhorn and colleagues [43] reported that recombinant human SOD improves oxygenation and pulmonary vasodilation at birth in lambs with PPHN induced by prenatal ligation of ductus arteriosus. SOD also improved the response to inhaled NO, suggesting that oxidant stress is a major cause of high PVR and impaired response to NO. An alternate approach is to reduce the oxidant stress from uncoupled eNOS with exogenous L-arginine to overcome the inhibition of NOS by ADMA and other endogenous arginine analogs [15]. Although L-arginine has been shown to improve vascular function and endothelium-dependent vasodilation in hyperlipidemia, the role of this therapy in PAH either alone or in combination with other drugs in the NO–cGMP system, such as sildenafil, has not been investigated.

Although the long-term administration of inhaled NO is not practical in IPAH/FPAH, the use of NO donors or nitrosothiols has not been tested in clinical trials. Other potential approaches, including endothelin and angiotensin receptor blockers and inhibitors of Rho kinase, target the contractile apparatus in vascular smooth muscle. Endothelin antagonists have been studied as monotherapy in PAH, but combining this therapy with other agents, such as PGI_2 and sildenafil, requires further study [45]. An inhaled form of Rho kinase inhibitor has been shown to ameliorate pulmonary hypertension induced by monocrotaline or chronic hypoxia in rats [93]. Statin drugs that lower cholesterol have been shown to improve NO-dependent vasodilation and endothelial function in patients who have hypertension and hyperlipidemias. Although these drugs are widely available and are logical candidates to reduce vascular remodeling, they have not been studied systematically in PAH [94,95]. Bone marrow–derived endothelial–like progenitor cells have been shown to engraft and repair the damage in pulmonary hypertension induced by monocrotaline in rats [96]. Gene therapy with intravenous infusion of syngenic smooth muscle cells loaded with vascular endothelial growth factor or eNOS gene has induced reversal of pulmonary hypertension in this rat model [97]. Gene therapy to selectively induce smooth muscle cell apoptosis in this model using a novel signaling molecule, survivin, has been shown to reverse established pulmonary hypertension in rats [98]. Although extrapolation of these approaches to human PAH from these animal models is not possible, they suggest future strategies to correct vascular remodeling and decrease pulmonary artery pressure.

Prognosis and natural history of the disease

Until the "modern era," marked by the use of pulmonary vasodilator agents, the diagnosis of pulmonary hypertension in children carried an extremely poor prognosis. In the 1960s, before the use of epoprostenol, a series of 35 patients who had primary pulmonary hypertension showed no

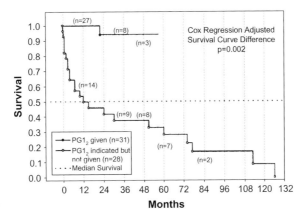

Fig. 6. Kaplan-Meier survival curves comparing survival of patients treated with long-term epoprostenol (Group 1, N = 31) with survival of patients for whom epoprostenol was indicated but unavailable (Group 2, N = 28). The 1-, 2-, 3-, and 4-year survival probabilities for Group 1 were 100%, 94%, 94%, and 94%, respectively, compared with 50%, 43%, 38%, and 38%, respectively, for Group 2 (P = .0002). (*From* Barst RJ, Maislin MS, Fishman AP. Vasodilator therapy for primary pulmonary hypertension in children. Circulation 1999;99:1197–208; with permission.)

survivors beyond 7 years from diagnosis, and 62% of the patients (22 of 35) died within the first year after the onset of symptoms [85]. Similarly, in 1995, the median survival in 18 children who had primary pulmonary hypertension was approximately 4 years (Figs. 6 and 7) [65,99]. Fig. 6 depicts the

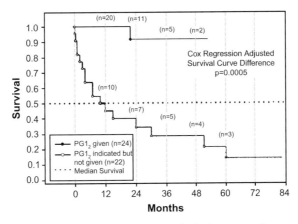

Fig. 7. Kaplan-Meier survival curves comparing survival of nonresponders treated with long-term epoprostenol (Group 1, n = 22) with survival of nonresponders for whom epoprostenol was indicated but unavailable (Group 2, n = 22). The 1-, 2-, 3-, and 4-year survival probabilities for Group 1 were 100%, 100%, 92%, and 92%, respectively, compared with 45%, 34%, 29%, and 29%, respectively, for Group 2 (P = .0005). (*From* Barst RJ, Maislin MS, Fishman AP. Vasodilator therapy for primary pulmonary hypertension in children. Circulation 1999;99:1197–208; with permission.)

survival curves of patients who had pulmonary hypertension treated with epoprostenol compared with those for whom epoprostenol was unavailable, and Fig. 7 shows the survival curves of nonresponders treated with epoprostenol compared with those for whom epoprostenol was unavailable. In both situations the group treated with epoprostenol had a significant survival advantage at 1, 2, 3, and 4 years [65].

Better understanding of the pulmonary vasculature and the advent of targeted therapies have improved the prognosis and altered the natural history of the diseases. Studies in children who had severe primary pulmonary hypertension treated with epoprostenol showed that intervention has a significant impact, with survival rates of 80% to 90% up to 4 years after diagnosis [65,83]. Future targeted and combination drug therapies are expected to continue to impact this field of study. In addition, the drugs and delivery modes described earlier are hoped to lessen the side-effects and complications of the therapy itself.

Summary

Understanding of idiopathic pulmonary hypertension, and pulmonary hypertension in general, has progressed over the years. A more succinct understanding of the pathophysiology of this disease has elucidated its mechanisms and facilitated a rational approach to its management. This approach has provided hope for patients who had a disease that was associated with significant morbidity and mortality shortly after diagnosis. Medications continue to evolve, providing this group of patients an improved outlook. Newer medications, especially in oral form, will continue to be developed and future studies will include combination medical therapy. Finally, the genomic approach to the study of pulmonary hypertension, including the identification of candidate genes, may allow manipulation of selected genes, further the understanding of the pathobiology of pulmonary hypertension, and allow this devastating disease to someday be prevented. Although recent advances have provided more options, further work is necessary to understand the role of the new treatment options and devise a rational approach to this disease entity.

Acknowledgments

This work is supported by grants from the AHA-Northland affiliate and HL57368 from NHLBI (GGK). The authors acknowledge that many other important observations made by several investigators could not be presented because of space limitations.

References

[1] Widlitz A, Barst R. Pulmonary artery hypertension in children. Eur Respir J 2003;21: 155–76.

[2] Rich S, Dantzker DR, Ayres SM, et al. Primary pulmonary hypertension: a national prospective study. Ann Intern Med 1987;107:216–23.

[3] Loyd JE, Primm RK, Newman JH. Familial primary pulmonary hypertension: clinical patterns. Am Rev Respir Dis 1984;129:194–7.

[4] Loyd JE, Atkinson JB, Pietra GG, et al. Heterogeneity of pathologic lesions in familial primary pulmonary hypertension. Chest 1986;98:497–503.

[5] Newman JH, Wheeler L, Lane KB, et al. Mutation in the gene for bone morphogenetic protein receptor II as a cause of primary pulmonary hypertension in a large kindred. N Engl J Med 2001;345:319–24.

[6] Trembath RC, Harrison R. Insights into the genetic and molecular basis of primary pulmonary hypertension. Pediatr Res 2003;53:883–8.

[7] Loyd JE, Butler MG, Faroud TM, et al. Genetic anticipation and abnormal gender ratio at birth in familial primary pulmonary hypertension. Am J Respir Crit Care Med 1995;152: 93–7.

[8] Shaul PW, Farrar MA, Magness RR. Pulmonary endothelial nitric oxide production is developmentally regulated in the fetus and newborn. Am J Physiol 1993;265:H1056–63.

[9] Brannon TS, MacRitchie AN, Jaramillo MA, et al. Ontogeny of cyclooxygenase-1 and cyclooxygenase-2 gene expression in ovine lung. Am J Physiol 1998;274(1 Pt 1):L66–71.

[10] Dawes GS, Mott JC, Widdicomb JG, et al. Changes in the lungs of the newborn lamb. J Physiol 1953;121:141–62.

[11] Cassin S, Dawes GS, Mott JC, et al. The vascular resistance of the foetal and newly ventilated lung of the lamb. J Physiol 1964;171:61–79.

[12] Velvis H, Moore P, Heymann MA. Prostaglandin inhibition prevents the fall in pulmonary vascular resistance as a result of rhythmic distension of the lungs in fetal lambs. Pediatr Res 1991;30:62–8.

[13] Abman SH, Chatfield BA, Hall SL, et al. Role of endothelium-derived relaxing factor during transition of pulmonary circulation at birth. Am J Physiol 1990;259:H1921–7.

[14] Tiktinsky MH, Morin FC III. Increasing oxygen tension dilates fetal pulmonary circulation via endothelium-derived relaxing factor. Am J Physiol 1993;265(1 Pt 2):H376–80.

[15] Wojciak-Stothard B, Haworth SG. Perinatal changes in pulmonary vascular endothelial function. Pharmacol Ther 2006;109(1–2):78–91.

[16] Shaul PW, Wells LB. Oxygen modulates nitric oxide production selectively in fetal pulmonary endothelial cells. Am J Respir Cell Mol Biol 1994;11(4):432–8.

[17] Shaul PW, Campbell WB, Farrar MA, et al. Oxygen modulates prostacyclin synthesis in ovine fetal pulmonary arteries by an effect on cyclooxygenase. J Clin Invest 1992;90(6): 2147–55.

[18] Konduri GG, Mattei J. Role of oxidative phosphorylation and ATP release in birth related pulmonary vasodilation in fetal lambs. Am J Physiol Heart Circ Physiol 2002;283(4): H1600–8.

[19] Konduri GG, Mital S, Gervasio CT, et al. Purine nucleotides contribute to pulmonary vasodilation caused by birth related stimuli in the ovine fetus. Am J Physiol 1997;272: H2377–84.

[20] Bloch KD, Filippov G, Sanchez LS, et al. Pulmonary soluble guanylate cyclase, a nitric oxide receptor, is increased during the perinatal period. Am J Physiol 1997;272(3 Pt 1): L400–6.

[21] Hanson KA, Burns F, Rybalkin SD, et al. Developmental changes in lung cGMP phosphodiesterase-5 activity, protein, and message. Am J Respir Crit Care Med 1998;158(1): 279–88.

[22] Travadi JN, Patole SK. Phosphodiesterase inhibitors for persistent pulmonary hypertension of the newborn: a review. Pediatr Pulmonol 2003;36(6):529–35.

[23] Manchester D, Margolis HS, Sheldon RE. Possible association between maternal indomethacin therapy and primary pulmonary hypertension of the newborn. Am J Obstet Gynecol 1976;126:467–9.

[24] Perkin RM, Levin DL, Clark R. Serum salicylate levels and right to left ductus shunts in newborn infants with persistent pulmonary hypertension. J Pediatr 1980;96:721–6.

[25] Vanmarter LJ, Leviton A, Allred EN. Persistent pulmonary hypertension of the newborn and smoking and aspirin and nonsteroidal anti-inflammatory drug consumption during pregnancy. Pediatrics 1996;97:658–62.

[26] Alano MA, Ngougmna E, Ostrea EM, et al. Analysis of nonsteroidal antiinflammatory drugs in meconium and its relation to persistent pulmonary hypertension of the newborn. Pediatrics 2001;107:519–23.

[27] Abman SH, Shanley PF, Accurso FJ. Failure of postnatal adaptation of the pulmonary circulation after chronic intrauterine pulmonary hypertension in fetal lambs. J Clin Invest 1989; 83:1849–58.

[28] Morin FC. Ligating the ductus arteriosus before birth causes persistent pulmonary hypertension in newborn lamb. Pediatr Res 1989;25:245–50.

[29] Shaul PW, Yuhanna IS, German Z, et al. Pulmonary endothelial NO synthase gene expression is decreased in fetal lambs with pulmonary hypertension. Am J Physiol Lung Cell Mol Physiol 1997;272:L1005–12.

[30] Villamor E, Le Cras TD, Horan MP, et al. Chronic intrauterine pulmonary hypertension impairs endothelial nitric oxide synthase in the ovine fetus. Am J Physiol 1997;272:L1013–20.

[31] Black SM, Johengen MJ, Soifer SJ. Coordinated regulation of genes of the nitric oxide and endothelin pathways during the development of pulmonary hypertension in fetal lambs. Pediatr Res 1998;44(6):821–30.

[32] Villanueva ME, Zaher FM, Svinarich DM, et al. Decreased gene expression of endothelial nitric oxide synthase in newborns with persistent pulmonary hypertension. Pediatr Res 1998;44:338–43.

[33] Pearson DL, Dawling S, Walsh W, et al. Neonatal pulmonary hypertension: Urea-cycle intermediates, nitric oxide production and carbamoylphosphate synthetase function. N Engl J Med 2001;344(24):1832–8.

[34] Brennan LA, Steinhorn RH, Wedgwood S, et al. Increased superoxide generation is associated with pulmonary hypertension in fetal lambs: a role for NADPH oxidase. Circ Res 2003; 92(6):683–91.

[35] The Neonatal Inhaled Nitric Oxide Study Group. Inhaled nitric oxide in full-term and nearly full-term infants with hypoxic respiratory failure. N Engl J Med 1997;336:597–604.

[36] Pierce CM, Krywawych S, Petros AJ. Asymmetric dimethyl arginine and symmetric dimethyl arginine levels in infants with persistent pulmonary hypertension of the newborn. Pediatr Crit Care Med 2004;5(6):517–20.

[37] Tzao C, Nickerson PA, Russell JA, et al. Pulmonary hypertension alters soluble guanylate cyclase activity and expression in pulmonary arteries isolated from fetal lambs. Pediatr Pulmonol 2001;31(2):97–105.

[38] Mueller CF, Laude K, McNally JS, et al. ATVB in focus: redox mechanisms in blood vessels. Arterioscler Thromb Vasc Biol 2005;25(2):274–8.

[39] Wedgwood S, Dettman RW, Black SM. ET-1 stimulates pulmonary arterial smooth muscle cell proliferation via induction of reactive oxygen species. Am J Physiol Lung Cell Mol Physiol 2001;281(5):L1058–67.

[40] Landmesser U, Dikalov S, Price SR, et al. Oxidation of tetrahydrobiopterin leads to uncoupling of endothelial cell nitric oxide synthase in hypertension. J Clin Invest 2003;111(8):1201–9.

[41] Konduri GG, Ou J, Shi Y, et al. Decreased association of HSP90 impairs endothelial nitric oxide synthase in fetal lambs with persistent pulmonary hypertension. Am J Physiol Heart Circ Physiol 2003;285(1):H204–11.

[42] Nandi M, Miller A, Stidwill R, et al. Pulmonary hypertension in a GTP-cyclohydrolase 1-deficient mouse. Circulation 2005;111(16):2086–90.

[43] Steinhorn RH, Albert G, Swartz DD, et al. Recombinant human superoxide dismutase enhances the effect of inhaled nitric oxide in persistent pulmonary hypertension. Am J Respir Crit Care Med 2001;164(5):834–9.

[44] The Task Force on Diagnosis and Treatment of Pulmonary Arterial Hypertension of the European Society of Cardiology. Guidelines on diagnosis and treatment of pulmonary arterial hypertension. Eur Heart J 2004;25:2243–78.

[45] Hoeper MM, Rubin LJ. Update in pulmonary hypertension 2005. Am J Respir Crit Care Med 2006;173(5):499–505.

[46] Humbert M, Deng Z, Simonneau G, et al. BMPR2 germline mutations in pulmonary hypertension associated with fenfluramine derivatives. Eur Respir J 2002;20(3):518–23.

[47] Cool CD, Rai PR, Yeager ME, et al. Expression of human herpesvirus 8 in primary pulmonary hypertension. N Engl J Med 2003;349(12):1113–22.

[48] Yuan JX, Rubin LJ. Pathogenesis of pulmonary arterial hypertension: the need for multiple hits. Circulation 2005;111(5):534–8.

[49] Harrison RE, Berger R, Haworth SG, et al. Transforming growth factor-beta receptor mutations and pulmonary arterial hypertension in childhood. Circulation 2005;111(4):435–41.

[50] Machado RD, James V, Southwood M, et al. Investigation of second genetic hits at the BMPR2 locus as a modulator of disease progression in familial pulmonary arterial hypertension. Circulation 2005;111:607–13.

[51] Yeager ME, Golpon HA, Voelkel NF, et al. Microsatellite mutational analysis of endothelial cells within plexiform lesions from patients with familial, pediatric, and sporadic pulmonary hypertension. Chest 2002;121(3 Suppl):61S.

[52] Eddahibi S, Humbert M, Fadel E, et al. Serotonin transporter overexpression is responsible for pulmonary artery smooth muscle hyperplasia in primary pulmonary hypertension. J Clin Invest 2001;108:1141–50.

[53] Yuan JX, Aldinger AM, Juhaszova M, et al. Dysfunctional voltage-gated K^+ channels in pulmonary artery smooth muscle cells of patients with primary pulmonary hypertension. Circulation 1998;98:1400–6.

[54] Giaid A, Saleh D. Reduced expression of endothelial nitric oxide synthase in the lungs of patients with pulmonary hypertension. N Engl J Med 1995;333:214–21.

[55] West J, Fagan K, Steudel W, et al. Pulmonary hypertension in transgenic mice expressing a dominant-negative BMPRII gene in smooth muscle. Circ Res 2004;94:1109–14.

[56] Grunig E, Dehnert C, Mereles D, et al. Enhanced hypoxic pulmonary vasoconstriction in families of adults or children with idiopathic pulmonary arterial hypertension. Chest 2005; 128(6 Suppl):630S–3S.

[57] Teichert-Kuliszewska K, Kutryk MJ, Kuliszewski MA, et al. Bone morphogenetic protein receptor-2 signaling promotes pulmonary arterial endothelial cell survival: implications for loss-of-function mutations in the pathogenesis of pulmonary hypertension. Circ Res 2006;98(2):209–17.

[58] Rabinovitch M, Keane JF, Fellows KG, et al. Quantitative analysis of the pulmonary wedge angiogram in congenital heart defects. Circulation 1981;63:152–64.

[59] Rich S, Kauffman E, Levy PS. The effect of high doses of calcium channel blockers on survival in pulmonary hypertension. N Engl J Med 1992;327:76–81.

[60] Fuster V, Peele PM, Edwards WD, et al. Primary pulmonary hypertension: natural history and the importance of thrombosis. Circulation 1984;70:580–7.

[61] Wagenvoort CA, Wagenvoort N. Pathology of pulmonary hypertension. New York: John Wiley and Sons; 1977.

[62] Barst RJ. Pharmacologically induced pulmonary vasodilatation in children and young adults with primary pulmonary hypertension. Chest 1986;98:497–503.

[63] Barst RJ, Hall JC, Gersony WM. Factors influencing survival among children with primary pulmonary hypertension treated with vasodilator agents. Circulation 1988; 78(Suppl 2):293.

[64] Barst RJ. Recent advances in the treatment of pediatric pulmonary artery hypertension. Pediatr Clin North Am 1999;46:331–45.

[65] Barst RJ, Maislin G, Fishman AP. Vasodilator therapy for primary pulmonary hypertension in children. Circulation 1999;99:1197–208.

[66] Sitbon O, Humbert M, Nunes H, et al. Long-term intravenous epoprostenol infusion in primary pulmonary hypertension: prognostic factors and survival. J Am Coll Cardiol 2002;40: 780–8.

[67] Simonneau G, Barst RJ, Galie N, et al. Continuous subcutaneous infusion of treprostinol, a prostacyclin analogue, in patients with pulmonary artery hypertension: a double-blind, randomized, placebo-controlled trial. Am J Respir Crit Care Med 2002;165: 800–4.

[68] Olschewski H, Simonneau G, Galie N, et al. Inhaled iloprost for severe pulmonary hypertension. N Engl J Med 2002;347:322–9.

[69] Max M, Rossaint R. Inhaled prostacyclin in the treatment of pulmonary hypertension. Eur J Pediatr 1999;158(Suppl 1):S23–6.

[70] Dahlem P, van Aalderen WM, de Neef M, et al. Randomized controlled trial of aerosolized prostacyclin therapy in children with acute lung injury. Crit Care Med 2004;32: 1055–60.

[71] Barst RJ, McGoon M, McLaughlin V, et al. Beroprost therapy for pulmonary artery hypertension. J Am Coll Cardiol 2003;41:2119–25.

[72] Rubin LJ, Badesch DB, Barst RJ, et al. Bosentan therapy for pulmonary artery hypertension. N Engl J Med 2002;346:896–903.

[73] Barst RJ, Ivy D, Dingemanse J, et al. Pharmacokinetics, safety, and efficacy of bosentan in pediatric patients with pulmonary artery hypertension. Clin Pharmacol Ther 2003;73: 372–82.

[74] Barst RJ, Langleben D, Frost A, et al. Sitaxsentan therapy for pulmonary artery hypertension. Am J Respir Crit Care Med 2004;169:441–7.

[75] Schulze-Neick IL, Reader JA, Shekerdemian L, et al. The endothelin antagonist BQ123 reduces pulmonary vascular resistance after surgical intervention for congenital heart disease. J Thorac Cardiovasc Surg 2002;124:435–41.

[76] Prendergast B, Newby DE, Wilson LE, et al. Early therapeutic experience with the endothelin antagonist BQ-123 in pulmonary hypertension after congenital heart surgery. Heart 1999; 82:505–8.

[77] Ivy D, Doran A, Claussen L, et al. Weaning and discontinuation of epoprostenol in children with idiopathic pulmonary hypertension receiving concomitant bosentan. Am J Cardiol 2004;93:943–6.

[78] Michelakis E, Tymchak W, Lien D, et al. Oral sildenafil is an effective and specific pulmonary vasodilator in patients with pulmonary artery hypertension: comparison with inhaled nitric oxide. Circulation 2002;105:2398–403.

[79] Atz A, Wessel DL. Sildenafil ameliorates effects of inhaled nitric oxide withdrawal. Anesthesiology 1999;91:307–10.

[80] Schulze-Neick I, Hartenstein P, Li J, et al. Intravenous sildenafil is a potent pulmonary vasodilator in children with congenital heart disease. Circulation 2003;108(Suppl 1): II167–73.

[81] Atz AM, Lefler AK, Fairbrother DL, et al. Sildenafil augments the effect of inhaled nitric oxide for postoperative pulmonary hypertensive crisis. J Thorac Cardiovasc Surg 2002; 124:628–9.

[82] Ghofrani HA, Wiedemann R, Rose F, et al. Sildenafil for the treatment of lung fibrosis and pulmonary hypertension: a randomized controlled trial. Lancet 2002;360:895–900.

[83] Rashid A, Ivy D. Severe paediatric pulmonary hypertension: new management strategies. Arch Dis Child 2005;90:92–8.

[84] Mathur PN, Powles RCP, Pugsley PO, et al. Effect of digoxin on right ventricular function in severe chronic airflow obstruction. Ann Intern Med 1981;95:283–8.

[85] Thilenius OG, Nadas AS, Jockin H. Primary pulmonary vascular obstruction in children. Pediatrics 1965;36:75–87.

[86] D'Alonzo GE, Barst RJ, Ayres SM, et al. Survival in patients with primary pulmonary hypertension: results from a national prospective registry. Ann Intern Med 1991;115:343–9.

[87] Thoele DG, Barst RJ, Gersong WM. Physiologic-based management of primary pulmonary hypertension in children and young adults [abstract]. J Am Coll Cardiol 1990;15:242A. Abstract.

[88] Nootens MT, Berarducci LA, Kauffman E, et al. Prevalence and hemodynamic implications of a patent foramen ovale in pulmonary hypertension [abstract]. J Am Coll Cardiol 1993;2: 402A. Abstract.

[89] Kerstein D, Garofano RO, Hsu DT, et al. Efficacy of blade balloon atrial septostomy in advanced pulmonary vascular disease [abstract]. Am Rev Respir Dis 1992;145:A717. Abstract.

[90] Kerstein D, Levy PS, Hsu DT, et al. Blade balloon atrial septostomy improves survival in patients with severe primary pulmonary hypertension. Circulation 1995;91:2028–35.

[91] Date H, Aoe M, Nagahiro I, et al. Improved survival after living-donor lobar lung transplantation. J Thorac Cardiovasc Surg 2004;128(6):933–40.

[92] Barr ML, Schenkel FA, Bowdish ME, et al. Living donor lobar lung transplantation: current status and future directions. Transplant Proc 2005;37(9):3983–6.

[93] Nagaoka T, Fagan KA, Gebb SA, et al. Inhaled Rho kinase inhibitors are potent and selective vasodilators in rat pulmonary hypertension. Am J Respir Crit Care Med 2005;171(5): 494–9.

[94] Kao PN. Simvastatin treatment of pulmonary hypertension: an observational case series. Chest 2005;127(4):1446–52.

[95] Taraseviciene-Stewart L, Scerbavicius R, Choe KH, et al. Simvastatin causes endothelial cell apoptosis and attenuates severe pulmonary hypertension. Am J Physiol Lung Cell Mol Physiol 2006; Epub ahead of print.

[96] Zhao YD, Courtman DW, Deng Y, et al. Rescue of monocrotaline-induced pulmonary arterial hypertension using bone marrow-derived endothelial-like progenitor cells: efficacy of combined cell and eNOS gene therapy in established disease. Circ Res 2005;96(4):442–50.

[97] Campbell AI, Zhao Y, Sandhu R, et al. Cell-based gene transfer of vascular endothelial growth factor attenuates monocrotaline-induced pulmonary hypertension. Circulation 2001;104(18):2242–8.

[98] McMurtry MS, Archer SL, Altieri DC, et al. Gene therapy targeting survivin selectively induces pulmonary vascular apoptosis and reverses pulmonary arterial hypertension. J Clin Invest 2005;115(6):1479–91.

[99] Sandoval J, Bauerle O, Gomez A, et al. Primary pulmonary hypertension in children: clinical characterization and survival. J Am Coll Cardiol 1995;25:466–74.

ELSEVIER
SAUNDERS

Pediatr Clin N Am
53 (2006) 989–1009

PEDIATRIC CLINICS
OF NORTH AMERICA

Molecular and Cellular Basis of Congenital Heart Disease

Tara L. Sander, PhD[a],*, Denise B. Klinkner, MD[b],
Aoy Tomita-Mitchell, PhD[c], Michael E. Mitchell, MD[d]

[a]Department of Surgery, Division of Pediatric Surgery, Cardiovascular Research Center,
Children's Research Institute and Medical College of Wisconsin, 8701 Watertown Plank Road,
Milwaukee, WI 53226, USA
[b]Department of General Surgery, Children's Research Institute and Medical College
of Wisconsin, 9200 W. Wisconsin Avenue, Milwaukee, WI 53226, USA
[c]Department of Surgery, Biotechnology and Bioengineering Center, Human and Molecular
Genetics Center, 8701 Watertown Plank Road, Milwaukee, WI 53226, USA
[d]Department of Surgery, Division of Cardiothoracic Surgery, Children's Hospital
of Wisconsin, Medical College of Wisconsin, 9000 W. Wisconsin Avenue, MS 715,
Milwaukee, WI 53226, USA

The incidence of congenital heart disease (CHD) affects 1 in 100 live births and is responsible for the majority of prenatal deaths [1,2]. The incidence of moderate and severe forms of CHD is approximately 3 to 6 per 1000 live births [2]. Therefore, approximately 1% of the newborn population have gross structural abnormalities of the heart, heart valves, or blood vessels with functional significance. This figure is likely an underestimate, because many common anomalies do not consistently present for specialized care, such as undiagnosed patent ductus arteriosus, aortic arch anomalies, bicuspid aortic valve, or small atrial or ventricular septal defects [2]. The severity of anomalies range from simple persistence of fetal circulation (patent foramen ovale, patent ductus arteriosus) to complex anatomic defects such as transposition of the great vessels, single ventricle anomalies, hypoplastic left heart syndrome, and the class of heterotaxy syndromes.

Although significant advances have been made in delineating the molecular mechanisms and genetic basis of heart formation and CHD [3], several

This work was supported in part by an award from the Children's Hospital of Wisconsin Research Foundation and Children's Research Institute, Milwaukee, Wisconsin (TLS) and by Grant # P20-RR/DE17702 (AT-M) from the National Center for Research Resources (NCRR), a component of the National Institutes of Health (NIH).

* Corresponding author.
E-mail address: sandert@mcw.edu (T.L. Sander).

unanswered questions remain regarding the complexity and progression of the disease. There are multiple known factors that can contribute to cardiac malformations. In addition, cardiac defects are a component of a number of genetic and phenotypic syndromes. Known causes include environmental exposures, exposure to medications during gestation, maternal diseases, chromosome disorders, and genetic factors. For the majority of children who have CHD, the cause is idiopathic or unknown. Although chromosomal abnormalities such as Down syndrome (trisomy 21) are clearly associated with CHD, particularly atrioventricular (AV) canal defects, the genetics is complex, and indeed many children who have trisomy 21 have normal hearts. Here the authors review the underlying mechanisms of heart development, and the cellular and molecular factors contributing to CHD.

Heart development

Defining the basic mechanisms of heart development is essential to understanding how disruptions in cardiac formation lead to the onset of CHD and provide insight into treatment. Heart development in vertebrates is an organized series of molecular and morphogenetic events that involves five primary steps: (1) migration of precardiac cells from the primitive streak and assembly of the paired cardiac crescents at the myocardial plate, (2) coalescence of the cardiac crescents to form the primitive heart tube, an event that establishes the definitive heart, (3) cardiac looping, a complex process that assures proper alignment of the future cardiac chambers, (4) septation and heart chamber formation, and (5) development of the cardiac conduction system and coronary vasculature [4,5]. Heart development in humans begins at 15 to 16 days of gestation with the migration of precardiac stem cells, which culminates in the development of the cardiac crescents or "cardiogenic plates" that fuse into the single heart tube having an arterial and a venous pole [4,6]. The first evident assembly of the mesoderm-derived myocardial (or cardiogenic) plate is seen at 18 days, followed by initiation of heart tube formation at 22 days.

Prior to and during looping, portions of the primitive heart tube undergo cellular specialization along the anterior-posterior axis, giving rise to specific segments that ultimately give rise to the chambers of the mature heart [4,7]. Segments of the heart tube differentiate and develop to consist of transitional zones and intervening primitive cardiac chambers that include the sinus venosus, sinoatrial ring, primitive atrium, AV ring encircling the AV canal, primitive left ventricle, primary fold or ring, primitive right ventricle, outflow tract ending at ventriculoarterial ring, and aortic sac (listed from venous to arterial pole) [4]. The transitional zones will give rise to the septa, valves, conduction system, and fibrous heart skeleton. The AV ring encircling the AV canal and the outflow tracts develop into endocardial cushions. At 23 days, the primary heart tube then begins its rightward looping, which brings all of the transitional zones together near the inner curvature of the heart tube.

By day 28 of development, the looping process is complete, which allows cardiac septation and chamber formation to begin [4,6]. Septation takes place at the atrium, ventricle (outflow tract), and arterial pole. During septation, the transitional zones are incorporated into the primitive chambers, leading to formation of the definitive cardiac atria and ventricles. During outflow tract septation, the outflow tract is lined on the inside by two endocardial cushions: the bulbar (proximal) cushions give rise to the muscular outflow tract septum, and the truncal (distal) cushions take part in semilunar valve formation. Neural crest cells enter the heart during fusion of the two cushions, in close contact with the myocardial cells, and begin to invade the myocardium. The myocardium then develops into a working myocardium and cardiac conduction system. After the proepicardium (PE) delaminates as a monolayer lining the myocardium, cells migrate from this lining, becoming the coronary vascular system, which is necessary for nutrition and oxygenation of the myocardium [4,8]. By day 49 of gestation, formation of the definitive heart is complete.

Cellular mechanisms of heart development

The process of transforming a tubelike structure into a four-chambered functional human heart requires a delicate balance of cellular growth, differentiation, and apoptosis. Specific signaling pathways and genetic mechanisms play a critical role in controlling these cellular processes and ensuring proper embryonic heart development. Disruptions in these cellular and molecular mechanisms often result in cardiac malformations and the onset of CHD. Common problems include defects in cardiac looping, septation, and chamber formation. Below the authors discuss the organization of specific cell types and their critical involvement in normal heart development. The authors identify key molecular mechanisms that control these cellular processes and introduce known mutations associated with human CHD.

Cardiac stem cells

Upon its appearance, the definitive heart essentially contains two primitive cardiac cell types, the myocardium and endocardium, both of which are derived from gastrulated precardiac mesoderm. These cells are capable of further division and growth, which shortly results in development of the working myocardium, and the endocardium. The remaining cell types of the heart, including "cardiac" fibroblasts, and smooth muscle and endothelial cells, which compose the coronary vasculature, concomitantly arise from a small, transient organ on the dorsal thoracic wall, the PE. Cells from the PE invade the newly developed definitive heart to form epicardium; continued migration gives rise to the coronary vasculature, and the cardiac fibroblasts, which ultimately become the predominant cell type in the heart.

By the time neonatal and adult stages are reached, cardiac stem cells are found within the heart. Although the origin of these cells is unclear, they have been classified according to specific antigens expressed on the cell surface [9,10]. For example, primitive progenitor and precursor stem cells express proteins v-kit Hardy-Zuckerman 4 feline sarcoma viral oncogene homolog (c-Kit), ATP-binding cassette subfamily B member 1 (ABCB1 or MDR1), and Sca-1 or caspase 3 (CASP3), whereas more differentiated cells do not [9,10].

Before their assembly into a recognizably definitive heart, myocardial and endocardial embryonic stem cells migrate within the precardiac mesoderm. These spread anteriorly and outward from the primitive streak to give rise to the bilateral cardiogenic plates of mesoderm [11]. Bone morphogenetic protein (BMP) and Wnt-mediated signals have been identified as important initiating factors that induce cardiomyocyte fate and activate the myocardial gene program [5]. At this stage, the cardiogenic plates express cardiac specific transcription factor genes, including NK2 transcription factor related locus 5 (*NKX2-5*), GATA binding protein 4 (*GATA4*), serum response factor (*SRF*), myocardin (*MYOCD*), and dickkopf homolog 1 (*DKK1*). Once the primitive heart tube is formed, a cascade of genes is expressed in an anterior (ventricular) and posterior (atrial) pattern, which helps regulate cellular processes that control cardiac looping, mechanisms guiding left-right symmetry, and chamber formation. When these genes are disturbed, there is insufficient remodeling of the inner curvature, leading to deficient leftward movement of the outflow tract over the AV canal that results in outflow tract abnormalities (eg, double-outlet right ventricle with ventricular septal defect). Other genes identified as important regulators of cardiac looping include MADS box transcription enhancer factor 2 polypeptide C (*MEF2C*), heart and neural crest derivatives expressed 2 (*HAND2*), T-box 5 (*TBX5*), and *NKX2-5* [5].

Endocardial cushions

Shortly after looping begins, the cardiac cushions begin to form, which are the primordia of the valves and membranous septae of the adult heart [12,13]. Endocardial cushions of the outflow tract contain mesenchymal cells that derive from endocardium that has undergone a cellular process referred to as endothelial-mesenchymal transformation (also called epithelial-mesenchymal transdifferentiation or transition [EMT]) [6,14]. Each segment of the primordial heart tube consists of two epithelial cell layers, an inner endothelium and an outer myocardium. The endothelial cells lining the AV canal and conotruncal segments are functionally distinct in that a subset are specified to delaminate, differentiate to mesenchymal cells, and migrate into the underlying extracellular matrix (called cardiac jelly). Locally expanded swelling of cardiac jelly and mesenchymal cells constitute the endocardial cushion tissue. Morphological signs of the transdifferentiation process include hypertrophy, loss of uniform cell shape, cell detachment, and extension of elongated cell processes into the adjoining extracellular matrix [14,15].

EMT within the AV regions and outflow tract of the developing heart is absolutely required for generation of the endocardial cushion tissue. Studies of avian valve development have demonstrated that a subset of endothelial cells from the endocardium is activated by a complex signal secreted by the myocardium [15,16]. The inductive signal causing EMT likely involves the interaction of various components expressed in a temporal and spatial manner during heart development. In the chicken, TGFβ2 and TGFβ3 are secreted by the myocardium and are present in the extracellular matrix, suggesting that the inductive signal for EMT includes TGFβ-signaling [16]. In addition, cardiac endothelial cells that undergo EMT express TGFβ receptor type III (TBRIII) and this may be a key mechanism regulating downstream TGFβ signaling in the target tissue [16].

In general, the molecular mechanisms regulating the selective expression and secretion of specific genes during discrete stages of cushion formation remain poorly understood. Differential patterns of gene expression within subpopulations of the cushion mesenchyme likely determine the fate of each cell in the developing heart, such as specification, delamination, proliferation, apoptosis, transdifferentiation, migration, and matrix invasion [12].

Mouse gene knockout models have identified molecules required for valve development that may function in endocardial cushion formation. For example, the loss of neurofibromin 1 (*NF1*), mothers against decapentaplegic homolog 6 (*SMAD6*), and epidermal growth factor receptor (*EGFR*) gene expression results in the formation of hyperplastic valves, suggesting that these genes serve as negative regulators of valve proliferation [17–19]. Furthermore, disruption of the retinoid X receptor alpha (*RXRα*), hyaluronan synthase-2 (*HAS2*), endoglin (*ENG*), sex determining region Y-box 4 (*SOX4*), vascular endothelial growth factor (*VEGF*), or nuclear factor of activated T-cells (*NFATc1*) results in the malformation or absence of valve development, suggesting that the expression of these genes is necessary for cardiac valve formation [20–25]. Other molecular markers of cushion development include fibroblast growth factor (FGF), Dell, v-erb-b2 erythroblastic leukemia viral oncogene homolog 3 (*ErbB3/HER3*), friend of GATA (*FOG*), forkhead box (*FOX*), msh homeobox homolog (*MSX*), neuroregulin, platelet-derived growth factor receptor (*PDGFR*), and Periostin [26,27]. Although the expression patterns and valve phenotypes observed in mice deficient for these genes are suggestive of an irreplaceable function, little is known about their roles in regulating the cellular and molecular events of the developing cushion mesenchyme during human cardiac development.

Proepicardium

Cells migrating from the PE contribute to the epicardium, which is essential for proper maturation of the myocardium, as well as for differentiation of cells comprising the coronary vasculature. The PE is a grapelike cluster of cells that are located on the pericardial side of the septum transversum in mammals, which lies directly dorsal to the developing heart [28]. The PE becomes visible on the dorsal body wall adjacent to the AV canal of the looped heart [8]. Each vesicle of the PE contains mesothelial cells that will migrate toward the developing heart and give rise to a mesothelium or epicardial monolayer that lines the myocardium of the heart. In avians, PE cells migrate across a transient extracellular matrix bridge structure, which has been termed the proepicardial organ (PEO), between the PE and myocardium and migrate radially from the point of attachment. In contrast in the mouse, clusters of cells detach from the PE and travel across the pericardial space to the AV myocardium. Upon attachment, clusters flatten into a monolayer and coalesce during initial epicardial formation. The epicardium generates multipotent epicardial-derived cells that accumulate in the subepicardial mesenchymal space that can undergo differentiation to cardiac fibroblasts, endothelial cells, and coronary smooth muscle cells, which will contribute to formation of the coronary vasculature. The epicardium also seems to be the source of a majority of the mesenchymal cells in the subepicardial space [8]. *TBX5* has been shown to play an important role in proepicardial cell migration during cardiogenesis [29]. In addition, the transcription factor serum response factor (*SRF*) regulates differentiation of coronary smooth muscle cells from PE-derived vascular precursor cells [30,31]. The Wilms tumor 1 (*WT1*) gene is another transcription factor that regulates epicardial-derived cell function and differentiation of the compact ventricular layer of the myocardium [28,32]. Furthermore, thin myocardium syndrome is characterized by a mutation in *WT1*, which takes place in association with the impaired function of various genes involved in epicardial development such as *FOG-2*, vascular cell adhesion molecule 1 (*VCAM-1*), integrins, erythropoietin (*EPO*) and its receptor (*EPOR*) [28].

Cardiac neural crest

The neural crest refers to a population of cells contained within the leading edge of the neural folds at the dorsal aspect of the developing spinal cord that migrate to various tissues in the developing embryo in a species and region dependent manner [11,33]. The neural crest is divided into two broad regions called the cranial and trunk, based on their ability to give rise to ectomesenchyme. Only the cranial neural crest has the capacity to give rise to ectomesenchyme, which gives rise to the bone, muscle, and connective tissue in the head. A subdivision of the cranial crest is defined as the "cardiac neural crest region" that forms the AP septum and smooth muscle tunica media of the great vessels of the head and neck. The cardiac crest originates from the middle of the otic placode to the caudal border of somite 3, corresponding to rhombomeres 6, 7, and 8. The cardiac crest may represent a transitional region between the cranial and trunk crest, because it shares properties with both regions. For example, it generates ectomesenchyme like the cranial crest, and lacks the ability for regeneration like the trunk.

Cells originating from the cardiac crest play an important role during heart development by participating in the septation of the cardiac outflow tract into the aorta and pulmonary trunk [11,34]. Several independent groups have monitored the migration and fate of neural crest cells in avian and murine models, often referred to as fate-mapping studies, to understand their contribution to heart development. The cardiac neural crest cells migrate through the pharyngeal arches and support development of the aortic arch arteries. A subpopulation of these cells continue on to the heart by invading the endocardial cushions of the cardiac outflow tract, in the form of two advancing columns of cells that later fuse to form the septum that divides the mature aorta from the pulmonary trunk [34].

A number of mouse models of CHD have been described, and many of these include primary or secondary defects of the cardiac neural crest. Animal models indicate that cardiac neural crest development is influenced by interactions between surrounding tissues including endothelium, pharyngeal endoderm and ectoderm, and cardiac myocardium. Specific murine genes have been implicated in cardiac neural crest development and include the following families of genes: bone morphogenic proteins (ie, *ALK2*, *BMPR1a*, *BMPR2* and *MSX2*), transforming growth factors *TGFβ2* and perlecan, *FGF8*, the *NOTCH* receptor, Jagged (*JAG*), *WNT*, endothelins, semaphorins, neurotropins, *VEGF165* and hypoxia-inducible factor 1 alpha (*HIF1A*), transcriptional regulators (ie, *SOX9, FOXC2, PAX3, NKX2-5*, snail homolog 1, and *TBX1*), and adhesion molecules (ie, neural cell adhesion molecule 1, N-cadherin, and connexin-43) [34]. Unfortunately, genetic mutations associated with disruptions in neural crest cell development that are directly related to human CHD are poorly understood; however, patients who have DiGeorge, Alagille, and Noonan syndrome have congenital heart defects that involve many structures influenced by cardiac neural crest cells, and some of these genes are directly associated with these syndromes (as described below).

Mechanisms associated with human congenital heart disease

CHD is the most common cause of infant deaths from birth defects; one in three infants who die from a birth defect have a heart defect [2,35–37]. Despite its clinical significance, the etiology of CHD remains largely unknown. Environmental risk factors for CHD have long been recognized, including exposure to organic compounds, maternal alcohol abuse, prenatal exposure to drugs, as well as conditions such as maternal diabetes, among others [38–42]. Genetic risk factors also contribute to CHD, evidenced by familial clustering, sibling recurrence risk, and the association of chromosomal abnormalities and clinical syndromes [38,43]. However, disease-related mutations in only a handful of human genes have been identified to date, contributing to just a small percentage of CHD. These mutations and chromosomal aberrations show variable expressivity and penetrance, and demonstrate that the disease cannot be explained by simple Mendelian inheritance, but must arise through more complex mechanisms [38,44]. Theories of multifactorial inheritance have long been proposed, whereby multiple genetic factors, perhaps interacting with environmental factors, combine to increase the risk for abnormal cardiac development [43]. Thus future investigations to define the genetic contribution to these malformations will likely require much larger populations to discover low frequency causal mutations and to quantitate low effect relationships between higher frequency single nucleotide polymorphisms (SNPs) and disease [45,46].

There are various molecular cascades that have been identified as playing roles in the cellular mechanisms of heart development. Many of these genetic pathways have been identified in various vertebrate model systems such as mouse, chick, and fly. Because murine models have been recognized as the closest mammalian equivalent for studies of human cardiac disease [47–49], the similarity of genomes and ability to modify or genetically engineer the mouse has led to its use in laboratory studies of CHD. As a result, multiple genetic pathways have been identified that contribute to heart development, and whose disruption results in phenotypes similar to CHD seen in humans. Some of these genetic mechanisms are discussed below, where focus is placed on genes in which human mutations have been identified and associated with CHD. The incidence and known mechanisms associated with human CHD are described below and summarized in Table 1. For clinicians, an overview is provided in the following reviews [3,5,50–52].

NKX2-5

The *NKX2-5* gene on chromosome 5q34 consists of two exons, which encode a 324 amino acid protein. This homeobox transcription factor is expressed during early cardiac morphogenesis and serves as a master regulatory protein [53–55]. Because of its critical role in cardiogenesis, *NKX2-5* has been a prime candidate in studies to identify the genetic basis of structural congenital heart defects. Mutations have been identified in patients who have a variety of congenital heart malformations, including atrial and ventricular septal defects, conotruncal abnormalities, and AV conduction defects, among others [44,56–58]. *NKX2-5* interacts with a number of different proteins and genes that also play critical roles in cardiovascular development and perhaps in disease. In particular, studies indicate that *NKX2-5,* GATA factors, and members of the T-box transcription factor (*TBX*) family participate in a transcriptional regulatory relationship during cardiogenesis [59–61].

Table 1
Types and incidence of human congenital heart defects

Defect	Incidence per 1000 live births [2]	Gene association
VSD	3.57	*NKX2-5* [29,112], *GATA4* [70,71], *TBX5* [64]
PDA	0.799	
ASD	0.941	*NKX2-5* [57,113], *GATA4* [70,71], *TBX5* [64,114], *MYHC* [115], *ACTC* [116]
AVSD	0.348	*CRELD1* [117]
PS	0.729	
AS	0.401	
CoA	0.409	
TOF	0.421	*NKX2-5* [58], *JAG1* [118]
d-TGA	0.315	*CFC1* [119], *ZIC3* [120]
HRH	0.222	
Ticuspid atresia	0.079	
Ebstein's anomaly	0.114	
Pul atresia	0.132	
HLH	0.266	*NKX2-5* [44,113]
Truncus	0.107	
DORV	0.157	*CFC1* [119], *NKX2-5* [44]
SV	0.106	
TAPVC	0.094	
All cyanotic	1.391	
All CHD[a]	9.596	
BAV	13.556	*Notch1* [121]
Syndromes		
Alagille	rare	*JAG1* [122]
Char		*TFAF2B* [123]
DiGeorge	14.1	Chomosome 22q11.2 [124], *TBX1* [125]
Holt-Oram	0.95	*TBX5* [126]
Jacobsen	1	Chromosome 11q [127]
Noonan	40[a]	*PTPN11* [128]
Williams[b]	13.3	Chromosome 7q11.23 [129]
Trisomy 13	3.44	[130]
Trisomy 18	14.2	[130]
Trisomy 21	100	[131]

Abbreviations: AS, aortic stenosis; ASD, atrial septal defect; AVSD, atrioventricular septal defect; BAV, bicuspid aortic valve; CoA, coarctation of the aorta; DORV, double-outlet right ventricle; d-TGA, complete transposition of the great arteries; HLH, hypoplastic left heart; HRH, hypoplastic right heart; PDA, patent ductus arteriosus; PS, pulmonary stenosis; SV, single ventricle; TAPVC, total anomalous pulmonary venous connection; TOF, tetralogy of Fallot; VSD, ventricular septal defect.

[a] Not population study.

[b] Up to 70% of patients have cardiovascular defects [132].

T-box transcription factors

Members of the *TBX* family also play a role in cardiac development, and mutations in some *TBX* genes are directly associated with CHD. For example, *TBX5* is a member of the *TBX* factor family and has a critical role in early forelimb and cardiac morphogenesis [62,63]. The gene maps to chromosome 12q24.1 and consists of nine exons. Germ-line *TBX5* mutations have been implicated in Holt-Oram syndrome (HOS), an autosomal-dominant disorder characterized by upper limb malformations and cardiac septation defects [53,64,65]. *TBX5* has been shown to interact with *NKX2-5* on a molecular level, and the two different types of transcription factors are thought to synergistically induce cardiac development [66,67]. Because of its complex regulation during normal heart development and its ability to partner with other cardiac transcription factors, *TBX5* is considered a strong candidate gene for understanding the genetic causes of congenital heart defects.

TBX1 is another member of the T-box transcription factor family linked to human syndromes with CHD [5]. A high percentage of patients who have conotruncal defects carry a 22q11 deletion, a region commonly deleted in DiGeorge syndrome. The gene *TBX1* is contained within this commonly deleted region and has been strongly implicated as a major contributor to DiGeorge syndrome. Interestingly, *TBX1* is not expressed in neural crest cells, but is expressed by pharyngeal endoderm, so *TBX1* may indirectly affect neural crest cell maturation. Although the etiology of the disease is unclear, other genes on 22q11 that are deleted in DiGeorge syndrome likely play a direct or indirect role in contributing to the disorder.

GATA4

Mouse and human data demonstrate that the zinc finger-containing transcription factors *GATA-4/5/6* play critical roles in cardiovascular development [68]. GATA4 interacts directly with NKX2-5 via the homeodomain of NKX2-5 and the zinc finger domain of GATA4, and is thought to regulate genes involved in embryogenesis and in myocardial differentiation and function [60,69]. GATA4 has also been demonstrated to form a complex with TBX5 that if disrupted can lead to CHD [70]. Mutations in *GATA4* have been identified in multiplex families to associate with septal defects [70–72].

Jagged 1

In addition to *TBX1*, the Jagged-1 (*JAG1*) gene has been clearly indicated to be associated with human CHD, although the expressivity of the disease is highly variable. Cardiac manifestations include abnormalities of the pulmonary vasculature, tetralogy of Fallot, atrial and ventricular septal defects, aortic stenosis, and coarctation of the aorta [73,74]. *JAG1* is found to be mutated in approximately 94% of patients who have Alagille syndrome, and encodes a protein for one of the five known ligands of the Notch signaling pathway [74,75]. The mechanism of how JAG1 mutations disrupt Jag1-Notch signaling and cause CHD is unknown, but there is some suggestion that functional haploinsufficiency is a possible mechanism [74,76].

Vascular endothelial growth factor/NFATc1 signaling

NFATc1 (or *NFAT2*) belongs to a family of calcium-sensitive transcription factors activated by calcineurin-dependent dephosphorylation that play important roles in human development [77,78]. Four *NFATc* genes have been identified, *NFATc1* through *c4*, but only *NFATc1* has a restricted pattern of expression in endocardial cells destined to the valve. Activation of NFATc1 protein results in exposure of nuclear localization sequences and translocation to the nucleus. Once nuclear, NFATc1 interacts with other transcription factors, including activator protein-1 (AP-1), nuclear factor-κB (NF-κB), and GATA4 (described above) to form regulatory complexes on DNA and control transcription.

NFATc1 is absolutely required for heart valve formation. This role was first discovered when null mutant mice lacking *NFATc1* gene expression failed to form aortic and pulmonary valves, resulting in embryonic death by day E13.5 [22,24,79]. These findings are consistent with recent studies demonstrating that valve malformation in the $NFATc1^{-/-}$ mouse embryo results in abnormal circulatory flow patterns and not primary myocardial dysfunction [79]. Although the *NFATc1* gene has not been directly associated with human CHD, mouse defects associated with loss of *NFATc1* function are similar to clinical cases of human CHD that have cardiac valve malformations [80]. Furthermore, gain-of-function germ-line mutations of the human protein tyrosine phosphatase, nonreceptor type 11 (PTPN11) gene that cause Noonan syndrome, a human development disorder with CHD present in approximately 85% of the cases, have been shown to disrupt Ca^{2+} oscillatory control and impair NFAT signaling [81]. This suggests that although NFATc1 mutations have not been identified in patients who have CHD, other genetic mechanisms directly associated with CHD, such as *PTPN11* and *GATA4*, might contribute to the development of congenital heart abnormalities by disrupting NFATc1 function. Therefore, a thorough knowledge of NFATc1 activation and function is important to understanding its potential role in CHD.

VEGF is an upstream regulator of calcineurin signaling and NFATc1 activation in the valve, resulting in increased proliferation of human pulmonary valve endothelial cells [82]. VEGF plays multiple roles in cardiac development. Disruption of *VEGF* expression is embryonic-lethal, caused by chamber malformations, septation defects, and underdeveloped endocardial cushions [83–85]. Normal cardiac valvular formation depends on not only the appropriate timing of *VEGF* expression [86], but also on the correct level of *VEGF* expression during development [83,84,87,88]. Recent work demonstrated failure to develop coronary arteries when quail embryos were exposed to VEGF-Trap at E6 or E7 [89], further supporting the hypothesis that VEGF must be finely regulated.

VEGF/NFATc1 signaling may be an important event during early stages of valve development, by promoting the proliferation of endothelial cells in the endocardial cushions. As a transcription factor, NFATc1 signaling likely leads to regulated expression of downstream target genes required for valve formation. Endothelin-1, tissue factor (*TF*) and the Down syndrome critical region 1 (*DSCR1*) have been identified as possible gene targets of NFATc1 in endothelium [90–93], but transcriptional targets of NFATc1 in the valve are not well-defined. Autoregulation of *NFATc1* may be required for maintaining high *NFATc1* expression in pro-valve endocardial cells [94]. Furthermore, NFATc signaling in the myocardium was shown to initiate heart valve morphogenesis at E9 by repressing *VEGF* expression, which is followed by NFATc1 playing a direct role in perpetuating the remodeling of the valvular leaflets at E11 [91]. This suggests that negative feedback control of VEGF/NFATc1 signaling might exist through NFATc-mediated repression of *VEGF* expression. In addition, negative regulators of VEGF/calcineurin/NFATc1 signaling in the valve might be effective modulators of valve morphogenesis. For example, cellular inhibitors of calcineurin phosphatase, as well as protein kinases, have the ability to block NFATc1 phosphorylation and nuclear translocation [77,78]. Interestingly, the authors recently found that the ligand-activated nuclear hormone receptor peroxisome proliferator activated receptor gamma (PPARγ) is a negative regulator of VEGF signaling and NFATc1 activation in human pulmonary valve endothelial cells [95], suggesting that PPARγ may be another important regulator of cushion development.

Diagnostics and therapeutics

Surgical intervention in neonates

Advances in anesthesia, echocardiography, and interventional catheterization techniques, along with the increased availability of prostaglandins in recent years, have resulted in significant modifications in the treatment of patients who have complex CHD in the neonatal period. Major trends include a shift to early primary and complete repair of complex defects (ie, transposition of the great vessels, interrupted-arch ventricular septal defect [VSD], congenital aortic stenosis, truncus arteriosus, tetralogy of Fallot with pulmonary atresia) and more aggressive palliation of the most complex single ventricle complexes, such as hypoplastic left heart syndrome and pulmonary atresia with intact ventricular septum. Understanding the genetic contributions to these disease processes may lead to early diagnosis in some cases, and to more informed counseling and preparation for the team and family embarking on neonatal cardiac surgical intervention.

Fetal intervention (in utero)

Surgical fetal interventions for CHD have been described [96]. Particular interest is currently focused on balloon dilation of the congenitally stenotic aortic valve annulus in some variants of hypoplastic left heart syndrome [97]. Fetal procedures have yet to demonstrate equivalent or improved outcomes compared with neonatal procedures. Nonetheless, intervening while on placental support and during a period of continued plasticity of development has numerous theoretical advantages. It has become clear that successful outcomes in fetal intervention in utero are absolutely dependent upon accurate prenatal diagnostics, clear understanding of developmental biology and fetal physiology, and patient selection. Understanding the genetic contributions to CHD combined with improvements in prenatal diagnostics will be critical to future success in this arena.

Microarray analysis

Microarray analysis has served has a useful tool to obtain a genetic profile of CHD. Genetic testing typically has required multiple affected family members or syndromic features. The technique of microarray analysis has been applied to CHD and other cardiovascular diseases [98]. A number of genes previously not associated with CHD were identified as being differentially expressed (either upregulated or downregulated) in disease. Recently, microarray analysis was used to identify genes expressed that contribute to the right ventricular hypertrophy and stunted angiogenesis in patients who had tetralogy of Fallot [99]. The specific roles of genes necessary for development need to be further delineated.

Gene therapy

Genetic therapies remain a process for laboratory development. Delivery of the correct gene may be done with nonviral or viral vectors [100]. These methods may lead to cytotoxity and do not necessarily correct the defect. Intracardiac injection of viral vectors did arrest cardiomyopathies in hamsters that would normally progress [101]. Ideally, a specific genetic defect would be corrected in the developing embryo. Modification of the heart has been possible in *Xenopus* embryos. By overexpression of conditional dominant-interfering eomesodermin (EOMES), hypoplastic left heart syndrome was created. Conversely, overexpressing the activity of a different EOMES led to increased heart size [102]. This technique demonstrates promise, yet little work has been performed in mammalian models. With this new capability, the development and potential treatments of HLHS and its variants will become more evident.

Stem cell therapy

Cardiac transplantation and surgical interventions are the most common treatments for end-stage heart failure; however, these procedures are constrained and complicated by the limited number of available donor organs and the lack of suitable autologous tissue to restore the injured heart. Thus, the development of new therapeutic approaches is necessary to advance the morbidity and mortality rate of patients who have heart failure.

Cell-based therapies using adult or embryonic stem cells constitute an exciting future approach for the treatment of CHD. As mentioned earlier, the embryonic heart, and perhaps even the adult heart, are self-renewing in the sense that they may contain primitive cardiac stem cells that may differentiate to form myocytes, smooth muscle cells, and endothelial cells [9,10]. Although present in exceedingly small numbers, the future ability to isolate cardiac stem cells for ex vivo amplification would have important implications toward understanding myocardial homeostasis, cardiac aging, and tissue repair. More importantly, amplification would provide a valuable source of cells for tissue engineering.

Stem cell treatment has promising therapeutic potential. Mouse embryonic stem cells have been cultured and induced to differentiate into cardiomyocytes [103]; however, because of several issues, including immune rejection, potential for teratoma, and the inability to demonstrate reproducibly pure and stable cardiac grafts in transplanted rodent hearts, embryonic stem cell use in humans remains an experimental area that has considerable challenges. By contrast, the use of adult stem cells for clinical purpose is currently underway. Putative endothelial and cardiomyocyte precursor cells from adult bone marrow have been isolated and injected into patients [100]. Also, mesenchymal stem cells have been injected directly into infarction sites or transfused as a blood product [104]. These cells find their way to the infarction site and appear to engraft in the injury site; however, the engraftment does not appear to be long-term. In addition, the politics and ethics surrounding human stem cell research are major challenges that need to be resolved before significant advancements are made.

Tissue engineering

The primary obstacle of stem cell therapy is the limited source of cells with the pluripotent potential to give rise to all cardiac cell types; however, stem cell technologies coupled with tissue engineering may provide a useful and plausible solution. Cardiac defects specific to the valve are the most common form of CHD, affecting 25% to 30% of patients who have CHD [2,12]. For many patients who have valvular disease, replacement of the diseased native heart valve with animal, mechanical, or synthetic tissue valve substitutes is required. Despite significant advances in valve replacement surgery, these substitute valves are prone to thrombosis and calcification, and often fail postoperatively because of progressive deterioration, thus requiring additional surgical intervention. Furthermore, major congenital malformations present significant challenges to pediatric cardiologists and cardiac surgeons, because children who require valve replacement procedures typically "outgrow" the replacement valve as they develop. Consequently, various efforts are underway to generate autologous, tissue-engineered heart valves that are functional, viable, and have the potential to grow with the child through adulthood.

Remarkably, many of the tissue-engineering achievements with blood vessels and valves have been made without a thorough understanding of the biology of native valve tissue [105,106]. One of the first successful attempts to tissue-engineer autologous semilunar heart valves involved the use of mesenchymal stem cells isolated from the bone marrow of sheep, which were seeded onto a biodegradable scaffold and then implanted back into sheep for a period of longer than 4 months [107]. The valves were functional and underwent extensive remodeling in vivo to resemble native heart valves, suggesting that stem cell-derived, tissue-engineered heart valves may be a real alternative form of therapy in the future for patients who have CHD in need of heart valve replacement. Unfortunately, technical challenges such as difficulties associated with re-endothelialization of the valve conduit have limited progress and advancement in the field of tissue-engineering [108]. A long-term goal of future studies is to develop novel tissue-engineering strategies for production of improved cardiac valve substitutes. Addressing such tissue-engineering challenges will require a fundamental knowledge of the molecular and cellular mechanisms regulating cardiac valve development.

Adult congenital heart defects

It should be noted that because of the advances in treatment of children who have even the most complex forms of CHD, these patients are now surviving into adulthood. As a direct consequence, there is an increasing number of adults who have moderate or severe forms of CHD. The population of adults with CHD is expected to increase by 5% each year [109–111], and Hoffman and colleagues [110] suggest that 320,000 to 600,000 adults are in need of specialized care now. Competent care requires an in-depth understanding of the molecular and cellular basis of CHD and the altered physiology that results from surgical correction [111].

Summary

The cellular and molecular basis of CHD is an evolving area of rapid discovery. This brief overview has introduced the basic mechanisms underlying cardiac development and CHD in order to permit a clear understanding of current diagnostics and therapeutics and their future development. It is clear that although significant advances have been made in understanding mechanisms controlling heart formation, the direct causes of CHD remain poorly defined. Future studies that delineate the complexity of these mechanisms are required to provide a comprehensive understanding of the etiologies of CHD. Such understanding will lead to the development of novel approaches to prevention and therapy.

Acknowledgments

The authors thank Drs. Ravi Misra, John Lough, Mary Hutson, and Raymond Runyan for expert advice on sections of this review in their specialty areas. We also apologize in advance for not including many excellent studies because of space limitations and the broad scope of this review.

References

[1] Hoffman JI. Incidence of congenital heart disease: I. Postnatal incidence. Pediatr Cardiol 1995;16(3):103–13.

[2] Hoffman JI, Kaplan S. The incidence of congenital heart disease. J Am Coll Cardiol 2002; 39(12):1890–900.

[3] Gruber PJ, Epstein JA. Development gone awry: congenital heart disease. Circ Res 2004; 94(3):273–83.

[4] Gittenberger-de Groot AC, Bartelings MM, Deruiter MC, et al. Basics of cardiac development for the understanding of congenital heart malformations. Pediatr Res 2005;57(2): 169–76.

[5] McFadden DG, Olson EN. Heart development: learning from mistakes. Curr Opin Genet Dev 2002;12(3):328–35.

[6] Fishman MC, Chien KR. Fashioning the vertebrate heart: earliest embryonic decisions. Development 1997;124(11):2099–117.

[7] Srivastava D, Olson EN. A genetic blueprint for cardiac development. Nature 2000; 407(6801):221–6.

[8] Bernanke DH, Velkey JM. Development of the coronary blood supply: changing concepts and current ideas. Anat Rec 2002;269(4):198–208.

[9] Anversa P, Kajstura J, Leri A, et al. Life and death of cardiac stem cells: a paradigm shift in cardiac biology. Circulation 2006;113(11):1451–63.

[10] Beltrami AP, Barlucchi L, Torella D, et al. Adult cardiac stem cells are multipotent and support myocardial regeneration. Cell 2003;114(6):763–76.

[11] Eisenberg LM, Markwald RR. Cellular recruitment and the development of the myocardium. Dev Biol 2004;274(2):225–32.

[12] Armstrong EJ, Bischoff J. Heart valve development: endothelial cell signaling and differentiation. Circ Res 2004;95(5):459–70.

[13] Person AD, Klewer SE, Runyan RB. Cell biology of cardiac cushion development. Int Rev Cytol 2005;243:287–335.

[14] Mjaatvedt CH, Yamamurs H, Wessels A, et al. Mechanisms of segmentation, septation, and remodeling of the tubular heart: Endocardial cushion fate and cardiac looping. In: Harvey RP, Rosenthal N, editors. Heart development. San Diego (CA): Academic Press; 1999. p. 159–77.

[15] Ramsdell AF, Markwald RR. Induction of endocardial cushion tissue in the avian heart is regulated, in part, by TGFbeta-3-mediated autocrine signaling. Dev Biol 1997;188(1): 64–74.

[16] Brown CB, Boyer AS, Runyan RB, et al. Requirement of Type III TGF-beta receptor for endocardial cell transformation in the heart. Science 1999;283(5410):2080–2.

[17] Chen B, Bronson RT, Klaman LD, et al. Mice mutant for Egfr and Shp2 have defective cardiac semilunar valvulogenesis. Nat Genet 2000;24(3):296–9.

[18] Galvin KM, Donovan MJ, Lynch CA, et al. A role for smad6 in development and homeostasis of the cardiovascular system. Nat Genet 2000;24(2):171–4.

[19] Lakkis MM, Epstein JA. Neurofibromin modulation of ras activity is required for normal endocardial-mesenchymal transformation in the developing heart. Development 1998; 125(22):4359–67.

[20] Bourdeau A, Dumont DJ, Letarte M. A murine model of hereditary hemorrhagic telangiectasia. J Clin Invest 1999;104(10):1343–51.

[21] Camenisch TD, Spicer AP, Brehm-Gibson T, et al. Disruption of hyaluronan synthase-2 abrogates normal cardiac morphogenesis and hyaluronan-mediated transformation of epithelium to mesenchyme. J Clin Invest 2000;106(3):349–60.

[22] de la Pompa JL, Timmerman LA, Takimoto H, et al. Role of the NF-ATc transcription factor in morphogenesis of cardiac valves and septum. Nature 1998;392(6672):182–6.

[23] Gruber PJ, Kubalak SW, Pexieder T, et al. RXR alpha deficiency confers genetic susceptibility for aortic sac, conotruncal, atrioventricular cushion, and ventricular muscle defects in mice. J Clin Invest 1996;98(6):1332–43.

[24] Ranger AM, Grusby MJ, Hodge MR, et al. The transcription factor NF-ATc is essential for cardiac valve formation. Nature 1998;392(6672):186–90.

[25] Schilham MW, Oosterwegel MA, Moerer P, et al. Defects in cardiac outflow tract formation and pro-B-lymphocyte expansion in mice lacking Sox-4. Nature 1996;380(6576): 711–4.

[26] Norris RA, Kern CB, Wessels A, et al. Identification and detection of the periostin gene in cardiac development. Anat Rec A Discov Mol Cell Evol Biol 2004;281(2):1227–33.

[27] Gitler AD, Lu MM, Jiang YQ, et al. Molecular markers of cardiac endocardial cushion development. Dev Dyn 2003;228(4):643–50.

[28] Munoz-Chapuli R, Macias D, Gonzalez-Iriarte M, et al. The epicardium and epicardial-derived cells: multiple functions in cardiac development. Rev Esp Cardiol 2002;55(10): 1070–82 [in Spanish].

[29] Hatcher CJ, Diman NY, Kim MS, et al. A role for Tbx5 in proepicardial cell migration during cardiogenesis. Physiol Genomics 2004;18(2):129–40.

[30] Landerholm TE, Dong XR, Lu J, et al. A role for serum response factor in coronary smooth muscle differentiation from proepicardial cells. Development 1999;126(10): 2053–62.

[31] Nelson TJ, Duncan SA, Misra RP. Conserved enhancer in the serum response factor promoter controls expression during early coronary vasculogenesis. Circ Res 2004;94(8): 1059–66.

[32] Carmona R, Gonzalez-Iriarte M, Perez-Pomares JM, et al. Localization of the Wilm's tumour protein WT1 in avian embryos. Cell Tissue Res 2001;303(2):173–86.

[33] Kirby ML, Hutson MR. Cardiac neural crest and conotruncal malformations. Semin Cell Dev Biol; in press.

[34] Stoller JZ, Epstein JA. Cardiac neural crest. Semin Cell Dev Biol 2005;16(6):704–15.

[35] Ferencz C, Rubin JD, McCarter RJ, et al. Congenital heart disease: prevalence at livebirth. The Baltimore-Washington Infant Study. Am J Epidemiol 1985;121(1):31–6.

[36] Gillum RF. Epidemiology of congenital heart disease in the United States. Am Heart J 1994;127(4 Pt 1):919–27.

[37] Thom T, Haase N, Rosamond W, et al. Heart disease and stroke statistics—2006 update: a report from the American Heart Association Statistics Committee and Stroke Statistics Subcommittee. Circulation 2006;113(6):e85–151.

[38] Ferencz C, Correa-Villasenor A, Loffredo CA, et al. Malformations of the cardiac outflow tract. Genetic and environmental risk factors of major cardiovascular malformations: the Baltimore-Washington Infant Study: 1981–1989, vol. 5. Armonk (NY): Futura Publishing Company, Inc.; 1997. p. 59–102.

[39] Ferencz C, Rubin JD, Loffredo CA, et al. Epidemiology of congenital heart disease: the Baltimore-Washington Infant Study, 1981–1989, vol. 4. Mt. Kisco (NY): Futura Publishing Company, Inc.; 1993. p. 33–62.

[40] Loffredo CA. Epidemiology of cardiovascular malformations: prevalence and risk factors. Am J Med Genet 2000;97(4):319–25.

[41] Loffredo CA, Silbergeld EK, Ferencz C, et al. Association of transposition of the great arteries in infants with maternal exposures to herbicides and rodenticides. Am J Epidemiol 2001;153(6):529–36.

[42] Loffredo CA, Wilson PD, Ferencz C. Maternal diabetes: an independent risk factor for major cardiovascular malformations with increased mortality of affected infants. Teratology 2001;64(2):98–106.

[43] Nora JJ, Nora AH. Recurrence risks in children having one parent with a congenital heart disease. Circulation 1976;53(4):701–2.

[44] McElhinney DB, Geiger E, Blinder J, et al. NKX2.5 mutations in patients with congenital heart disease. J Am Coll Cardiol 2003;42(9):1650–5.

[45] Pritchard JK. Are rare variants responsible for susceptibility to complex diseases? Am J Hum Genet 2001;69(1):124–37.

[46] Tabor HK, Risch NJ, Myers RM. Opinion: candidate-gene approaches for studying complex genetic traits: practical considerations. Nat Rev Genet 2002;3(5):391–7.

[47] Gruber PJ. Cardiac development: new concepts. Clin Perinatol 2005;32(4):845–55 [vii].

[48] Rossant J. Mouse mutants and cardiac development: new molecular insights into cardiogenesis. Circ Res 1996;78(3):349–53.

[49] Wessels A, Sedmera D. Developmental anatomy of the heart: a tale of mice and man. Physiol Genomics 2003;15(3):165–76.

[50] Gibbons GH, Liew CC, Goodarzi MO, et al. Genetic markers: progress and potential for cardiovascular disease. Circulation 2004;109(Suppl 1):IV47–58.

[51] Liew CC, Dzau VJ. Molecular genetics and genomics of heart failure. Nat Rev Genet 2004; 5(11):811–25.

[52] Olson EN. A decade of discoveries in cardiac biology. Nat Med 2004;10(5):467–74.

[53] Lints TJ, Parsons LM, Hartley L, et al. Nkx-2.5: a novel murine homeobox gene expressed in early heart progenitor cells and their myogenic descendants. Development 1993;119(2): 419–31 [erratum: Development 1993;119(3):969].

[54] Lyons I, Parsons LM, Hartley L, et al. Myogenic and morphogenetic defects in the heart tubes of murine embryos lacking the homeo box gene Nkx2-5. Genes Dev 1995;9(13): 1654–66.

[55] Tanaka M, Chen Z, Bartunkova S, et al. The cardiac homeobox gene Csx/Nkx2.5 lies genetically upstream of multiple genes essential for heart development. Development 1999; 126(6):1269–80.

[56] Benson DW, Silberbach GM, Kavanaugh-McHugh A, et al. Mutations in the cardiac transcription factor NKX2.5 affect diverse cardiac developmental pathways. J Clin Invest 1999; 104(11):1567–73.

[57] Schott JJ, Benson DW, Basson CT, et al. Congenital heart disease caused by mutations in the transcription factor NKX2-5. Science 1998;281(5373):108–11.

[58] Goldmuntz E, Geiger E, Benson DW. NKX2.5 mutations in patients with tetralogy of fallot. Circulation 2001;104(21):2565–8.

[59] Davis DL, Wessels A, Burch JB. An Nkx-dependent enhancer regulates cGATA-6 gene expression during early stages of heart development. Dev Biol 2000;217(2):310–22.

[60] Jiang Y, Drysdale TA, Evans T. A role for GATA-4/5/6 in the regulation of Nkx2.5 expression with implications for patterning of the precardiac field. Dev Biol 1999;216(1): 57–71.

[61] Molkentin JD, Antos C, Mercer B, et al. Direct activation of a GATA6 cardiac enhancer by Nkx2.5: evidence for a reinforcing regulatory network of Nkx2.5 and GATA transcription factors in the developing heart. Dev Biol 2000;217(2):301–9.

[62] Horb ME, Thomsen GH. Tbx5 is essential for heart development. Development 1999; 126(8):1739–51.

[63] Liberatore CM, Searcy-Schrick RD, Yutzey KE. Ventricular expression of tbx5 inhibits normal heart chamber development. Dev Biol 2000;223(1):169–80.

[64] Basson CT, Bachinsky DR, Lin RC, et al. Mutations in human TBX5 [corrected] cause limb and cardiac malformation in Holt-Oram syndrome. Nat Genet 1997;15(1):30–5.

[65] Li QY, Newbury-Ecob RA, Terrett JA, et al. Holt-Oram syndrome is caused by mutations in TBX5, a member of the Brachyury (T) gene family. Nat Genet 1997;15(1):21–9.

[66] Habets PE, Moorman AF, Clout DE, et al. Cooperative action of Tbx2 and Nkx2.5 inhibits ANF expression in the atrioventricular canal: implications for cardiac chamber formation. Genes Dev 2002;16(10):1234–46.

[67] Hiroi Y, Kudoh S, Monzen K, et al. Tbx5 associates with Nkx2–5 and synergistically promotes cardiomyocyte differentiation. Nat Genet 2001;28(3):276–80.

[68] Parmacek MS, Leiden JM. GATA transcription factors and cardiac development. In: Harvey RP, Rosenthal N, editors. Heart development. Toronto: Academic Press; 1999. p. 291–306.

[69] Shiojima I, Komuro I, Oka T, et al. Context-dependent transcriptional cooperation mediated by cardiac transcription factors Csx/Nkx-2.5 and GATA-4. J Biol Chem 1999;274(12): 8231–9.

[70] Garg V, Kathiriya IS, Barnes R, et al. GATA4 mutations cause human congenital heart defects and reveal an interaction with TBX5. Nature 2003;424(6947):443–7.

[71] Hirayama-Yamada K, Kamisago M, Akimoto K, et al. Phenotypes with GATA4 or NKX2.5 mutations in familial atrial septal defect. Am J Med Genet A 2005;135(1):47–52.

[72] Okubo A, Miyoshi O, Baba K, et al. A novel GATA4 mutation completely segregated with atrial septal defect in a large Japanese family. J Med Genet 2004;41(7):e97.

[73] Krantz ID, Smith R, Colliton RP, et al. Jagged1 mutations in patients ascertained with isolated congenital heart defects. Am J Med Genet 1999;84(1):56–60.

[74] Warthen DM, Moore EC, Kamath BM, et al. Jagged1 (JAG1) mutations in Alagille syndrome: increasing the mutation detection rate. Hum Mutat 2006;27(5):436–43.

[75] Kadesch T. Notch signaling: a dance of proteins changing partners. Exp Cell Res 2000; 260(1):1–8.

[76] Morrissette JD, Colliton RP, Spinner NB. Defective intracellular transport and processing of JAG1 missense mutations in Alagille syndrome. Hum Mol Genet 2001;10(4):405–13.

[77] Crabtree GR, Olson EN. NFAT signaling: choreographing the social lives of cells. Cell 2002;109(Suppl):S67–79.

[78] Schulz RA, Yutzey KE. Calcineurin signaling and NFAT activation in cardiovascular and skeletal muscle development. Dev Biol 2004;266(1):1–16.

[79] Phoon CK, Ji RP, Aristizabal O, et al. Embryonic heart failure in NFATc1 −/− mice: novel mechanistic insights from in utero ultrasound biomicroscopy. Circ Res 2004;95(1):92–9.

[80] Nolan GP. Cardiac development. Transcription and the broken heart. Nature 1998; 392(6672):129–30.

[81] Uhlen P, Burch PM, Zito CI, et al. Gain-of-function/Noonan syndrome SHP-2/Ptpn11 mutants enhance calcium oscillations and impair NFAT signaling. Proc Natl Acad Sci U S A 2006;103(7):2160–5.

[82] Johnson EN, Lee YM, Sander TL, et al. NFATc1 mediates vascular endothelial growth factor-induced proliferation of human pulmonary valve endothelial cells. J Biol Chem 2003;278(3):1686–92.

[83] Carmeliet P, Ferreira V, Breier G, et al. Abnormal blood vessel development and lethality in embryos lacking a single VEGF allele. Nature 1996;380(6573):435–9.

[84] Ferrara N, Carver-Moore K, Chen H, et al. Heterozygous embryonic lethality induced by targeted inactivation of the VEGF gene. Nature 1996;380(6573):439–42.

[85] Stalmans I, Lambrechts D, De Smet F, et al. VEGF: a modifier of the del22q11 (DiGeorge) syndrome? Nat Med 2003;9(2):173–82.

[86] Dor Y, Camenisch TD, Itin A, et al. A novel role for VEGF in endocardial cushion formation and its potential contribution to congenital heart defects. Development 2001;128(9):1531–8.

[87] Ferrara N. Vascular endothelial growth factor. Eur J Cancer 1996;32A(14):2413–22.

[88] Miquerol L, Langille BL, Nagy A. Embryonic development is disrupted by modest increases in vascular endothelial growth factor gene expression. Development 2000;127(18):3941–6.

[89] Tomanek RJ, Ishii Y, Holifield JS, et al. VEGF family members regulate myocardial tubulogenesis and coronary artery formation in the embryo. Circ Res 2006;98(7):947–53.

[90] Armesilla AL, Lorenzo E, Gomez del Arco P, et al. Vascular endothelial growth factor activates nuclear factor of activated T cells in human endothelial cells: a role for tissue factor gene expression. Mol Cell Biol 1999;19(3):2032–43.

[91] Chang CP, Neilson JR, Bayle JH, et al. A field of myocardial-endocardial NFAT signaling underlies heart valve morphogenesis. Cell 2004;118(5):649–63.

[92] Lange AW, Molkentin JD, Yutzey KE. DSCR1 gene expression is dependent on NFATc1 during cardiac valve formation and colocalizes with anomalous organ development in trisomy 16 mice. Dev Biol 2004;266(2):346–60.

[93] Nemer G, Nemer M. Cooperative interaction between GATA5 and NF-ATc regulates endothelial-endocardial differentiation of cardiogenic cells. Development 2002;129(17):4045–55.

[94] Zhou B, Wu B, Tompkins KL, et al. Characterization of Nfatc1 regulation identifies an enhancer required for gene expression that is specific to pro-valve endocardial cells in the developing heart. Development 2005;132(5):1137–46.

[95] Sander TL, Noll L, Klinkner DB, et al. Rosiglitazone antagonizes VEGF signaling and NFATc1 activation in cardiac valve endothelium. Endothelium 2006;13(3):181–90.

[96] Park HK, Park YH. Fetal surgery for congenital heart disease. Yonsei Med J 2001;42(6):686–94.

[97] Makikallio K, McElhinney DB, Levine JC, et al. Fetal aortic valve stenosis and the evolution of hypoplastic left heart syndrome: patient selection for fetal intervention. Circulation 2006;113(11):1401–5.

[98] Archacki S, Wang Q. Expression profiling of cardiovascular disease. Hum Genomics 2004;1(5):355–70.

[99] Sharma HS, Peters TH, Moorhouse MJ, et al. DNA microarray analysis for human congenital heart disease. Cell Biochem Biophys 2006;44(1):1–9.

[100] Melo LG, Pachori AS, Kong D, et al. Gene and cell-based therapies for heart disease. FASEB J 2004;18(6):648–63.

[101] Kawada T, Nakazawa M, Nakauchi S, et al. Rescue of hereditary form of dilated cardiomyopathy by rAAV-mediated somatic gene therapy: amelioration of morphological findings, sarcolemmal permeability, cardiac performances, and the prognosis of TO-2 hamsters. Proc Natl Acad Sci U S A 2002;99(2):901–6.

[102] Ryan K, Russ AP, Levy RJ, et al. Modulation of eomes activity alters the size of the developing heart: implications for in utero cardiac gene therapy. Hum Gene Ther 2004;15(9):842–55.

[103] Wei H, Juhasz O, Li J, et al. Embryonic stem cells and cardiomyocyte differentiation: phenotypic and molecular analyses. J Cell Mol Med 2005;9(4):804–17.

[104] Pittenger MF, Martin BJ. Mesenchymal stem cells and their potential as cardiac therapeutics. Circ Res 2004;95(1):9–20.

[105] Hoerstrup SP, Sodian R, Daebritz S, et al. Functional living trileaflet heart valves grown in vitro. Circulation 2000;102(Suppl 3):III44–9.

[106] Nugent HM, Edelman ER. Tissue engineering therapy for cardiovascular disease. Circ Res 2003;92(10):1068–78.

[107] Sutherland FW, Perry TE, Yu Y, et al. From stem cells to viable autologous semilunar heart valve. Circulation 2005;111(21):2783–91.

[108] Schoen FJ, Levy RJ. Founder's award, 25th annual meeting of the Society for Biomaterials, perspectives. Providence, RI, April 28–May 2, 1999. Tissue heart valves: current challenges and future research perspectives. J Biomed Mater Res 1999;47(4):439–65.

[109] Brickner ME, Hillis LD, Lange RA. Congenital heart disease in adults. First of two parts. N Engl J Med 2000;342(4):256–63.

[110] Hoffman JI, Kaplan S, Liberthson RR. Prevalence of congenital heart disease. Am Heart J 2004;147(3):425–39.

[111] Sanders SP. We know how many—but how? Am Heart J 2004;147(3):398–400.

[112] Sarkozy A, Conti E, Neri C, et al. Spectrum of atrial septal defects associated with mutations of NKX2.5 and GATA4 transcription factors. J Med Genet 2005;42(2):e16.

[113] Elliott DA, Kirk EP, Yeoh T, et al. Cardiac homeobox gene NKX2-5 mutations and congenital heart disease: associations with atrial septal defect and hypoplastic left heart syndrome. J Am Coll Cardiol 2003;41(11):2072–6.

[114] Hatcher CJ, Basson CT. Getting the T-box dose right. Nat Med 2001;7(11):1185–6.

[115] Ching YH, Ghosh TK, Cross SJ, et al. Mutation in myosin heavy chain 6 causes atrial septal defect. Nat Genet 2005;37(4):423–8.

[116] Kirk EP, Hyun C, Thomson PC, et al. Quantitative trait loci modifying cardiac atrial septal morphology and risk of patent foramen ovale in the mouse. Circ Res 2006;98(5):651–8.

[117] Robinson SW, Morris CD, Goldmuntz E, et al. Missense mutations in CRELD1 are associated with cardiac atrioventricular septal defects. Am J Hum Genet 2003;72(4):1047–52.

[118] Eldadah ZA, Hamosh A, Biery NJ, et al. Familial tetralogy of Fallot caused by mutation in the jagged1 gene. Hum Mol Genet 2001;10(2):163–9.

[119] Bamford RN, Roessler E, Burdine RD, et al. Loss-of-function mutations in the EGF-CFC gene CFC1 are associated with human left-right laterality defects. Nat Genet 2000;26(3): 365–9.

[120] Ware SM, Peng J, Zhu L, et al. Identification and functional analysis of ZIC3 mutations in heterotaxy and related congenital heart defects. Am J Hum Genet 2004;74(1):93–105.

[121] Garg V, Muth AN, Ransom JF, et al. Mutations in NOTCH1 cause aortic valve disease. Nature 2005;437(7056):270–4.

[122] Heritage ML, MacMillan JC, Colliton RP, et al. Jagged1 (JAG1) mutation detection in an Australian Alagille syndrome population. Hum Mutat 2000;16(5):408–16.

[123] Satoda M, Zhao F, Diaz GA, et al. Mutations in TFAP2B cause Char syndrome, a familial form of patent ductus arteriosus. Nat Genet 2000;25(1):42–6.

[124] Oskarsdottir S, Vujic M, Fasth A. Incidence and prevalence of the 22q11 deletion syndrome: a population-based study in Western Sweden. Arch Dis Child 2004;89(2):148–51.

[125] Yagi H, Furutani Y, Hamada H, et al. Role of TBX1 in human del22q11.2 syndrome. Lancet 2003;362(9393):1366–73.

[126] Vaughan CJ, Basson CT. Molecular determinants of atrial and ventricular septal defects and patent ductus arteriosus. Am J Med Genet 2000;97(4):304–9.

[127] Grossfeld PD, Mattina T, Lai Z, et al. The 11q terminal deletion disorder: a prospective study of 110 cases. Am J Med Genet A 2004;129(1):51–61.

[128] Tartaglia M, Gelb BD. Noonan syndrome and related disorders: genetics and pathogenesis. Annu Rev Genomics Hum Genet 2005;6:45–68.

[129] Stromme P, Bjornstad PG, Ramstad K. Prevalence estimation of Williams syndrome. J Child Neurol 2002;17(4):269–71.

[130] Goldstein H, Nielsen KG. Rates and survival of individuals with trisomy 13 and 18. Data from a 10-year period in Denmark. Clin Genet 1988;34(6):366–72.

[131] Bishop J, Huether CA, Torfs C, et al. Epidemiologic study of Down syndrome in a racially diverse California population, 1989–1991. Am J Epidemiol 1997;145(2):134–47.

[132] Eronen M, Peippo M, Hiippala A, et al. Cardiovascular manifestations in 75 patients with Williams syndrome. J Med Genet 2002;39(8):554–8.

ELSEVIER
SAUNDERS

Pediatr Clin N Am
53 (2006) 1011–1028

PEDIATRIC CLINICS
OF NORTH AMERICA

The Molecular Basis of Pediatric Hypertension

Julie R. Ingelfinger, MD[a,b,*]

[a]Pediatric Nephrology, Yawkey 6C, MassGeneral Hospital for Children at Massachusetts General Hospital, 55 Fruit Street, Boston, MA 02114, USA
[b]Harvard Medical School, 25 Shattuck Street, Boston, MA 02115, USA

Blood pressure, the product of cardiac output and peripheral vascular resistance, follows a circadian rhythm and is altered by numerous circulating and local substances and by many physiologic events (Fig. 1) [1,2]. During the course of the 24-hour day, systolic blood pressure varies considerably [3]. It is hardly surprising, then, that the factors controlling blood pressure, including its molecular determinants, are complex. With infants, children, and adolescents increasingly being identified with elevated blood pressure, considering different aspects of pathogenesis has become ever more important for pediatricians.

Why do children develop hypertension? Clearly, some have definable causes, which may include monogenic forms of hypertension, although these are rare [4]. It has become clear that many children have primary (essential) hypertension. Simplistically, their blood pressures become elevated when those factors that control cardiac output or peripheral vascular resistance are altered, resulting in hypertension [4]. Classically, cardiac output is determined by stroke volume, the condition of the cardiac muscle, the sympathetic nervous system, and local vasoactive factors within the heart, kidneys, and vasculature [5,6]. Peripheral vascular resistance is determined by vascular tone, circulating factors, and nerves. All of these variables are affected by afferent input from the brain, kidneys, and other organs. The number of genes, signaling pathways, and systems that are involved in blood pressure regulation is enormous, and dissecting those factors that are most important in hypertension has proven challenging. This article briefly considers molecular mechanisms of hypertension in those several conditions

---

* Pediatric Nephrology, Yawkey 6C, MassGeneral Hospital for Children, 55 Fruit Street, Boston, MA 02114.

E-mail address: jingelfinger@partners.org

0031-3955/06/$ - see front matter © 2006 Elsevier Inc. All rights reserved.
doi:10.1016/j.pcl.2006.08.005

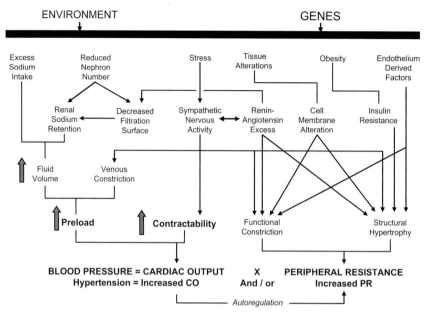

Fig. 1. A number of physical, environmental, genetic, and hormonal factors act together to influence both cardiac output and peripheral vascular resistance.

in which mutations in a single gene give rise to hypertension and then considers the contribution of these and other genes to essential hypertension.

Monogenic forms of hypertension

Specific mutations in a small number of genes have elucidated abnormalities in several forms of heritable hypertension, because the aberrant gene product or function leads to a specific and definable cause of hypertension in each case. Such conditions, classified as monogenic hypertension, often are associated with severe elevations in blood pressure, frequently presenting early in childhood [7,8].

Positional cloning (in the past called "reverse genetics") has been successful in leading to the discovery of genes that are mutated in these disorders [9–11]. Using this approach, informative pedigrees with a large number of family members are phenotyped, and the mode of inheritance is analyzed (autosomal recessive, dominant, sex-linked, codominant, and so forth). Linkage analysis then can be performed with microsatellite markers or other highly polymorphic genetic markers that are evenly spaced throughout the genome (at approximately 10-cM intervals). Because about 70% of people are heterozygous, allele inheritance can be followed through large pedigrees. If a linkage study is successful, a specific chromosomal region in the genome is found to be linked to the trait being studied. The LOD (logarithm of the odds) score is used to describe such a region as present or absent. An LOD score greater than 3.3 (corresponding to a genomewise significance level of 4.5×10^{-5}) generally is considered significant [10]. A search for known genes of interest can begin following discovery of a relevant chromosomal region.

Because several types of monogenic hypertension are associated with low plasma renin levels or activity, profiling renin levels or activity against sodium excretion can be invaluable in directing a patient's hypertension evaluation. Table 1 lists the best-characterized forms of monogenic hypertension, each of which is considered briefly. Children and adolescents with hypertension who have a suggestive family history, severe hypertension from an early age, or hypertension that is difficult to control should be evaluated for monogenic hypertension.

Glucocorticoid-responsive aldosteronism

In the late 1960s Sutherland and colleagues [13] and New and coworkers [14] observed that some hypertensive patients who had increased aldosterone secretion and suppressed renin levels improved when they were given dexamethasone. (See Online Mendelian Inheritance in Man [OMIM] #103900 at http://www.ncbi.nlm.nih.gov/Omim.) A large number of affected families with this condition [15–20], now known as glucocorticoid-responsive aldosteronism or GRA, have been reported. The hypertension in this disease is attributable to the effects of a chimeric gene (fusion of the 11 β-hydroxylase and aldosterone synthase genes by way of an unequal crossing-over event) [21,22], which results in stimulation of aldosterone synthesis by corticotropin rather than by angiotensin II or potassium. Aldosterone synthesis and secretion in people who have GRA is generally high [20,23–25], with resultant salt and water retention and plasma volume expansion.

Urine and plasma (or serum) aldosterone levels are often but not invariably elevated in GRA. Because the protein product of the chimeric gene converts cortisol to 18-hydroxy and 18-oxo metabolites, these can be measured in urine [26–29]. In people who have this condition the urinary levels of 18-Ftetrahydrocortisol (TH18oxoF) and 18-hydroxycortisol are high, and the ratio of TH18oxoF/urinary tetrahydroaldosterone (THAD) is increased. Genetic testing is both sensitive and specific in this disorder.

GRA should be considered as a potential cause of hypertension if a child who has elevated blood pressure has a family history of severe resistant essential hypertension or if family members have had serious cardiovascular events, such as stroke and myocardial infarction, early in life. A case series that reviewed the findings in 20 children who had established GRA indicated that 16 were hypertensive, some as early as the first month of life [30]. The 4 children who were not hypertensive were diagnosed in the course

Table 1
Monogenic forms of hypertension

Signs and Sx	Hormonal findings	Mutation	Genetics	Comment
Steroidogenic enzyme defects				
Steroid 11β-hydroxylase deficiency	⇓ PRA and aldo; high serum androgens/urine 17 ketosteroids; elevated DOC and 11-deoxycortisol	CYP11B1 mutation (encodes cytochrome P$_{450}$11β/18 of ZF); impairs synthesis of cortisol and ZF 17-deoxysteroids	Most cases are autosomal recessive Adrenal: Zona fasciculata	Hypertensive virilizing CAH; most patients identified by time they are hypertensive. Increased BP may also occur from medication side effects
Steroid 11α-hydroxylase/ 17, 20-lyase deficiency	⇓ PRA and aldo; low serum/urinary 17-hydroxysteroids; decreased cortisol; ⇑ corticosterone (B) and DOC in plasma; serum androgens and estrogens very low; serum gonadotrophins very high	CYP17 mutation (encodes cytochrome P$_{450}$C17) impairs cortisol and sex steroid production	Adrenal: zona fasciculata; Gonadal: interstitial cells (Leydig in testis; theca in ovary)	CAH with male pseudohermaphroditism; female external genital phenotype in males; primary amenorrhea in females
Dexamethasone-suppressible hypertension				
Glucocorticoid-remediable aldosteronism (GRA)	Plasma and urinary aldo responsive to corticotropin; dexamethasone suppressible within 48 hr; ⇑ urine and plasma 18OHS, 18-OHF, and 18 oxoF	Chimeric gene that is expressed at high level in ZF (regulated like CYP11B1) and has 18-oxidase activity (CYP11B2 functionality)	Adrenal: abnormal presence of enzymatic activity in adrenal ZF, allowing completion of aldo synthesis from 17-deoxy steroids	Hypokalemia in sodium-replete state

Apparent mineralocorticoid excess AME	⇑ plasma corticotropin and secretory rates of all corticosteroids; nl serum F (delayed plasma clearance)	Mutation in 11βOHSD type 2	⇑ plasma F bioact in periphery (F→E) of bi-dir. 11βOHSD or slow clearance by 5 α/β reduction to allo dihydro-F	Cardiac conduction changes; LVH, vessel remodeling; some calcium abnormalities; nephrocalcinosis; rickets
Non-steroidal defects Liddle's syndrome	Low plasma renin, low or normal K⁺; negligible urinary aldosterone	Mutations in the epithelial sodium channel, ENaC	Autosomal dominant ENaC channel is constitutively active in this disorder	Responds to triamterene, other distal agents, low-salt diet
Pseudohypoaldosteronism II — Gordon syndrome	Low plasma renin, normal or elevated K⁺	Mutations in WNK1 or WNK4	Autosomal dominant	Responds to thiazides
Hypertension and brachydactyly	Short metacarpals, short stature, hypertension	Linkage to chromosome 12p	Autosomal dominant	??

Abbreviations: **B,** corticosterone or Compound B; bi-dir, bidirectional; bioact, bioactive; CAH, congenital adrenal hyperplasia; DOC, deoxycorticosterone; **F,** cortisol, or Compound F; LVH, left ventricular hypertrophy; nl, normal; OHSD, hydroxysteroid dehydrogenase; PRA, plasma renin activity; Sx, symptoms; ZF, zona fasciculate.

Adapted from Ingelfinger JR. Low renin hypertension in childhood. In: Lifshitz F, editor. Pediatric Endocrinology. 4th edition. New York: Marcel Dekker; 2003.

of family evaluations. Half of the children who had hypertension required multiple antihypertensive medications to bring their blood pressure levels under control; 3 children did not achieve blood pressure control, even with multiple agents [30].

Apparent mineralocorticoid excess

Apparent mineralocorticoid excess (AME, OMIM # 218030) also is characterized by low-renin hypertension with hypokalemia and metabolic alkalosis [31]. New and colleagues first described this condition in the late 1970s [32,33]. The hypertension in AME is often severe, presents early in life, and may already be accompanied by end-organ damage by the time of diagnosis [34].

Affected patients have low levels of 11-β-hydroxysteroid dehydrogenase, the enzyme that converts cortisol to cortisone. Normally, the microsomal enzyme 11β-hydroxysteroid dehydrogenase converts active 11-hydroxyglucocorticoids to their inactive keto-metabolites. Because aldosterone and cortisol bind to the mineralocorticoid receptor, there is delayed conversion of cortisol to the biologically inactive compound, cortisone [35,36]. The increased cortisol can then bind and activate the mineralocorticoid receptor [37–41]. In AME patients, high levels of cortisol, acting by way of the mineralocorticoid receptor, exert effects usually reserved for potent mineralocorticoids.

AME is attributable to a mutation in 11-β-hydroxysteroid dehydrogenase 2 (11-β-HSD2), which is important in epithelial sodium transport. The clinical picture of classical AME is severe hypertension, failure to thrive, and often persistent polydipsia. Dietary sodium restriction may be useful as patients are volume expanded. Plasma renin levels and activity are markedly decreased.

Similar physiology occurs in the severe hypertension that has been reported in people who have ingested large amounts of licorice. The active component of licorice, glycyrrhetinic acid, inhibits 11-β-hydroxysteroid dehydrogenase, increasing the available cortisol and stimulation of the mineralocorticoid receptor [42]. The pathogenesis of licorice-induced hypertension is similar to that seen genetically in AME [39,40,43].

Liddle syndrome

Liddle syndrome (OMIM # 177200) is named for the clinical investigator who described a unique family with an autosomal-dominant form of severe hypertension accompanied by hypokalemia and both low renin and low aldosterone levels [44,45]. The affected family members presented with a clinical picture of aldosterone excess, yet the biochemical picture was marked by extremely low renin and aldosterone levels [46,47]. Some, but not all, affected patients have hypokalemia. Early studies demonstrated that inhibiting the aldosterone receptor had no effect on the hypertension. In contrast, a low-salt diet and inhibitors of the distal nephron sodium transporters were effective. Furthermore, red blood cell transport studies suggested an abnormality in membrane sodium transport [48]. These observations, taken together, suggested that there was a sodium transport abnormality that involved renal handling of salt and water. The primary role of the kidneys in this syndrome was demonstrated when a patient who had this syndrome required a renal transplant, after which hypertension and hypokalemia rapidly resolved [49].

The cloning of the epithelial sodium channel, ENaC, which contains α, β, and γ subunits, is integral to mineralocorticoid-dependent sodium transport within the renal epithelia. It is now known that activating mutations in the β and γ subunits of ENaC (which lie in close proximity on chromosome 16) lead to Liddle syndrome.

Gordon syndrome or pseudohypoaldosteronism type II

Gordon syndrome, or familial hyperkalemia (OMIM #145260), also called pseudohypoaldosteronism type II, is an autosomal-dominant form of hypertension associated with hyperkalemia that is present in the face of normal glomerular filtration rate [50–53]. In addition, increased renal salt reabsorption and acidemia may be present [50–53]. PHAII is attributable to mutations in the WNK1 and WNK4 kinase genes located on human chromosomes 12 and 17, respectively [54,55]. The name WNK derives from a molecular description: the absence of a key lysine in kinase subdomain II (with no K kinases) [56,57]. Immunohistochemical analysis has revealed that WNK1 and WNK4 are expressed predominantly in the distal convoluted tubule and collecting duct. WNK1 is a cytoplasmic protein, and WNK4 is found in tight junctions in the distal portion of the nephron.

Mutations in the introns of WNK1 lead to PHA II, whereas the mutations in WNK 4 are missense mutations [54–56]. Normally, WNK4 downregulates the activity of ion transport pathways expressed in these nephron segments, such as the apical thiazide-sensitive Na^+-Cl^- cotransporter and apical secretory K^+ channel ROMK, and upregulates paracellular chloride transport and phosphorylation of tight junction proteins, such as claudins. In addition, WNK4 downregulates other Cl^- influx pathways, such as the basolateral Na^+-K^+-$2Cl^-$ cotransporter and Cl^-/HCO_3^- exchanger. Considering the normal functions, it is understandable that WNK4 mutations behave as a loss-of-function for the Na^+-Cl^- cotransporter and yet a gain-of-function when it comes to ROMK and claudins. These dual effects of WNK4 mutations fit with proposed mechanisms for the electrolyte abnormalities and hypertension in PHA-II and point to WNK4 as a multifunctional regulator of diverse ion transporters.

Some, but not all, patients have hyperchloremia, metabolic acidosis, and suppressed plasma renin activity. The hypertension and electrolyte abnormalities generally improve when the patient is treated with triamterene or thiazide diuretics. In contrast, aldosterone receptor antagonists do not correct the clinical abnormalities.

PHAII genes were mapped initially to chromosomes 17, 1, or 12 [54–57]. One kindred with large intronic deletions that increase WNK1 expression was described, as was another with missense mutations in WNK4, located on chromosome 17. Of note, WNK 1 is expressed in various tissues, whereas WNK4 is expressed primarily in the kidney. In the renal collecting duct WNKs regulate the handling of potassium and hydrogen, increasing salt resorption and intravascular volume. Mutations in WNKs lead to relatively increased salt resorption and high intravascular volume. Current research suggests that WNK1 may play important roles in BP regulation within the general population [58,59].

Other types of monogenic hypertension

Hypertension with brachydactyly, also called Bilginturan syndrome (OMIM #112410), is a familial syndrome in which affected individuals have short metacarpals, hypertension, and short stature. Linkage studies have suggested that the gene lies on chromosome 12p in a region defined by markers D12S364 and D12S87 [60,61]. Neither a responsible gene nor a specific mutation in this region has been identified.

Molecular basis of primary hypertension

Abundant evidence suggests that primary hypertension develops as a result of multiple interacting genes and environmental influences. In the premolecular era it was well recognized that primary hypertension had a genetic component. It was suggested in the decade before the millennium that genetic factors account for 60% to 70% of familial hypertension [62]. Although it was originally estimated that 5 to 10 genes might be involved in determining blood pressure level, it now seems more likely that more genes are involved [63–65]. OMIM currently notes many genes or chromosome regions that may be involved in primary hypertension (Table 2).

It has been estimated that more than 1 billion people worldwide have essential hypertension [64]. Although the contributions of interacting genes and gene products to blood pressure level will be delineated more completely in the future, much is presently unknown. Attempts to understand the contribution of genes to primary (essential) hypertension go back to the mid-twentieth century. Familial aggregation of blood pressure (and hypertension) has been reported for decades. Within the molecular era, the search for genes that control blood pressure has widened greatly. It was estimated that variation in genetic makeup accounted for half of the phenotypic variation in blood pressure [62].

Despite the recognition that genes are involved in essential hypertension, identifying the involved genetic mechanisms for hypertension, even in the

Table 2
Partial list of genes possibly involved in primary hypertension

OMIM number	Gene	Function	Gene map locus
106180	ACE, angiotensin converting enzyme; kininase 2	Converts Ang I to Ang II and involved in bradykinin breakdown	17q23
601699.0001	PTGIS, prostaglandin I2 synthase or prostacyclin synthase	Vasodilator and inhibitor of platelet aggregation	20q13.11-q13.13
106150	Angiotensinogen, AGT	Substrate of renin angiotensin system; source of angiotensins	1q42-q43
106165	AGTR1, angiotensin receptor 1	Vascular receptor for angiotensin II	3q21-q25
139130	GNB3, the beta unit of guanine nucleotide binding protein	Abnormalities in gene may be responsible for G-protein hyperresponsiveness in hypertension	12p13
191191	TNFR2, tumor necrosis factor receptor 2	May be linked with hypertension? how	1p36.3-p36.2
600423	Endothelin-converting enzyme 1, ECE1	Involved in processing of endothelin	1p36.1
102680	Adducin-1, ADD-1	Cytoskeletal protein	4p16.3
605325.0001	CYP3A5, cytochrome P450, subfamily IIIA, polypeptide 5	CYP3A5*1/*3 polymorphism is associated with hypertension	7q22.1
163729.0001	NOS3, nitric oxide synthase 3	Mutation associated with therapy-resistant hypertension	7q36
171190	Phenylethanolamine N-methyltransferase, PNMT, PENT	May be involved in essential hypertension	17q21-q22

Additionally, listed in OMIM, susceptibility loci for essential hypertension have been mapped to chromosomes 17 (HYT1; 603918), 15q (HYT2; 604329), 2p25-p24 (HYT3; 607329), 12p (HYT4; 608742), 20q (HYT5; 610261), and 5p (HYT6; 610262).

present post-genomic era, remains problematic. Both animal models of experimental hypertension and human studies have been important in what is known to date. At this point, examining potential risk alleles and candidate genes in children who have hypertension remains a research tool with promise.

Investigating polygenic hypertension: experimental models

Animal models have been central to better understanding of hypertension. A few years ago, summarizing studies in rats, Rapp [66] noted that 24 regions on 19 chromosomes might be associated with elevated blood pressure. Since then, further refinement using congenic animals (a fully congenic strain is one in which all animals are identical at all loci except for a transferred locus, such as a linked segment of a given chromosome) and consomic strains (two rat strains are consomic when they differ by just one chromosome pair) to isolate specific similarities in the genome have resulted in the identification of additional chromosomal areas of interest. Mouse models also have helped identify and study many candidate genes. Targeted gene deletion studies in murine models have indicated that more than a dozen genes contribute to blood pressure. Not surprisingly, these include the angiotensin type 2 receptor (and other members of the renin-angiotensin system), insulin receptor substrate, the dopamine receptor, endothelial nitric oxide synthase, the bradykinin receptor, and apolipoprotein E [67].

The roles of several candidate genes, in particular renin-angiotensin system genes, have been addressed by genetic manipulation in murine models (reviewed in [68]). Particularly useful studies have been made possible by increasing expression of a given gene (using transgenic approaches or other means of overexpressing a given gene) or deleting gene function (with knockouts). In a transgenic model, naked DNA that contains the regulatory and coding region of a gene is injected into the pronucleus of a fertilized egg [69]. The naked DNA then randomly integrates into the genome of the mouse. The effects of the transgene vary, because the location of integration and copy number may not be the same. The phenotypic change from deleting or knocking out a gene may clarify the gene's importance. Gene targeting by way of embryonic stem ES cell cultures also is useful [70,71].

The value of inbred strains is also important in hypertension research [72]. For example, Hilbert and coworkers [73] and Jacob and colleagues [74] used linkage studies in the stroke-prone spontaneously hypertensive rat that indicated that the angiotensin converting enzyme (ACE) gene was involved in determining hypertension. The interested reader is referred to recent reviews [75,76].

Human hypertension

Studies in humans are more difficult. Most people who have common conditions, such as high blood pressure, possess susceptibility alleles rather than disease alleles per se, and not all people who have a given susceptibility allele have the disease in question. Either the necessary environmental exposure to cause the condition is absent, or another necessary complementary allele (or alleles) is lacking. Given the multiple potential interactions, and the fact that susceptibility alleles are generally common, it is difficult to trace a given allele through most pedigrees. In a recent case-control analysis concerning the heritability of primary and secondary hypertension in children, Robinson and colleagues [77] observed that primary hypertension in children, as in adults, is likely influenced heavily by contributions of multiple genes, whereas, in contrast, secondary hypertension was related to few genes.

Many susceptibility alleles confer only a small effect on blood pressure levels, which means that segregation analysis is difficult. As of 2004, linkage studies in humans suggested areas of 15 chromosomes associated with hypertension [78–84]. Additional studies are adding new regions at a considerable rate [85–102]. Certain candidate genes, such as members of the renin-angiotensin system, have been associated with hypertension in humans for some time [103,104]. Some loci that have been uncovered in linkage studies also point to their importance.

Although linkage analysis often is used as a first step [9–11], it is not as powerful in this setting as in conditions with clear Mendelian inheritance, because many people who do not have the condition being studied also may carry the susceptibility allele. Consequently, another approach is to use sets of affected siblings (sib pairs). When sibs are affected by a given health problem, such as hypertension, they would be expected to share more than half of their alleles near or at the susceptibility locus, the chance of which is then calculated [9–11]. A linked locus is likely to have an LOD score of greater than 3.6; such loci tend to be large (in the range of 20–40 cM), so that further study will be required. After a replicate study confirms linkage, fine mapping can be performed, narrowing the region where the gene may be. Linkage disequilibrium or association testing between disease and genetic markers then may be performed, often using single nucleotide polymorphisms (SNPs), which are randomly present roughly every 1000 base pairs, making them amenable to automated testing. With the SNP approach, which requires high throughput sequencing and bioinformatics, one can narrow a large region (10–40 cM) to a much smaller region of roughly 1×10^6 base pairs (9107) [105].

To date, the genomewide screens that have been performed to identify hypertension genes in humans have comprised subjects from diverse ethnic groups, with different phenotypes, selected by various criteria. Genomewide studies have led to at least 27 loci of interest. Some studies have employed single, large pedigrees, whereas others have used more than 2000 sib pairs from roughly 1500 families [106–108]. The United States Family Blood Pressure Program (FBPP) [107] used genomic scan data obtained by way of four partner networks. The FBPP aimed to select phenotypes that would reflect the ethnic diversity of the United States. Disappointingly, however, no genomewide significance has been reported from the USFBP Program. The Medical Research Council British Genetics of Hypertension study reported the phenotyping of 2010 sib pairs drawn from 1599 families with severe hypertension and then performing a 10-cM genomewide scan [108]. This strategy led to a locus on chromosome 6q with an LOD score of 3.21 with a genomewide significance of 0.042. One should be circumspect, however, in interpreting these results, because this locus is at the end of chromosome 6, a chromosomal location that may generate errors. Three additional loci with LOD scores greater than 1.57 [108] were also reported by this group, and one of them was similar to that reported in Finnish and Chinese studies [108].

Candidate genes

Focusing on genes of already-known interest that are close to the peak of observed genetic linkage is another strategy—the candidate gene approach. It is easier to proceed with further study when the full sequence of a given candidate gene is known.

Several candidate genes were present within areas on chromosomes 2 and 9 that had been identified by the linkage analysis [108]. Various genes of interest have merited attention, including serine-threonine kinases STK39 and STK17B on chromosome 2q, a protein kinase on chromosome 9q called PKNBETA, a G-protein–coupled receptor on chromosome 9 called GPR107 9q, GPR21 on 9q33, and a potassium channel, KCNJ3, noted on 2q24.1.

Several candidate genes have been considered as susceptibility genes before study, especially those that encode proteins of the renin-angiotensin system, because these already were associated with hypertension and cardiovascular regulation during the pre-genomic era. Izawa and coworkers [109] selected a group of 27 candidate genes by reviewing physiologic and genetic data that concerned vascular biology, leukocyte and platelet biology, and glucose and lipid metabolism. Having chosen these candidate genes, they then chose 33 SNPs within these genes, most of which were located within promoter regions, exons, or spliced donor or acceptor sites in introns. They then examined relationships to hypertension in a cohort of 1940 individuals. The results suggested that polymorphisms in the TNF alpha gene were associated with hypertension in women and that polymorphisms in the CC chemokine receptor 2 gene were associated with hypertension in men [109].

Presently, the candidate genes noted in the OMIM as being involved in primary hypertension include members of the renin-angiotensin system, the strongest evidence of which exists for angiotensinogen and the angiotensin II type I receptor. Other genes of interest listed include prostacyclin synthase, the beta unit of guanine nucleotide binding protein, tumor necrosis factor receptor 2, endothelin-converting enzyme 1, adducin-1, CYP3A5, nitric oxide synthase 3, and phenylethanolamine N-methyltransferase. Of these, there are now fairly robust data that adducin is important in salt-sensitive hypertension [110].

Variants or subphenotypes

Analysis of so-called "subphenotypes" by way of positional cloning may be potentially illuminating when a variant of a complex disease is clinically distinct [9–11,110]. Fewer susceptibility genes are likely to be involved in this situation. The physiology involved in examining and distinguishing subphenotypes may be intricate, however, as in the case of salt-sensitive hypertension [12]. Careful metabolic studies will be critical for confirming the subphenotype (hypertension with salt sensitivity) and will be needed for such studies.

Genes and hypertension in the individual pediatric patient

An infant, child, or teenager who has hypertension plus a history or signs and symptoms consistent with a form of monogenic hypertension should be evaluated with the known syndromes in mind. Specific therapy always should be sought in young children who have hypertension, which implies the need for accurate diagnosis of a secondary form of hypertension that can lead to curative therapy (dilation of renal artery stenosis) or disease-specific therapy (diuretics for excess volume). Most children who have elevated blood pressure, however, have essential hypertension. Despite the promise of future genetic diagnosis, currently no standard diagnostic testing for polygenic primary hypertension is available.

References

[1] Hall JE, Guyton AC, Brands MW. Pressure-volume regulation in hypertension. Kidney Int Suppl 1996;55:S35–41.

[2] Coleman TG, Guyton AC, Cowley AW Jr, et al. Feedback mechanisms of arterial pressure control. Contrib Nephrol 1977;8:5–12.

[3] Hadtstein C, Wuhl E, Soergel M, et al. German Study Group for Pediatric Hypertension. Normative values for circadian and ultradian cardiovascular rhythms in childhood. Hypertension 2004;43(3):547–54.

[4] National High Blood Pressure Education Program Working Group on High Blood Pressure in Children and Adolescents. The fourth report on the diagnosis, evaluation and treatment of high blood pressure in children and adolescents. Pediatrics 2004;114:555–76.

[5] Jones JE, Natarajan AR, Jose PA. Cardiovascular and autonomic influences on blood pressure. In: Portman RJ, Sorof JM, Ingelfinger JR, editors. Pediatric hypertension. New Jersey: Humana Press; 2004. p. 23–43.

[6] Segar JL, Robillard JE. Neurohumoral regulation of blood pressure. In: Portman RJ, Sorof JM, Ingelfinger JR, editors. Pediatric hypertension. New Jersey: Humana Press; 2004. p. 3–21.

[7] Yiu VW, Dluhy RG, Lifton RP, et al. Low peripheral plasma renin activity as a critical marker in pediatric hypertension. Pediatr Nephrol 1997;11:343–6.

[8] New MI, Geller DS, Fallo F, et al. Monogenic low renin hypertension. Trends Endocrinol Metab 2005;16(3):92–7.

[9] Bogardus C, Baier L, Permana P, et al. Identification of susceptibility genes for complex metabolic diseases. Ann NY Acad Sci 2002;967:1–6.

[10] Lander E, Kruglyak L. Genetic dissection of complex traits: guidelines for interpreting and reporting linkage results. Nat Genet 1995;11:241–7.

[11] Wang DG, Fan J-B, Siao C-J, et al. Large-scale identification, mapping and genotyping of single-nucleotide polymorphisms in the human genome. Science 1998;280:1077–82.

[12] Reudelhuber TL. Salt-sensitive hypertension: if only it were as simple as rocket science. J Clin Invest 2003;111:1115–6.

[13] Sutherland DJ, Ruse JL, Laidlaw JC. Hypertension, increased aldosterone secretion and low plasma renin activity relieved by dexamethasone. Can Med Assoc J 1966;95:1109–19.

[14] New MI, Peterson RE. A new form of congenital adrenal hyperplasia. J Clin Endocrinol Metab 1967;27:300–5.

[15] New MI, Oberfield SE, Levine LS, et al. Demonstration of autosomal dominant transmission and absence of HLA linkage in dexamethasone-suppressible hyperaldosteronism. Lancet 1980;1:550–1.

[16] Miura K, Yoshinaga K, Goto K, et al. A case of glucocorticoid-responsive hyperaldosteronism. J Clin Endocrinol Metab 1968;28(12):1807–15.

[17] New MI, Siegal EJ, Peterson RE. Dexamethasone-suppressible hyperaldosteronism. J Clin Endocrinol Metab 1973;37:93–100.

[18] Giebink GS, Gotlin RW, Biglieri EG, et al. A kindred with familial glucocorticoid-suppressible aldosteronism. J Clin Endocrinol Metab 1973;36:715–23.

[19] Grim CE, Weinberger MH. Familial dexamethasone-suppressible hyperaldosteronism. Pediatrics 1980;65:597–604.

[20] Oberfield SE, Levine LS, Stoner E, et al. Adrenal glomerulosa function in patients with dexamethasone-suppressible normokalemic hyperaldosteronism. J Clin Endocrinol Metabl 1981;53:158–64.

[21] Lifton RP, Dluhy RG, Powers M, et al. Chimeric 11β-hydroxylase/aldosterone synthase gene causes GRA and human hypertension. Nature 1992;355:262–5.

[22] Lifton RP, Dluhy RG, Powers M, et al. Hereditary hypertension caused by chimeric gene duplications and ectopic expression of aldosterone synthetase. Nat Genet 1992;2:66–74.

[23] Gill JR Jr, Bartter FC. Overproduction of sodium-retaining steroids by the zona glomerulosa is adrenocorticotropin-dependent and mediates hypertension in dexamethasone-suppressible aldosteronism. J Clin Endocrinol Metab 1981;53:331–7.

[24] Gomez-Sanches CE, Gill JR Jr, Ganguly A, et al. Glucocorticoid-suppressible aldosteronism: a disorder of the adrenal transitional zone. J Clin Endocrinol Metab 1988;67:444–8.

[25] Ulick S, Chan CK, Gill JR Jr, et al. Defective fasciculate zone function as the mechanims of glucocorticoid-remediable aldosteronism. J Clin Endocrinol Metab 1990;71:1151–7.

[26] Ulick S, Chu MD. Hypersecretion of a new cortico-steroid, 18-hydroxycortisol in two types of adrenocortical hypertension. Clin Exp Hypertens 1982;(Suppl 9/10):1771–7.

[27] Ulick S, Chu MD, Land M. Biosynthesis of 18-oxocortisol by aldosterone-producing adrenal tissue. J Biol Chem 1983;258:5498–502.

[28] Gomez-Sanchez CE, Montgomery M, Ganguly A, et al. Elevated urinary excretion of 18-oxocortisol in glucocorticoid-suppressible aldosteronism. J Clin Endocrinol Metab 1984;59:1022–4.

[29] Shackleton CH. Mass spectrometry in the diagnosis of steroid-related disorders and in hypertension research. J Steroid Biochem Mol Biol 1993;45:127–40.

[30] Dluhy RG, Anderson B, Harlin B, et al. Glucocorticoid-remediable aldosteronism is associated with severe hypertension in early childhood. J Pediatr 2001;138(5):715–20.

[31] Cerame BI, New MI. Hormonal hypertension in children: 11b-hydroxylase deficiency and apparent mineralocorticoid excess. J Pediatr Endocrinol 2000;13:1537–47.

[32] New MI, Levine LS, Biglieri EG, et al. Evidence for an unidentified ACTH-induced steroid hormone causing hypertension. J Clin Endocrinol Metab 1977;44:924–33.

[33] New MI, Oberfield SE, Carey RM, et al. A genetic defect in cortisol metabolism as the basis for the syndrome of apparent mineralocorticoid excess. In: Mantero F, Biglieri EG, Edwards CRW, editors. Endocrinology of hypertension. Serono Symposia No. 50. New York: Academic Press; 1982. p. 85–101.

[34] Downey MK, Riddick L, New MI. Apparent mineralocorticoid excess: a genetic form of fatal low-renin hypertension. Program and Abstracts, Merican Society of Hypertension, Second World Congress on Biologically Active Atrial Peptides. New York, May 1987.

[35] Ulick S, Ramirez LC, New MI. An abnormality in steroid reductive metabolism in a hypertensive syndrome. J Clin Endocrinol Metab 1977;44:799–802.

[36] Ulick S, Levine LS, Gunczler P, et al. A syndrome of apparent mineralocorticoid excess associated with defects in the peripheral metabolism of cortisol. J Clin Endocrinol Metab 1979;44:757–64.

[37] White PC, Munte T, Agarwal AK. 11β-hydroxysteroid dehydrogenase and the syndrome of apparent mineralocorticoid excess. Endocr Rev 1997;18:135–56.

[38] Ferrari P, Lovati E, Frey FJ. The role of the 11β-hydroxysteroid dehydrogenase type 2 in human hypertension. J Hypertens 2000;18:241–8.

[39] Obeyesekere VR, Ferrari P, Andrews RK, et al. The R337C mutation generates a high Km 11 beta-hydroxysteroid dehydrogenase type II enzyme in a family with apparent mineralocorticoid excess. J Clin Endo Metab 1995;80:3381–3.

[40] Ferrari P, Obeyesekere VR, Li K. Point mutations abolish 11 beta-hydroxysteroid dehydrogenase type II activity in three families with the congenital syndrome of apparent mineralocorticoid excess. Mol Cell Endocrinol 1996;119:21–4.

[41] Mune T, Rogerson FM, Nikkila H, et al. Human hypertension caused by mutations in the kidney isozyme of 11 beta-hydroxysteroid dehydrogenase. Nat Genet 1995;10:394–9.

[42] Stewart PM, Wallace AM, Valentino R, et al. Mineralocorticoid activity of liquorice: 11β-hydroxysteroid dehydrogenase deficiency comes of age. Lancet 1987;2:821–3.

[43] Moudgil A, Rodich G, Jordan SC, et al. Nephrocalcinosis and renal cysts associated with apparent mineralocorticoid excess syndrome. Pediatr Nephrol 2000;15(1–2):60–2.

[44] Liddle GW, Bledsoe T, Coppage WS. A familial renal disorder simulating primary aldosteronism but with negligible aldosterone secretion. Trans Assoc Phys 1963;76:199–213.

[45] Shimkets RA, Warnock DG, Bositis CM, et al. Liddle's syndrome: heritable human hypertension caused by mutations in the b subunit of the epithelial sodium channel. Cell 1994;79:407–14.

[46] Hansson JH, Nelson-Williams C, Suzuki H, et al. Hypertension caused by a truncated epithelial sodium channel gamma subunit: genetic heterogeneity of Liddle syndrome. Nat Genet 1995;11:76–82.

[47] Rossier BC. 1996 Homer Smith Award Lecture: cum grano salis: the epithelial sodium channel and the control of blood pressure. J Am Soc Nephrol 1997;8:980–92.

[48] Wang C, Chan TK, Yeung RT, et al. The effect of triamterene and sodium intake on renin, aldosterone, and erythrocyte sodium transport in Liddle's syndrome. J Clin Endocrinol Metabl 1981;52:1027–32.

[49] Botero-Velez M, Curtis JJ, Warnock DG. Brief report: Liddle's syndrome revisited—a disorder of sodium reabsorption in the distal tubule. N Engl J Med 1994;330:178–81.

[50] Paver W, Pauline G. Hypertension and hyperpotassaemia without renal disease in a young male. Med J Aust 1964;2:305–6.

[51] Gordon RD. The syndrome of hypertension and hyperkalemia with normal glomerular filtration rate: Gordon's syndrome. Aust N Z J Med 1986;16(2):183–4.

[52] Take C, Ikeda K, Kurasawa T, et al. Increased chloride reabsorption as an inherited renal tubular defect in familial type II pseudohypoaldosteronism. Engl J Med 1991;324:472–6.

[53] Erdogan G, Corapciolgu D, Erdogan MF, et al. Furosemide and dDAVP for the treatment of pseudohypoaldosteronism type II. J Endocrinol Invest 1997;20:681–4.

[54] Mansfield TA, Simon DB, Farfel Z, et al. Multilocus linkage of familial hyperkalaemia and hypertension, pseudohypoaldosteronism type II, to chromosomes 1q31–42 and 17p11-q21. Nat Genet 1997;16:202–5.

[55] Wilson FH, Disse-Nicodeme S, Choate KA, et al. Human hypertension caused by mutations in WNK kinases. Science 2001;293:1107–12.

[56] Cope G, Golbang A, O'Shaughnessy KM. WNK kinases and the control of blood pressure. Pharmacol Ther 2005;106(2):221–31.

[57] Faure S, Delaloy C, Leprivey V, et al. WNK kinases, distal tubular ion handling and hypertension. Nephrol Dial Transplant 2003;18(12):2463–7.

[58] Tobin MD, Raleigh SM, Newhouse S, et al. Association of WNK1 gene polymorphisms and haplotypes with ambulatory blood pressure in the general population. Circulation 2005;112(22):3423–9. Epub 2005 Nov 21.

[59] Hadchouel J, Delaloy C, Faure S, et al. Familial hyperkalemic hypertension. J Am Soc Nephrol. 2006 Jan;17(1):208–17. Epub 2005 Oct 12.

[60] Schuster H, Wienker TF, Toka HR, et al. Autosomal dominant hypertension and brachydactyly in a Turkish kindred resembles essential hypertension. Hypertension 1996;28: 1085–92.

[61] Bilginturan N, Zileli S, Karacadag S, et al. Hereditary brachydactyly associated with hypertension. J Med Genet 1973;10(3):253–9.

[62] Ward R. Familial aggregation and genetic epidemiology of blood pressure. In: Laragh JH, Brenner BM, editors. Hypertension: pathophysiology, diagnosis and management. New York: Raven Press; 1990. p. 81–100.

[63] Garcia EA, Newhouse JM, Caulfield MJ, et al. Genes and hypertension. Curr Pharm Des 2003;9:1679–89.

[64] Mein CA, Caulfield MJ, Dobson RJ, et al. Genetics of essential hypertension. Hum Mol Genet 2004;13(Review Issue 1):R169–75.

[65] Staessen JA, Wang J, Bianchi G, et al. Essential hypertension. Lancet 2003;361:1629–41.

[66] Rapp JP. Genetic analysis of inherited hypertension in the rat. Physiol Rev 2000;80:135–72.

[67] Doris PA. Hypertension genetics, SNPs, and the common disease: common variant hypothesis. hypertension 2002;39(Part 2):323–31.

[68] Cvetkovic B, Sigmund CD. Understanding hypertension through genetic manipulation in mice. Kidney Int 2000;57:863–74.

[69] Gordon JW, Ruddle FH. Gene transfers into mouse embryos: production of transgenic mice by pronuclear integration. Methods Enzymol 1983;101:411–33.

[70] Evans MJ, Kaufman MH. Establishment in culture of pluripotential cells from mouse embryos. Nature 1981;292:154–6.

[71] Capecchi MR. Altering the genome by homologous recombination. Science 1989;244: 1288–92.

[72] Stoll M, Kwitek-Black AE, Cowley AW, et al. New target regions for human hypertension via comparative genomics. Genome Res 2000;10:473–82.

[73] Hilbert P, Lindpaintner K, Beckmann JS, et al. Chromosomal mapping of two genetic loci associated with blood-pressure regulation in hereditary hypertensive rats. Nature 1991; 353(6344):521–9.

[74] Jacob HJ, Lindpaintner K, Lincoln SE, et al. Genetic mapping of a gene causing hypertension in the stroke-prone spontaneously hypertensive rat. Cell 1991;67:213–24.

[75] Mullins LJ, Bailey MA, Mullins JJ. Hypertension, kidney, and transgenics: a fresh perspective. Physiol Rev 2006;86(2):709–46.

[76] Lerman LO, Chade AR, Sica V, et al. Animal models of hypertension: an overview. J Lab Clin Med 2005;146(3):160–73.

[77] Robinson RF, Batisky DL, Hayes JR, et al. Significance of heritability in primary and secondary pediatric hypertension. Am J Hypertens 2005;18:917–21.

[78] Rice T, Rankinen T, Province MA, et al. Genome-wide linkage analysis of systolic and diastolic blood pressure: the Quebec family study. Circulation 2000;102:1956–63.

[79] Perola M, Kainulainen K, Pajukanta P, et al. Genome-wide scan of predisposing loci for increased diastolic blood pressure in Finnish siblings. J Hypertens 2000;18:1579–85.

[80] Pankow JS, Rose KM, Oberman A, et al. Possible locus on chromosome 18q influencing postural systolic blood pressure changes. Hypertension 2000;36:471–6.

[81] Krushkal J, Ferrell R, Mockrin SC, et al. Genome-wide linkage analyses of systolic blood pressure using highly discordant siblings. Circulation 1999;99:1407–10.

[82] Levy D, DeStefano AL, Larson MG, et al. Evidence for a gene influencing blood pressure on chromosome 17: genome scan linkage results for longitudinal blood pressure phenotypes in subjects from the Framingham Heart Study. Hypertension 2000;36:477–83.

[83] Sharma P, Fatibene J, Ferraro F, et al. A genome-wide search for susceptibility loci to human essential hypertension. Hypertension 2000;35:1291 6.

[84] Xu X, Rogus JJ, Terwedow HA, et al. An extreme-sib-pair genome scan for genes regulating blood pressure. Am J Hum Genet 1999;64:1694–701.

[85] Munroe PB, Wallace C, Xue MZ, et al. Medical Research Council British Genetics of Hypertension Study. Increased support for linkage of a novel locus on chromosome 5q13 for essential hypertension in the British Genetics of Hypertension Study. Hypertension 2006; 48(1):105–11.

[86] Ciullo M, Bellenguez C, Colonna V, et al. New susceptibility locus for hypertension on chromosome 8q by efficient pedigree-breaking in an Italian isolate. Hum Mol Genet 2006;15(10):1735–43.

[87] Bell JT, Wallace C, Dobson R, et al. Two-dimensional genome-scan identifies novel epistatic loci for essential hypertension. Hum Mol Genet 2006;15(8):1365–74.

[88] Cheung BM, Leung RY, Man YB, et al. Association of hypertension with single nucleotide polymorphisms in the quantitative trait locus for abdominal obesity-metabolic syndrome on chromosome 17. J Hum Hypertens 2006;20(6):419–25.

[89] Laramie JM, Wilk JB, Hunt SC, et al. Evidence for a gene influencing heart rate on chromosome 5p13–14 in a meta-analysis of genome-wide scans from the NHLBI Family Blood Pressure Program. BMC Med Genet 2006;7:17.

[90] Padmanabhan S, Wallace C, Munroe PB, et al. Chromosome 2p shows significant linkage to antihypertensive response in the British Genetics of Hypertension Study. Hypertension 2006;47(3):603–8.

[91] Pausova Z, Gaudet D, Gossard F, et al. Genome-wide scan for linkage to obesity-associated hypertension in French Canadians. Hypertension 2005;46(6):1280–5. Epub 2005 Oct 10.

[92] Benjafield AV, Wang WY, Speirs HJ, et al. Genome-wide scan for hypertension in Sydney Sibships: the GENIHUSS study. Am J Hypertens 2005;18(6):828–32.

[93] Pankow JS, Dunn DM, Hunt SC, et al. Further evidence of a quantitative trait locus on chromosome 18 influencing postural change in systolic blood pressure: the Hypertension Genetic Epidemiology Network (HyperGEN) Study. Am J Hypertens 2005;18(5 Pt 1): 672–8.

[94] Lynch AI, Arnett DK, Atwood LD, et al. A genome scan for linkage with aortic root diameter in hypertensive African Americans and whites in the Hypertension Genetic Epidemiology Network (HyperGEN) study. Am J Hypertens 2005;18(5 Pt 1):627–32.

[95] Chen W, Li S, Srinivasan SR, et al. Autosomal genome scan for loci linked to blood pressure levels and trends since childhood: the Bogalusa Heart Study. Hypertension 2005;45(5): 954 9.

[96] Cheung BM, Leung RY, Man YB, Wong LY, Lau CP. Association of essential hypertension with a microsatellite marker on chromosome 17. J Hum Hypertens 2005;19(5):407–11.

[97] Zhu X, Luke A, Cooper RS, et al. Admixture mapping for hypertension loci with genome-scan markers. Nat Genet 2005;37(2):177–81.

[98] Liu W, Zhao W, Chase GA. Genome scan meta-analysis for hypertension. Am J Hypertens 2004;17(12 Pt 1):1100–6.

[99] de Lange M, Spector TD, Andrew T. Genome-wide scan for blood pressure suggests linkage to chromosome 11, and replication of loci on 16, 17, and 22. Hypertension 2004;44(6): 872–7.

[100] Wilk JB, Djousse L, Arnett DK, et al. Genome-wide linkage analyses for age at diagnosis of hypertension and early-onset hypertension in the HyperGEN study. Am J Hypertens 2004; 17(9):839–44.

[101] Morrison AC, Cooper R, Hunt S, et al. Genome scan for hypertension in nonobese African Americans: the National Heart, Lung, and Blood Institute Family Blood Pressure Program. Am J Hypertens 2004;17(9):834–8.

[102] Gu F, Ge D, Huang J, et al. Genetic susceptibility loci for essential hypertension and blood pressure on chromosome 17 in 147 Chinese pedigrees. J Hypertens 2004;22(8):1511–8.

[103] Lalouel J-M, Rohrwasser A, Terreros D, et al. Angiotensinogen in essential hypertension: from genetics to nephrology. J Am Soc Nephrol 2001;12:606–15.

[104] Zhu X, Yen-Pei CC, Yan D, et al. Associations between hypertension and genes in the renin-angiotensin system. Hypertension 2003;41:1027–34.

[105] The International SNP Map Working Group. A map of human genome sequence variation containing 1.42 million single nucleotide polymorphisms. Nature 2001;409:928–33.

[106] Harrap SB. Where are all the blood pressure genes? Lancet 2003;361:2149–51.

[107] Province MA, Kardia SLR, Ranade K, et al. A meta-analysis of genome-wide linkage scans for hypertension: the National Heart Lung and Blood Institute Family Blood Pressure Program. Am J Hypertens 2003;16:144–7.

[108] Caulfield M, Munroe P, Pembroke J, et al. Genome-wide mapping of human loci for essential hypertension. Lancet 2003;361:2118–23.

[109] Izawa H, Yamada Y, Okada T, et al. Prediction of genetic risk for hypertension. Hypertension 2003;41:1035–40.

[110] Manunta P, Bianchi G. Pharmacogenomics and pharmacogenetics of hypertension: update and perspectives–the adducin paradigm. J Am Soc Nephrol 2006;17(4,Suppl 2):S30–5.

ELSEVIER
SAUNDERS

Pediatr Clin N Am
53 (2006) 1029–1037

PEDIATRIC CLINICS

OF NORTH AMERICA

Reactive Oxygen Species Cerebral Autoregulation in Health and Disease

Maia Terashvili, PhD[a,b],
Phillip F. Pratt, PhD[c], Debebe Gebremedhin, PhD[a,b],
Jayashree Narayanan, MS[a,b], David R. Harder, PhD[a,b,*]

[a]*Department of Physiology, Medical College of Wisconsin, 8701 Watertown Plank Road, Milwaukee, WI 53226, USA*
[b]*Cardiovascular Research Center, Medical College of Wisconsin, 8701 Watertown Plank Road, Milwaukee, WI 53226, USA*
[c]*Department of Anesthesiology and Pharmacology and Toxicology, Medical College of Wisconsin, 8701 Watertown Plank Road, Milwaukee, WI 53226, USA*

Superoxide and other oxygen radicals (ROS) derived from the oxidative metabolism of L-arginine influence cell signaling and gene expression. In some tissues ROS stimulate structural changes, such as proliferation, hypertrophy, or remodeling. ROS production within the developing CNS stimulates excitation and in vascular tissue causes contraction. The effects of ROS-induced autoregulatory failure in the CNS following hypoxic-ischemic encephalopathy, seizures, trauma, or stroke in children leads to acute mortality and chronic morbidity.

Production and effects of ROS on the cerebral vasculature

Regulation of nutritive blood flow to metabolically active tissue is a vital process supplying substrate for enzymatic production of intermediates to maintain cellular homeostasis. In the brain, neuronal metabolism relies almost exclusively on oxidative pathways requiring adequate delivery of oxygen and glucose. Under normal ranges of physiologic blood pressure, cerebral blood flow to the brain remains constant despite fluctuations in transmural pressure. This autoregulation is largely a function of signaling

This article was support by NIH/NHLBI grants PO1 HL6876, PO1 HL59996, and RO1 HL33833 and the Veterans Administration grant 3440-06P.

* Corresponding author.

E-mail address: dharder@mcw.edu (D.R. Harder).

0031-3955/06/$ - see front matter © 2006 Elsevier Inc. All rights reserved.
doi:10.1016/j.pcl.2006.08.003

events in the vessel wall such that increasing arterial pressure depolarizes and activates arterial muscle keeping flow relatively constant [1–4].

Reactive oxygen species are believed to be involved in cellular signaling in blood vessels in both normal and pathologic states. The major pathway for the production of ROS is by way of the one-electron reduction of molecular oxygen to form an oxygen radical, the superoxide anion ($O_2 \cdot^-$). Within the vasculature there are several enzymatic sources of $O_2 \cdot^-$, including xanthine oxidase, the mitochondrial electron transport chain, and nitric oxide (NO) synthases [5]. Studies in recent years, however, suggest that the major contributor to $O_2 \cdot^-$ levels in vascular cells is the membrane-bound enzyme NADPH-oxidase [6]. Produced $O_2 \cdot^-$ can react with other radicals, such as NO, or spontaneously dismutate to produce hydrogen peroxide (H_2O_2) [7]. In cells, the latter reaction is an important pathway for normal $O_2 \cdot^-$ breakdown and is usually catalyzed by the enzyme superoxide dismutase (SOD). Once formed, H_2O_2 can undergo various reactions, both enzymatic and nonenzymatic. The antioxidant enzymes catalase and glutathione peroxidase act to limit ROS accumulation within cells by breaking down H_2O_2 to H_2O. Metabolism of H_2O_2 can also produce other, more damaging ROS [8]. For example, the endogenous enzyme myeloperoxidase uses H_2O_2 as a substrate to form the highly reactive compound hypochlorous acid. Alternatively, H_2O_2 can undergo Fenton or Haber-Weiss chemistry, reacting with Fe^{2+}/Fe^{3+} ions to form toxic hydroxyl radicals (^-OH) [8].

ROS are involved in oxidation of lipoproteins, modulation of apoptosis, upregulation of adhesion molecule expression, and activation of the processes involved in vascular remodeling, such as enhancement of vascular smooth muscle growth and activation of matrix metalloproteinases [9]. In addition, one of the most powerful acute effects of ROS in the vasculature is the alteration of vascular smooth muscle tone. There is evidence that $O_2 \cdot^-$ can not only constrict [10] but also dilate cerebral arteries [11]. Moreover, several studies have demonstrated clearly that small cerebral arterioles relax in response to the $O_2 \cdot^-$ metabolite H_2O_2 [12,13]. H_2O_2 thus causes powerful dilatation of cerebral arterioles whether applied exogenously or generated endogenously within the vascular wall in response to agonists, such as bradykinin or arachidonic acid [14,15]. These dilator responses seem to be mediated primarily by cyclooxygenase-derived ROS, which open potassium channels in the vascular smooth muscle cell membrane to cause hyperpolarization and thus relaxation [14–16]. In the cerebral circulation, therefore, ROS such as $O_2 \cdot^-$ and H_2O_2 could possibly either dilate or even exert opposing effects on vascular tone. The balance between $O_2 \cdot^-$ and H_2O_2 in the vascular wall is regulated by the expression and activity of endogenous SOD.

The role of cytochrome P450 enzymes for the production of ROS

The cytochrome P450 (CYP) enzymes are membrane-bound, heme-containing terminal oxidases that are found in organisms from

Archaebacteria to humans. These enzymes are responsible for the metabolic activation or inactivation of most types of drugs and toxins. CYP enzymes are capable of metabolizing endogenous arachidonic acid (AA) into vaso-reactive products and therefore are often referred to as the third pathway of AA metabolism (cyclooxygenases and lipoxygenases being the other two pathways). Much attention thus has been focused on the role of CYP enzymes in vascular homeostasis [17]. In addition to the production of vasoreactive AA metabolites, CYP enzymes also generate ROS, such as $O_2 \cdot^-$ and H_2O_2. For example, released free AA following stimulation of as-trocytes with glutamate is converted to epoxyeicosatrienoic acid (EETs) by microsomal epoxygenases (CYP 2C11) or PGI2/Tx by cyclooxygenases. Both these processes generate $O_2 \cdot^-$, which is further metabolized to H_2O_2 by superoxide dismutase (SOD). Similarly, stimulation of vascular smooth muscle cell by pressure, stretch, flow, and so forth, triggers the release of AA, which is metabolized to 20-HETE by CYP 4A enzyme that can also generate $O_2 \cdot^-$, which is further metabolized to H_2O_2 by SOD. ROS thus are produced during metabolism of AA by CYP enzymes and may play an important role in regulation of the tyrosine kinase pathways. Addition-ally, another recent report provides strong evidence that $O_2 \cdot^-$ participates in the endothelium-derived hyperpolarizing factor (EDHF) response of CYP-derived EETs, suggesting that an endothelial epoxygenase homolo-gous to human CYP 2C8/9 is the source of $O_2 \cdot^-$ in coronary arteries [17]. Release of inhibitory radical species would be expected to inhibit pres-sure-induced myogenic tone. On the other hand, $O_2 \cdot^-$ has been shown to inhibit NO production, which would enhance myogenic tone [18]. Given the potential sources of ROS formation in the form of NADPH P450 oxidases in the cerebral arterial wall, it is important that we define the role of ROS on myogenic mechanisms in the cerebral circulation.

Action of ROS on ion channels

Maintenance of cellular ionic gradients is essential to cell survival and function. Apart from maintaining osmotic equilibrium, ion channels are co-transporters that mediate the movement of ions against electrical and con-centration gradients and regulate plasma and mitochondrial membrane potential. Plasma membrane potential controls many cell-specific processes. In the brain, the membrane potential controls the active state of arterial muscle, release of paracrine substances from vascular and capillary endo-thelial cells, neuronal activity, and multiple processes in astrocytes. With respect to arteriolar muscle there are four major K^+ channel isoforms: Ca^{2+}-activated K^+ channels, delayed rectifier K^+ channels, inwardly recti-fying K^+ channels, and ATP-sensitive K^+ channels [19]. On patch clamping freshly isolated cerebral arteriolar muscle the major K^+ channel isoform present is K_{Ca}. If analogy with other excitable cells is assumed, it is the inwardly rectifying K^+ channel that is largely responsible for setting the level of membrane potential [19,20]. Inhibition of K^+ channels depolarizes cerebral vascular muscle as defined by the K^+ equilibrium potential, however [21,22]. The major voltage-sensitive Ca^{2+} channel in cerebral arterial muscle is the L-type Ca^{2+} channel [23]. To date we have little evidence for rapidly inactivating T-type Ca^{2+} channels in cerebral arterial muscle. There are also several Cl^- channels in cerebral arteriolar muscle, and there is increased interest in them with respect to regulation of membrane potential and other cellular processes [24]. In this review we focus on K_{Ca} channel.

Free radicals exert direct and indirect actions on ion channels. The redox status of channel proteins has been hypothesized to affect the ion channel activity in arterial muscle [25,26]. This hypothesis states that the balance between oxygen and its reactive species functions as an oxygen sensor through actions on ion channels [26,27]. In this regard K^+ channels have been shown to be sensitive to H_2O_2 [26,28–31]. H_2O_2 has been demonstrated to hyperpolarize arterial muscle by way of activation of maxi K_{Ca} by direct and indirect mechanisms [15,26,28–31]. In cat, H_2O_2 has been shown to activate ATP-sensitive K^+ channels [11]. A recent report provides evidence that H_2O_2 can function as an EDHF [31]. ROS repeatedly have been demonstrated to modulate $[Ca^{2+}]_i$ on agonist stimulation of L-type Ca^{2+} channels, which could be either the primary or secondary target [32]. The literature on free radicals and direct action on ion channels as determined by patch clamp or direct measurement of membrane potential is not extensive. Given the importance of membrane potential on cellular control mechanisms, however, this is an area of active investigation.

There are many indirect actions of ROS on vascular membrane potential. Activation/inhibition of ion channels to a large extent depends on channel protein phosphorylation. Both upstream regulators of protein/tyrosine kinases and direct effects on their translocation and activation have been shown to be sensitive to reactive radical species. Tyrosine kinases and phosphatases are targets of H_2O_2 as activators and inhibitors [33]. H_2O_2 can activate ERK1/2 and p38 MAPK in the presence of agents such as angiotensin [9,34]. H_2O_2 also can mediate EGF-induced activation of phospholipase C (PLC) [35]. In general, phospholipases are targets of ROS. PLC activity regulates diacylglycerol (DAG) level, which in turn activates and induces translocation of protein kinase C (PKC) [36]. Recent literature demonstrates that ion channel phosphorylation is mediated by kinase activity [37,38]. Alteration of PKC, either through DAG or directly, and tyrosine kinase activities induced by ROS would be expected to modulate ion channel activity, resulting in membrane potential responses with downstream modulation of cell functions under membrane potential influence. Similarly, modification of PLC activity changes levels of intracellular inositol triphosphate (IP_3) affecting Ca^{2+} release from internal stores.

Action of ROS on K_{Ca} channel activity in cerebral arterial muscle cells

Activation of arterial smooth muscle is regulated largely by the level of membrane potential. The plasma membrane potential is set by unequal distribution of ions. Ion species with high relative conductance set the membrane potential in accordance to specific charge and concentration gradients (ie, Nernst potential); in vascular muscle cells K^+ is the dominant species in this regard. Vascular smooth muscle membrane potential is a major influence in defining the level of activation, and in cerebral arterial muscle cells the major determinant of activation and contraction. Indeed, a 1.0-mV reduction in membrane potential initiates a significant increase in active tension with a correlation coefficient relating change in membrane potential to change in active tension of 0.98 [2,3]. The mechanisms by which ROS modulate ion channels, including K_{Ca} channel activity in vascular muscle, remain largely unexplored. We have shown that the K_{Ca} is a target for $O_2 \cdot^-$ [39]. At this time we do not know how $O_2 \cdot^-$ enhances K_{Ca} activity; it could act directly on channel proteins or on second messengers, which include PKC and tyrosine kinase, that mediate phosphorylation of K_{Ca} channels. Generation of H_2O_2 also seems to activate K_{Ca} (Debebe Gebremedhin, PhD, and David R. Harder, PhD, unpublished data, 2005). Both H_2O_2 and $O_2 \cdot^-$ thus act to increase single-channel K_{Ca} activity in cerebral vascular muscle cells.

ROS in the brain: actions on functional hyperemia

The source of ROS in the brain may require CYP enzyme activity and is supported further by data obtained recently in our laboratory using samples of cerebrospinal fluid (CSF) containing the spin trap N-tert-butyl hydroxylamine, which is selective for $O_2 \cdot^-$ (Debebe Gebremedhin, PhD, and David R. Harder, PhD, unpublished data, 2005) and support a recent report that an endothelial CYP isoform (C8/C9) generates $O_2 \cdot^-$ in coronary arteries [40]. Given the many cell types in the brain, it is certain that there is no single source of ROS. Whatever the source of ROS, these free radicals appear to impinge chronically on mechanisms regulating blood flow in the brain; for example, infusion of scavengers, such as SOD, into the CSF increased blood flow as measured by laser-Doppler flowmetry (Debebe Gebremedhin, PhD, and David R. Harder, PhD, unpublished data, 2005). The effect of SOD on baseline blood flow is most likely attributed to removal of $O_2 \cdot^-$, which potentially enhances nitric oxide. The increase in blood flow was reversed after the infusion was completed (Debebe Gebremedhin, PhD, and David R. Harder, PhD, unpublished data, 2005). The literature would suggest that the source of cerebral $O_2 \cdot^-$ produced would be by way of nitric oxide synthase (NOS) through NAD(P)H-dependent reductase activity. The CYP NAD(P)H reductase, however, is virtually the same as NOS (NOS is a heme-containing protein similar to CYP enzyme system). In summary, scavenging of $O_2 \cdot^-$ by infusion of SOD modulates the cerebral blood flow in vivo (Debebe Gebremedhin, PhD, and David R. Harder, PhD, unpublished data, 2005), demonstrating that these molecules participate in the regulation of nutritive blood flow in the brain. Even more dramatic is the action of 30-minute subdural infusion of a cocktail of xanthine/xanthine oxidase/catalase (X/XO/Cat, 0.2 mM xanthine/20 mU xanthine oxidase/500 U catalase). We have shown that under control conditions there is significant autoregulation of CSF; however, there is complete inhibition of CSF autoregulation on elevation of arterial pressure following infusion of a cocktail designed to generate excess $O_2 \cdot^-$ as shown by increased fluorescent intensity of ethidium bromide produced by $O_2 \cdot^-$ from dihydroethidium [39].

When a membrane-enriched homogenate is exposed to H_2O_2 (xanthine/XO) there is a marked and significant reduction in 20-HETE formation by way of CYP ω-hydroxylase (Debebe Gebremedhin, PhD, and David R. Harder, PhD, unpublished data, 2005), which is one of the primary mediators of pressure-induced activation of cerebral arteries [41,42]. The action of $O_2 \cdot^-$ in inhibiting 20-HETE production in a membrane-enriched solution in which all conditions are optimized is most likely attributable to a direct action on CYP ω-hydroxylase activity.

Possible pathogenetic role of intracisternally generated ROS

Subarachnoid hemorrhage (SAH) results in a high mortality rate; 15% of patients who have SAH die before reaching the hospital and 30% die within 24 hours of onset [43]. Patients who survive the initial hemorrhage and overcome vasospasms frequently experience persistent cognitive deficits, psychosocial impairments, and a decrease in quality of life as a result of acute brain injury [44]. Most research in this area has focused on the late phase, however, when vasospasm occurs, whereas the mechanisms of acute brain injury are poorly understood.

Lipid peroxidation and other consequences of increased levels of ROS have been implicated in the cause of cerebral vasospasm after SAH [45,46]. The primary contributor to ROS production after SAH is the autooxidation within the subarachnoid space of oxyhemoglobin to met-Hb [47]. As a direct product of this redox reaction, $O_2 \cdot^-$ is converted to highly reactive hydroxide anion (^-OH) through the metal-catalyzed Haber-Weiss and Fenton reactions [48,49]. In support of this theory that ROS are primary pathogens for SAH, various antioxidants have been shown to attenuate cerebral vasospasm in animals and humans [50–54]. It also has been shown that intracisternal overproduction of $O_2 \cdot^-$ may initiate or mediate cerebral arterial vasoconstriction and subsequent structural damage [46]. Moreover, administration of ferrous (Fe^{2+}) or ferric (Fe^{3+}) iron chelators was shown to mitigate against cerebral vasospasm, providing evidence that the iron-catalyzed Haber-Weiss and Fenton reactions are involved in the mechanism of ROS generation leading to the occurrence of cerebral vasospasm [55,56]. These studies further support the pathogenic role of ROS in cerebral vasospasm after SAH.

In summary, cerebral blood flow is maintained at a constant rate despite fluctuations in arterial pressure. The ability of the cerebral vasculature to autoregulate is primarily the function of the activities of the native K_{Ca} channel. The K_{Ca} channel is also a target for several paracrine factors and various physical forces, which alter cerebral tone. Astrocytes are intermediary cell types that function to increase cerebral blood flow to match the metabolic demand of activated neurons. Channelopathy coupled with functional alteration of the mechanisms regulating cerebral blood flow could lead to episodic stroke or cerebral vasospasm. Knowledge of the mechanism by which the functions of the cerebral circulation are regulated will help to develop new therapies for the treatment of pediatric patients suffering from hypoxic injury, trauma, stroke, and other cerebral disorders, including acute infections such as meningitis and encephalitis [57].

References

[1] Bohlen HG, Harper SL. Evidence of myogenic vascular control in the rat cerebral cortex. Cir Res 1984;55:554–9.

[2] Harder DR. Comparison of electrical properties of middle cerebral and mesenteric artery in cat. Am J Physiol 1980;239:C23–6.

[3] Harder DR, Gilbert R, Lombard JH. Vascular muscle cell depolarization and activation in renal arteries on elevation in transmural pressue. Am J Physiol 1998;253: F778–81.

[4] McCarron JG, Osol G, Halpern W. Myogenic responses is independent of endothelium in rat pressurized posterior cerebral arteries. Blood Vessels 1989;26:315–9.

[5] Cai H, Harrison DG. Endothelial dysfunction in cardiovascular diseases: the role of oxidant stress. Circ Res 2000;87:840–4.

[6] Griendling KK, Sorescu D, Ushio-Fukai M. NAD (P) H oxidase. Role in cardiovascular biology and disease. Circ Res 2000;86:494–501.

[7] Griendling KK, Sorescu D, Lassegue B, et al. Modulation of protein kinase activity and gene expression by reactive oxygen species and their role in vascular physiology and pathophysiology. Arterioscler Thromb Vasc Biol 2000;20:2175–83.

[8] Wolin MS. Interaction of oxidants with vascular signaling systems. Arterioscler Thromb Vasc Biol 2000;20:1430–42.

[9] Cheeseman KH, Slater TF. An introduction to free radical biochemistry. Br Med Bull 1993; 49:481–93.

[10] Cosentino F, Sill JC, Katusic ZS. Role of superoxide anions in the mediation of endothelium-dependent contractions. Hypertension 1994;23:229–35.

[11] Wei EP, Kontos HA, Beckman JS. Mechanisms of cerebral vasodilation by superoxide, hydrogen peroxide and peroxynitrite. Am J Physiol 1996;271:H1262–6.

[12] Leffler CW, Busija DW, Armstead WM, et al. H_2O_2 effect on cerebral prostanoids and pial arteriolar diameter in piglets. Am J Physiol 1990;258:H1382–7.

[13] Wei EP, Kontos HA. H_2O_2 and endothelium-dependent cerebral arteriolar dilation. Implications for the identity of endothelium-derived relaxing factor generated by acetylcholine. Hypertension 1990;16:162–9.

[14] Sobey CG, Heistad DD, Faraci FM. Potassium channels mediate dilatation of cerebral arterioles in response to arachidonate. Am J Physiol 1998;275:H1606–12.

[15] Sobey CG, Heistad DD, Faraci FM. Mechanisms of bradykinin-induced cerebral vasodilatation in rats. Evidence that reactive oxygen species activate K^+ channels. Stroke 1997;28: 2290–5.

[16] Iida Y, Katusic ZS. Mechanisms of cerebral arterial relaxations to hydrogen peroxide. Stroke 2000;31:2224–30.

[17] Fleming I, Michaelis UR, Bredenkotter D, et al. Endothelium-derived hyperpolarizing factor synthase (cytochrome P450 2C9) is functionally significant source of reactive oxygen species in coronary arteries. Circ Res 2001;88:44–51.

[18] Kojda G, Harrison D. Interaction between NO and reactive oxygen species: pathophysiological importance in atherosclerosis, hypertension, diabetes and heart failure. Cardiovasc Res 1999;43:562–71.

[19] Nelson MT, Quayle JM. Physiological roles and properties of potassium channels in arterial smooth muscle. Am J Physiol 1995;268:C799–822.

[20] Trieschmann U, Isenberg G. Ca^{2+}-activated K^+ channels contribute to the resting potential of vascular myocytes. Ca^{2+}-sensitivity is increased by intracellular Mg^{2+}-ions. Pflugers Archv 1989;414:S183–4.

[21] Brayden JE, Nelson MT. Regulation of arterial tone by activation of calcium-dependent potassium channels. Science 1992;256:532–5.

[22] Marshal JJ, Kontos HA. Endothelium-derived relaxing factor: A prospective from in vivo data. Hypertension 1990;16:371–86.

[23] Gebremedhin D, Lange AR, Narayanan J, et al. Cat cerebral arterial smooth muscle cells express cytochrome P450 4A2 enzyme and produce the vasoconstrictor 20-HETE which enhances L-type Ca2+current. J Physiol 1998;507:771–81.

[24] Nelson MT, Conway MA, Knot HJ, et al. Chloride channel blockers inhibit myogenic tone in rat cerebral arteries. J Physiol 1997;502:259–64.

[25] Berzezinska AK, Gebremedhin D, Chilian WM, et al. Peroinitrite inhibits large conductance Ca^{2+}-activated K^+ channels in rat cerebral arterial muscle cells. Am J Physiol 2000;278: H1883–90.

[26] Bychkov R, Pieper K, Ried C, et al. Hydrogen peroxide, potassium currents and membrane potential in human endothelial cells. Circulation 1999;99:1719–25.

[27] Bychkov R, Gollasch M, Stienke T, et al. Calcium-activated potassium channels and nitrate-induced vasodilation in human coronary arteries. J Pharmacol Exp Ther 1998;285:293–8.

[28] Barlow RS, El-mowafey AM, White RE. H_2O_2 opens BK_{Ca} channels via the PLA2-arachidonic acid signaling cascade in coronary artery smooth muscle. Am J Physiol 2000;279: H475–83.

[29] Barlow RS, White RE. Hydrogen peroxide relaxes porcine coronary arteries by stimulating Bk_{Ca} channel activity. Am J Physiol 1998;275:H1283–9.

[30] Hayabuchi Y, Nakaya Y, Matsuoka S, et al. Hydrogen peroxide-induced vascular relaxation in porcine coronary arteries is mediated by Ca^{2+}-activated K^+ channels. Am J Physiol 1998; 13:9–17.

[31] Metoba T, Shimokawa H, Nakashima M, et al. Hydrogen peroxide is an endothelium-derived hyperpolarizing factor in mice. J Clin Invest 2000;106:1521–30.

[32] Graier WF, Hoebel BG, Paltauf-Doburzynska J, et al. Effect of superoxide anions on endothelial Ca^{2+} signaling pathways. Arteriosc Thromb Vasc Biol 1998;18:1470–9.

[33] Wolin MS. Interaction of oxidants with vascular signaling systems. Arterioscle Thromb Vasc Biol 2000;20:1430–42.

[34] Zafari AM, Ushio-Fukai M, Akers M, et al. Role of NADPH/NADPH oxidase-derived H_2O_2 in angiotensin II-induced vascular hypertrophy. Hypertension 1998;32:4888–95.

[35] Servitja JM, Masgrau R, Pardo R, et al. Effects of oxidative stress on phospholipid signaling in rat cultured astrocytes and brain slices. J Neurochem 2000;75:788–94.

[36] Gopalakrishna R, Jaken S. Protein kinase C signaling and oxidative stress. Free Radic Biol Med 2000;28:1349–61.

[37] Shubert R, Noack T, Serebrykov VN. Protein kinase C reduces K_{Ca} current of rat tail artery smooth muscle cells. Am J Physiol 1999;276:C648–58.

[38] Shipston MJ, Armstrong DL. Activation of protein kinase C inhibits calcium-activated potassium channels in rat pituitary tumor cells. J Physiol 1996;493:665–72.

[39] Zagorac D, Yamaura K, Zhang C, et al. The effect of superoxide anion on autoregulation of cerebral blood flow. Stroke 2005;36:2589–94.

[40] Fleming I, Michaelis UR, Bredenkotter D, et al. Endothelium-derived hyperpolarizing factor synthase (cytochrome P450 2C9) is functionally significant source of reactive oxygen species in coronary arteries. Circ Res 2001;88:44–51.

[41] Gebremedhin D, Lange AR, Lowry TF, et al. Production of 20-HETE and its role in autoregulation of cerebral blood flow. Circ Res 2000;87:60–5.

[42] Kauser K, Clark JE, Masters BS, et al. Inhibitors of cytochrome P450 attenuate the myogenic response of dog renal arcuate arteries. Circ Res 1991;68:1154–63.

[43] Boderick JP, Brott T, Tomsick T, et al. Intracerebral hemorrhage more than twice as common as subarachnoid hemorrhage. J Neurosurg 1993;78:188–91.

[44] Hutter BO, Kreitschmann-Andermahr I, Gilsbach JM. Health-related quality of life after aneurismal subarachnoid hemorrhage: impacts of bleeding severity, computerized tomography findings, surgery, vasospasm and neurological grade. J Neurosurg 2001;94:241–51.

[45] Asano T, Sasaki T, Koide T, et al. Experimental evaluation of the beneficial effect of an antioxidant on cerebral vasospasm: the effect of an antioxidant on cerebral vasospasm. Neurol Res 1984;6:49–53.

[46] Mori T, Nagata K, Ishida T, et al. Superoxide anions in the pathogenesis of talc-induced cerebral vasocontraction. Neuropathol Appl Neurobiol 1995;21:378–85.

[47] MacDonald RL, Weir BKA. A review of hemoglobin and the pathogenesis of chronic cerebral vasospasm. Stroke 1991;22:971–82.

[48] Haber F, Weiss J. The catalytic decomposition of hydrogen peroxidase by iron salts. Proc R Soc Lond A 1934;147:332–51.

[49] Fenton HJH. Oxidation of tartaric acid in the presence of ion. J Chem Soc 1894;23:899–910.

[50] Shishido T, Suzuki R, Qian L, et al. The role of superoxide anions in the pathogenesis of cerebral vasospasm. Stroke 1994;25:864–8.

[51] Fadel MM, Foley PL, Kassell NF, et al. Histidine attenuates cerebral vasospasm in a rabbit model of subarachnoid hemorrhage. Surg Neurol 1995;43:52–8.

[52] Watanabe T, Nishiyama M, Hori T, et al. Ebselen ameliorates delayed cerebral vasospasm in a canine two-hemorrhage model. Neurol Res 1997;19:563–5.

[53] Germano A, Imperatore C, D'Avella D, et al. Antivasospastic and brain-protective effects of a hydroxyl radical scavenger (AVS) after experimental subarachnoid hemorrhage. J Neurosurg 1998;88:1075–81.

[54] Saito I, Asano T, Sano K, et al. Neuroprotective effect of an antioxidant, ebselen, in patients with delayed neurological deficits after aneurysmal subarachnoid hemorrhage. Neurosurgery 1998;42:269–77.

[55] Arthur AS, Fergus AH, Lanzino G, et al. Systemic administration of the iron chelator deferiprone attenuates subarachnoid hemorrhage-induced cerebral vasospasm in the rabbit- Neurosurgery 1997;41:1385–91.

[56] Horky LL, Pluta RM, Boock RJ, et al. Role of ferrous iron chelator 2, 2′-dipyridyl in preventing delayed vasospasm in a primate model of subarachnoid hemorrhage. J Neurosurg 1998;88:298–303.

[57] Potts MB, Koh SE, Whetstone WD, et al. Traumatic injury to the immature brain: potential therapeutic targets. Neuro RX 2006;3:143–53.

ELSEVIER
SAUNDERS

Pediatr Clin N Am
53 (2006) 1039–1051

PEDIATRIC CLINICS
OF NORTH AMERICA

Index

Note: Page numbers of article titles are in **boldface** type.

A

ABCA3 protein, deficiency of, 914–921
  evaluation of, 918
  postmortem diagnosis of, 921
  treatment of, 919–921

ABI TaqMan method, 809

Achondroplasia, 867–868

ACTC gene, in heart development and defects, 997

Activin-like kinase-1, defects of, in pulmonary hypertension, 969

Adenosine, for pulmonary hypertension, 972

ADMA protein, in pulmonary hypertension pathogenesis, 967

Affymetrix platform, for genomewide association studies, 810–811

Alagille syndrome, 997–999

Aldosteronism, glucocorticoid-responsive, 1013–1015

Alpha-satellite DNA, 844–847, 849

Aneurysms, in polycystic kidney disease, 893

Anthrax, laboratory diagnosis of, 822–823, 825, 834

Anticoagulants, for pulmonary hypertension, 973

Antiviral drugs, for respiratory infections
  coronavirus NL63, 945–946
  parainfluenza virus, 941–943
  respiratory syncytial virus, 935–937

Aorta
  abnormalities of, in polycystic kidney disease, 893
  coarctation of, 997–998

Aortic stenosis, 997–998, 1001

Aortic valve, bicuspid, 997

Apert syndrome, 867

Apparent mineralocorticoid excess, 1015–1016

Arachidonic acid, metabolism of, reactive oxygen species in, 1031

Arboviruses, laboratory diagnosis of, 822, 831–832, 834

Arenaviruses, laboratory diagnosis of, 822, 830–831, 834

Arginine, for pulmonary hypertension, 980

Artificial chromosomes. *See* Human artificial chromosomes.

Association mapping, 810

Asthma, bronchiolitis and, 946

Atrial septal defect, 996–998

Atrial septostomy, for pulmonary hypertension, 979

Atrioventricular conduction defects, 996

Atrioventricular septal defect, 997

Autoregulation, cerebral, reactive oxygen species in, **1029–1037**

Autosomal dominant polycystic kidney disease. *See* Polycystic kidney disease, inherited.

Autosomal recessive polycystic kidney disease. *See* Polycystic kidney disease, inherited.

Avian influenza, laboratory diagnosis of, 822–823, 826, 832–833

AXIN2 protein, defects of, 863–865

Bacillus anthracis, laboratory diagnosis of, 822–823, 825, 827, 834

B

Bacterial artificial chromosomes, versus human artificial chromosomes, 846, 849–850

doi:10.1016/S0031-3955(06)00131-3

United States Postal Service
Statement of Ownership, Management, and Circulation

1. Publication Title	2. Publication Number	3. Filing Date
Pediatric Clinics of North America	4 2 4 - 6 6 6 0	9/15/06

4. Issue Frequency	5. Number of Issues Published Annually	6. Annual Subscription Price
Feb, Apr, Jun, Aug, Oct, Dec	6	$125.00

7. Complete Mailing Address of Known Office of Publication *(Not printer)* *(Street, city, county, state, and ZIP+4)*

Elsevier Inc.
360 Park Avenue South
New York, NY 10010-1710

Contact Person
Sarah Carmichael
Telephone
(215) 239-3681

8. Complete Mailing Address of Headquarters or General Business Office of Publisher *(Not printer)*

Elsevier Inc., 360 Park Avenue South, New York, NY 10010-1710

9. Full Names and Complete Mailing Addresses of Publisher, Editor, and Managing Editor *(Do not leave blank)*
Publisher *(Name and complete mailing address)*

John Schrefer, Elsevier Inc., 1600 John F. Kennedy Blvd., Suite 1800, Philadelphia, PA 19103-2899

Editor *(Name and complete mailing address)*

Carla L. Holloway, Elsevier Inc., 1600 John F. Kennedy Blvd., Suite 1800, Philadelphia, PA 19103-2899

Managing Editor *(Name and complete mailing address)*

Catherine Bewick, Elsevier Inc., 1600 John F. Kennedy Blvd., Suite 1800, Philadelphia, PA 19103-2899

10. Owner *(Do not leave blank. If the publication is owned by a corporation, give the name and address of the corporation immediately followed by the names and addresses of all stockholders owning or holding 1 percent or more of the total amount of stock. If not owned by a corporation, give the names and addresses of the individual owners. If owned by a partnership or other unincorporated firm, give its name and address as well as those of each individual owner. If the publication is published by a nonprofit organization, give its name and address.)*

Full Name	Complete Mailing Address
Wholly owned subsidiary of	4520 East-West Highway
Reed/Elsevier Inc., US holdings	Bethesda, MD 20814

11. Known Bondholders, Mortgagees, and Other Security Holders Owning or Holding 1 Percent or More of Total Amount of Bonds, Mortgages, or Other Securities. If none, check box ☐ None

Full Name	Complete Mailing Address
N/A	

12. Tax Status *(For completion by nonprofit organizations authorized to mail at nonprofit rates)* *(Check one)*
The purpose, function, and nonprofit status of this organization and the exempt status for federal income tax purposes:
☐ Has Not Changed During Preceding 12 Months
☐ Has Changed During Preceding 12 Months *(Publisher must submit explanation of change with this statement)*

(See Instructions on Reverse)

PS Form 3526, October 1999

---

13. Publication Title	14. Issue Date for Circulation Data Below
Pediatric Clinics of North America	August 2006

15.	Extent and Nature of Circulation		Average No. Copies Each Issue During Preceding 12 Months	No. Copies of Single Issue Published Nearest to Filing Date
a.	Total Number of Copies *(Net press run)*		7,583	7,100
b. Paid and/or Requested Circulation	(1)	Paid/Requested Outside-County Mail Subscriptions Stated on Form 3541. *(Include advertiser's proof and exchange copies)*	3,923	3,646
	(2)	Paid In-County Subscriptions Stated on Form 3541 *(Include advertiser's proof and exchange copies)*		
	(3)	Sales Through Dealers and Carriers, Street Vendors, Counter Sales, and Other Non-USPS Paid Distribution	2,303	2,206
	(4)	Other Classes Mailed Through the USPS		
c.	Total Paid and/or Requested Circulation *(Sum of 15b. (1), (2), (3), and (4))*	▶	6,226	5,852
d. Free Distribution by Mail *(Samples, compliment-ary, and other free)*	(1)	Outside-County as Stated on Form 3541	182	165
	(2)	In-County as Stated on Form 3541		
	(3)	Other Classes Mailed Through the USPS		
e.	Free Distribution Outside the Mail *(Carriers or other means)*			
f.	Total Free Distribution *(Sum of 15d. and 15e.)*	▶	182	165
g.	Total Distribution *(Sum of 15c. and 15f.)*	▶	6,408	6,017
h.	Copies not Distributed		1,175	1,083
i.	Total *(Sum of 15g. and h.)*	▶	7,583	7,100
j.	Percent Paid and/or Requested Circulation *(15c. divided by 15g. times 100)*		97.16%	97.26%

16. Publication of Statement of Ownership
Publication required. Will be printed in the **October 2006** issue of this publication. ☐ Publication not required

17. Signature and Title of Editor, Publisher, Business Manager, or Owner

[signature] Jean Francei – Executive Director of Subscription Services

Date 9/15/06

I certify that all information furnished on this form is true and complete. I understand that anyone who furnishes false or misleading information on this form or who omits material or information requested on the form may be subject to criminal sanctions (including fines and imprisonment) and/or civil sanctions (including civil penalties).

Instructions to Publishers

1. Complete and file one copy of this form with your postmaster annually on or before October 1. Keep a copy of the completed form for your records.

2. In cases where the stockholder or security holder is a trustee, include in items 10 and 11 the name of the person or corporation for whom the trustee is acting. Also include the names and addresses of individuals who are stockholders who own or hold 1 percent or more of the total amount of bonds, mortgages, or other securities of the publishing corporation. In item 11, if none, check the box. Use blank sheets if more space is required.

3. Be sure to furnish all circulation information called for in item 15. Free circulation must be shown in items 15d, e, and f.

4. Item 15h, Copies not Distributed, must include (1) newsstand copies originally stated on Form 3541, and returned to the publisher, (2) estimated returns from news agents, and (3), copies for office use, leftovers, spoiled, and all other copies not distributed.

5. If the publication had Periodicals authorization as a general or requester publication, this Statement of Ownership, Management, and Circulation must be published; it must be printed in any issue in October or, if the publication is not published during October, the first issue printed after October.

6. In item 16, indicate the date of the issue in which this Statement of Ownership will be published.

7. Item 17 must be signed.

Failure to file or publish a statement of ownership may lead to suspension of Periodicals authorization.

PS Form 3526, October 1999 *(Reverse)*

Moving?

Make sure your subscription moves with you!

To notify us of your new address, find your **Clinics Account Number** (located on your mailing label above your name), and contact customer service at:

E-mail: elspcs@elsevier.com

800-654-2452 (subscribers in the U.S. & Canada)
407-345-4000 (subscribers outside of the U.S. & Canada)

Fax number: 407-363-9661

Elsevier Periodicals Customer Service
6277 Sea Harbor Drive
Orlando, FL 32887-4800

*To ensure uninterrupted delivery of your subscription, please notify us at least 4 weeks in advance of move.